Review of Preventive and Social Medicine for NEET

Amithab Arora MD (Std)

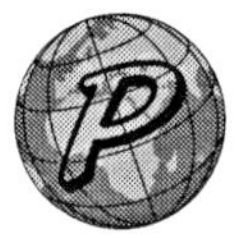

PEEPEE

PUBLISHERS AND DISTRIBUTORS (P) LTD.

Review of Preventive and Social Medicine for NEET

Published by
Pawaninder P. Vij and Anupam Vij
Peepee Publishers and Distributors (P) Ltd.
Head Office: 160, Shakti Vihar, Pitam Pura,
Delhi-110 034 (India)
Correspondence Address:
7/31, First Floor, Ansari Road, Daryaganj
New Delhi-110 002 (India)
Ph: 65195868, 23246245, 9811156083
e-mail: peepee160@yahoo.co.in
e-mail: peepee160@rediffmail.com
e-mail: peepee160@gmail.com
www.peepeepub.com

First Edition: **2015**

ISBN: 978-81-8445-009-5

Contents

C•H•A•P•T•E•R **ONE**

Man and Medicine Towards Health for All

DIRECTION: Following MCQ's are provided with a few suggestive answers/completions. Only one answer is correct. You have to identify the *BEST* one in each case.

1. **Who is acknowledged as the first great Indian physician and teacher?**
   A. Atreya
   B. Vaghbhata
   C. Charaka
   D. Sushruta

2. **Who said, "Every culture had developed a system of medicine, and medical history is but one aspect of the history of culture"?**
   A. John Snow
   B. Henry Siegerist
   C. Charles Smith
   D. Lamuhar Kalakki
   E. Dubos

3. **The medical systems that are truly Indian in origin and development includes:**
   A. Ayurveda
   B. Unani
   C. Siddha
   D. All of the above
   E. Both A and C but not 'B' above

4. **The Hindu God of Medicine was:**
   A. Atreya
   B. Vaghbhata
   C. Charaka
   D. Dhanwantri

5. **"Ayurveda" means:**
   A. Healing touch
   B. Cures of disease
   C. Knowledge of life
   D. All of the above
   E. Both A and B above

6. **Out of the four *Vedas,* which ultimately developed into the science of Ayurveda?**
   A. Atharvaveda
   B. Samaveda
   C. Rigveda
   D. All of the above

7. **Following are recognised celebrated authorities in Ayurvedic medicine:**
   I. Atreya
   II. Charaka
   III. Sushruta
   IV. Vaghbhata
   Select the true answer from the code given below:
   A. I only
   B. I and II only
   C. I, II and III only
   D. I, II, III and IV all

8. "Sushruta Samhita" deals with the following:
A. Medicine
B. Surgery
C. Naturopathy
D. Acupuncture

9. Egyptians worshipped whom as their "God of medicine"?
A. Hippocrates
B. Horus
C. Imhotep
D. Homer

10. Who were known as the early pioneers of immunization?
A. Indian
B. French
C. Greek
D. German
E. Chinese

11. To whom it is associated .... "the great doctor is one who treats not someone who is already ill but someone not yet ill".
A. Indian
B. Chinese
C. Greek
D. French
E. Egyptian

12. Specialization prevailed in Egyption times as they had the following speciality doctors...
I. Eye doctors
II. Head doctors
III. Tooth doctors
...of these
A. I and II are correct
B. II and III are correct
C. II is correct
D. I, II and III all correct

13. "Horus" was regarded as "God of health" for:
A. Chinese
B. Egyptian
C. Mesopotamian
D. Greek

14. Match the following:

Countries	*Contribution/ Associations*
I. India	**A. Samuel Hahnemann**
II. Chinese	**B. Edwin Smith Papyrus**
III. Egyptian	**C. "Baré-foot doctors"**
IV. German	**D. "Tridosha theory of diseases**

A. I-D; II-C; III-B; IV-A
B. I-A; II-B; III-C; IV-D
C. I-B; II-A; III-C; IV-A
D. I-D; II-C; III-A; IV-B

15. Which is the best known medical manuscripts belonging to the Egyptian times?
A. Edwin Smith Papyrus
B. Ebers Papyrus
C. Cannon of Medicine
D. All of these
E. Both A and B

16. To whom we called "Father of Indian Surgery"?
A. Atreya
B. Sushruta
C. Charaka
D. Vaghbhata

17. Who was the court physician to a Budhist king "Kanishka"?
A. Atreya
B. Sushruta
C. Charaka
D. Baghbhata

18. The "laws of Manu" were regarded as the code of:
A. Conduct
B. Personal hygiene
C. Personal relation
D. Upper caste and lower caste among Hindus

19. Which system of medicine has been introduced by Muslim rulers in India?
A. Alopathic
B. Mesopotamian
C. Unani-Tibbi
D. Sidha system
E. Greek system

20. On whose work did Charaka based his famous treatise "Charaka Samhita"?
A. Atreya
B. Sushruta
C. Himself
D. Vaghbhata

21. Following are the recognised "Tridoshas in Ayurveda" *except* for one:
A. Kapha
B. Shankha
C. Vata
D. Pitta

22. Who was the founder of "Homeopathy"?
A. Galen
B. Imhotep
C. Homer
D. Samuel Hainemann
E. Samuel Shettuck

23. The two principles on which Chinese medicine is based are the following:
A. Tung and Sung
B. Tsang and Tsing
C. Yan and Yin
D. Mong and Ming
E. Yun and Yuon

24. The oldest medical prescription comes to us from:
A. Indian
B. Mesopotamian
C. Chinese
D. Greek
E. Egyptian

25. The very first "codification of medical practice" was given by whom?
A. Atreya
B. Manu
C. Hammurabi
D. Galen

26. The greatest physician in Greek medicine was:
A. Aesculapius
B. Galen
C. Avicenna
D. Hippocrates

27. Who is still regarded as "Father of medicine"?
A. Atreya
B. Hippocrates
C. Avicenna
D. Douglas Guthrie

28. Who said, "Where there is love for mankind, there is love for the art of healing"?
A. Hippocrates
B. Douglas Guthrie
C. Avicenna
D. Galen
E. Aesculapius

29. Who wrote the book, "Airs, Water and Places"?
A. Avicenna
B. Galen
C. Hippocrates
D. Aesculapius

30. Which is not included in the four humors of the Greek medicine?
A. Phlegm
B. Vatta
C. Yellow bile
D. Blood only
E. Black bile only

31. "Since both, in importance and in time, health precedes disease, so we ought to consider first how health may be preserved and then how one may best cure disease" was said by whom?
A. Galen
B. Sushruta
C. Hippocrates
D. Avicenna

32. Who is regarded as the Greek goddess of curative medicine?
A. Hippocrates
B. Panacea
C. Galen
D. Hygiea

33. Who is regarded as the Greek goddess of preventive medicine?
A. Hippocrates
B. Panacea
C. Hygiea
D. Rhazes

34. Which was regarded as the "dark age of medicine"?
A. 100 to 550 AD
B. 550 to 750 AD
C. 500 to 100 AD
D. 500 to 1500 AD
E. 1500 to 2000 AD

35. To which language the words drug, alcohol, syrup, sugar belong?
A. Arabian
B. Sanskrit
C. Hebrews
D. Chinese
E. Greek

36. Who compiled the 21 volume encyclopedia, the "Canon of Medicine"?
A. Avicenna
B. Abu-Becr
C. Charaka
D. Galen only

37. Who was the 1st to observe pupillary reaction to light?
A. Parcelsus
B. Avicenna
C. Galen
D. Rhazes

38. Who wrote the first known book on disease of children"
A. Atreya
B. Hippocrates
C. Rhazes
D. Galen

39. The physician who publicly burnt the works of Galen and Avicenna was:
A. Fracastorius
B. Parcelsus
C. Rhazes only
D. Galen
E. None of the above

40. The physician credited with the discovery that syphilis is sexually transmitted is:
A. Aesculapius
B. Parcelsus
C. Fracastorius
D. Galen

41. Who is considered as the "father of art of surgery"?
A. Ambroise Pare
B. Sushruta
C. Galen
D. John Hunter

42. Who is considered as the "father of science of surgery"?
A. Galen
B. John Hunter
C. Sushruta only
D. Ambroise Pare

43. Medicine was revived by whom?
A. Aesculapius
B. Galen
C. Parcelsus
D. Vesalius

44. Who enunciated, "the theory of contagion"?
A. Andreas Vesalius
B. Galen
C. Parcelsus
D. Fracastorius
E. None of the above

45. Who has been called "the man of modern science"?
A. Andreas vesalius

B. Fracastorius
C. Galen
D. Parcelsus
E. Louis Pasteur

46. Who was given the name of English Hippocrates?
A. Andreas Vesalius
B. Thomas Sydenham
C. Galen
D. Fracastorius
E. John Hunter

47. Who made the D/d of "scarlet fever", "malaria", "dysentery" and "cholera"?
A. Fracastorius
B. Vesalius
C. John Hunter
D. Thomas Sydenham
E. Galen only

48. Which is often called the "father of public health"?
A. Malaria
B. Brucellosis
C. Cholera
D. Dengue haemorrhagic fever
E. All the above

49. Who was the non-physician epidemiologist who first established the role of polluted water in the spread of cholera?
A. John Snow
B. John Hunter
C. John Major
D. John Ryle

50. Who was the first person to demonstrate the role of drinking water in transmission of enteric fever (typhoid)?
A. Galen
B. Atreya
C. William Budd
D. John Snow

51. The "Public Health Act of 1848 of England" goes to the credit of whom?
A. Virchow
B. Sir John Simon
C. Ronald Ross
D. William Budd
E. John Snow

52. Which is the 1st disease conclusively proved to be caused by bacterias?
A. Anthrax
B. Tuberculosis
C. Cholera
D. Typhoid

53. Edward Jenner of Great Britain, who discovered vaccination against smallpox, was a pupil of:
A. Galen
B. John Hunter
C. Louis Pasteur
D. Robert Koch
E. All of the above

54. If smallpox vaccine was credited to Edward Jenner then anti-rabies vaccine to whom?
A. Robert Koch
B. Von Behring
C. Louis Pasteur
D. Enders
E. Both A and B above

55. The concept of social medicine was revived by whom?
A. Neumann
B. Virchow
C. John Ryle
D. Alfred Grotjahn
E. Rene Sand

56. The triad of disease factors postulated by Galen includes the following, *save* for one:
A. Contributory
B. Predisposing
C. Exciting
D. Environmental
E. None of these

57. "Medicine is a social science and politics is medicine on large scale" was said by whom?
A. Galen

B. Virchow
C. Rene Sand
D. Pasteur

58. "The science and art of preventing disease, prolonging life and promoting health and efficiency through organized community effort". This is the definition of public health given in 1920 by whom?
A. Rene Sand
B. John Ryle
C. C.E.A. Winslow
D. Lord Dawson
E. Leavell and Clark

59. "Disease prevention, health promotion and study of man as a social being in relation to his total environment". This statement defines:
A. Society
B. Social medicine
C. Sociology
D. Socialized medicine
E. None of the above

60. The "concept of health centre" was 1st mooted by:
A. Lord Dawson
B. John Ryle
C. Joseph Bhore
D. CEA Winslow
E. Mckeown

61. Who said, "Large numbers of the world's people, perhaps more than half, have no access to health care at all, and for many of the rest the care they receive does not answer the problems they have".
A. Lord Dawson
B. John Ryle
C. John Bryant
D. Joseph Bhore
E. CEA Winslow

Answers

1 A	2 B	3 E	4 D	5 C	6 A	7 D	8 B	9 C	10 E
11 B	12 D	13 B	14 A	15 E	16 B	17 C	18 B	19 C	20 A
21 B	22 D	23 C	24 B	25 C	26 D	27 B	28 A	29 C	30 B
31 A	32 B	33 C	34 D	35 A	36 A	37 D	38 C	39 B	40 C
41 A	42 B	43 C	44 D	45 A	46 B	47 D	48 C	49 A	50 C
51 B	52 A	53 B	54 C	55 D	56 A	57 B	58 C	59 B	60 A
61 C									

C•H•A•P•T•E•R TWO

Concepts of Health and Disease

DIRECTION: Following MCQ's are provided with a few suggestive answers/completions. Only one answer is correct. You have to identify the *BEST* one in each case.

1. **W.H.O. adopted the goal of health for all by 2000 AD:**
   A. In 1977
   B. In 1981
   C. In 1983
   D. In 1985
2. **While the understanding of health and disease improved, the concept about health changed, *except:***
   A. Holistic
   B. Biomedical
   C. Economic
   D. Socio-economic
   E. Ecological
3. **"Health implies the relative absence of pains and discomfort and a continuous adaptation and adjustment to the environment to ensure optimal function". This definition of Health is given by:**
   A. WHO
   B. UNESCO
   C. UNICEF
   D. Dubos
4. **The quantification of the following dimension(s) of health is considered very-very difficult or impossible:**
   I. Physical
   II. Social
   III. Mental
   IV. Spiritual
   V. Vocational
   VI. Emotional
   VII. Environmental
   Select the true answer from the code given below:
   A. I, II, III and IV
   B. II, III, IV and VI
   C. I, II, III, V and VII
   D. I, III, V and III
5. **The "Operational definition of health" as defined by WHO includes the following:**
   A. Health is a state of complete physical, mental and social well-being and not merely an absence of disease or infirmity
   B. A condition or quality of the human organism expressing the adequate functioning of the organism in given conditions, genetic or environemental
   C. The condition of being sound in body, mind or spirit, especially freedom from physical disease or pain

D. A state of relative equilibrium of body from and function which results from it successful dynamic adjustment to forces tending to disturb it, it is not passive interplay between body substances and forces impinging upon it but an active response of body forces working toward readjustment

E. All of the above

6. At the community level, the state of health may be assessed by the following indicators, *except:*

A. Birth rate

B. Death rate

C. Infant mortality rate

D. Expectation of life

E. None of these

7. Recently, mental health has been defined as:

A. A state of balance between the individual and the surrounding world

B. A state of harmony between oneself and others

C. A coexistence between the realities of the self and that of other people and that of the environment

D. All of the above

E. Both A and B above

8. Criticism is also levelled against WHO definition of health because it considers health as:

A. Positive

B. State

C. Spiritual

D. Social

E. Physical

9. Following disease are due to psychological factors:

A. Peptic ulcer

B. Bronchial asthma only

C. Essential hypertension

D. Both A and C above

E. All of the above

10. Most important component of level of living includes:

I. Housing

II. Health

III. Occupation

IV. Education

Select the true response from the following code given below:

A. I and IV only

B. II only

C. III and IV only

D. I, II and III

E. I, II, III and IV All

11. How many components are included under the level of living?

A. Three

B. Six

C. Nine

D. Twelve

E. Eleven

12. Statement (S): Health is the most important component of the level of living. Reason (R): Because its impairment always means impairment of the level of living.

A. Both (S) and (R) are true and (R) is the true explanation of (S)

B. Both (S) and (R) are true (R) is not the true explanation of (S)

C. (S) is true but (R) is false

D. Both (S) and (R) are false

13. The condition of life resulting from the combination of the effects of the complete range of factors like those determining health, happiness, education, social and intellectual attainments, freedom of action, justice and freedom of expressions. This definition defines quality of life, which is given by:

A. National Health Council of India

B. UNICEF

C. WHO

D. National Health Council of USA

14. The physical quality of life index (PQLI) is associated with the following three indicators:
   I. Infant mortality
   II. Measure economic growth
   III. Literacy only
   IV. Life expectancy at age one
Select the true response from the code given below:
A. I only
B. I, II and IV only
C. I, III and IV
D. II, III and IV
E. I, II, III and IV

15. The PQLI describes quality of life and takes into consideration the following, *except* for one:
A. Expectancy of life at birth
B. Infant mortality
C. Life expectancy at one year
D. Education

16. Which state in India has got the highest figure in respect of PQLI?
A. Andhra Pradesh
B. Bihar
C. Punjab
D. Kerala
E. Maharashtra only

17. If the PQLI value in Kerala State is 70, then what is the figure for the rest of the Indian States?
A. 70 **B.** 80
C. 50 **D.** 20
E. 43

18. Statement (S): In Indian States, the infant mortality is lowest in Kerala. Reason (R): Because Kerala has got highest female literacy in India.
A. Both (S) and (R) are true and (R) is the true explanation of (S)
B. Both (S) and (R) are true and (R) is not the true explanation of (S)
C. (S) is true but (R) is false
D. Both (S) and (R) are false

19. To achieve the goal of HFA by 2000 AD, the WHO target for expenditure of each nation's GNP on health care should be at least how much?
A. 2.5%
B. 5%
C. 7.5%
D. 10%

20. Following health problems in developed countries are associated with lifestyle changes:
A. Coronary heart disease
B. Obesity
C. Lung Cancer
D. Drug addiction
E. All of the above

21. Following diseases enumerated below are said to be due to hazard of affluence society, *except:*
A. Obesity
B. Coronary heart disease
C. Diabetes mellitus
D. None of these

22. The female literacy rate in Kerala is:
A. 39.42%
B. 49.42%
C. 59.42%
D. 69.42%
E. 86.93%

23. At present, India is spending how much of its GNP on health care and family welfare?
A. 1% **B.** 2%
C. 3% **D.** 0.5%
E. 5%

24. The greatest threat to human health in India today is the ever increasing:
A. Unplanned urbanization
B. Growth of slums
C. Deterioration of environment
D. All of these
E. Both A and B

25. "Everyone has the right to a standard of living adequate for the health and well being of himself and his family ...". This was stated in which article of the Universal Declaration of Human Rights?

A. Article 6
B. Article 25
C. Article 52
D. Article 60
E. Article 35

26. "The people's health ought to be the concern of the people themselves. They must struggle for it and plan for it. The war against disease and for health can not be fought by physicians alone. It is a people's war in which the entire population must be mobilised permanently". This statement was said by whom?

A. Henry Sigerist
B. Rene Dubos
C. Charles Olive
D. CEA Winslow
E. Rene Sand

27. Which part of Constitution of India provides that health is a state responsibility and its relevant portions are to be found in the Directive Principles of State Policy?

A. Part I **B.** Part II
C. Part III **D.** Part IV
E. Part V

28. In which year, the National Health Policy was approved by Parliament clearly indicates India's commitment to the goal of health for all by the year 2000 AD?

A. 1978 **B.** 1981
C. 1983 **D.** 1985
E. 1990

29. Following abbreviations are correctly described, *except:*

A. HFA—High Frequency Antenna
B. TCDC—Technical Cooperation in Developing Countries
C. ASEAN—Association of South-East Asian Nations
D. SAARC—South Asia Association for Regional Cooperation

30. The state of KERALA exceeds the rest of the country (INDIA) in providing the following, *except:*

A. Rural birth rate
B. Per capita income
C. IMR
D. Doctor-population ratio

31. Statement (S): The WHO is a major factor in fostering international health.

Reason (R): Because in keeping with its constitutional mandate, WHO acts as a directing and coordinating authority on international health work.

A. Both (S), (R) are true and related to cause and effect
B. Both (S) and (R) are true but not related to cause and effect
C. (S) is true, (R) is false
D. Both (S) and (R) are false

32. Kerala has surpassed all the Indian states in the following important measures of health and social development:

I. Female literacy rate
II. Life expectancy at birth
III. Annual growth rate
IV. Death rate

Select the true answer from the code given below:

A. I only
B. I and II only
C. I, II and IV only
D. I, II, III and IV All

33. Statement (S): Health Services are no longer considered merely as a complex of solely medical measures but a "sub-

system" from overall socio-economic system.

Reason (R): Because, in the final analysis, human health and well-being are the ultimate goals of development.

A. Both (S) and (R) are true but (R) is not the true explanation of 'S'
B. Both (S) and (R) are true but (R) is the true explanation of 'S'
C. (S) true, (R) false
D. (R) true, (S) false
E. Both false

34. Which state in India is considered a "Yardstick" for judging health status in the country?

A. Andhra Pradesh
B. Bihar only
C. Rajasthan only
D. Kerala
E. Madhya Pradesh

35. Which of the following statements are true in respect of health development?

A. It is defined as "the process of continuous progressive improvement of the health status of a population
B. It is based on the fundamental principle that governments have a responsibility for the health of their people and at the same time people should have the right as well as the duty, individually and collectively to participate in the development of their own health
C. It contributes to and results from social and economic development
D. UNO, UNDP and World Bank has shown a growing interest in it
E. All of the above

36. It has been suggested that in relation to health trends which term is more appropriate?

A. Health indicator
B. Health index
C. Health indices
D. All of the above
E. Both B and C above

37. In WHO's guidelines for health programme evaluation "INDICATORS" are defined as:

A. Indicator as such
B. Variables
C. Indices
D. Index
E. Any of the above

38. Following are recognised characteristics of an ideal indicator:

I. Should be valid
II. Should be reliable and objective
III. Should be sensitive
IV. Should be specific

Select the true answer from the code given below:

A. I only
B. I and II only
C. I, II, III and IV All
D. I, II and III only

39. Statement (S): When used for international comparison, the usefulness of the crude death rate (CDR) is restricted.
Reason (R): Because it is influenced by age-sex composition of the population.

A. Both (S) and (R) are true and related to cause and effect
B. Both (S) and (R) are true but unrelated to cause and effect
C. (S) true, (R) untrue
D. Both (S) and (R) untrue

40. Following statements are true regarding expectation of life:

I. Life expectancy at birth is used most frequently
II. It is a good indicator of socio-economic development
III. It can be considered as a positive health indicator
IV. It has not been adopted as a global health indicator

Select the false statements from the code given below:

A. I, II and III only
B. IV only
C. I and III only
D. I and II only
E. II and IV

41. **A minimum life expectancy at birth should be how much is the goal of health for all by 2000 AD?**
A. 60 years
B. 62 years
C. 64 years
D. 70 years

42. **Statement (S): The global strategy of HFA has suggested and IMR of not more than 50/1000 live births by 2000 AD.**
Reason (R): Because the IMR is a sensitive indicator of the availability, utilization and effectiveness of health care, particularly perinatal care.
A. Both (S) and (R) are true, but not related to cause and effect
B. Both (S) and (R) are true, and related to cause and effect
C. (S) true, (R) false
D. Both (S) and (R) false

43. **The most sensitive indicators of health and level of living of a people is:**
A. Proportional mortality ratio
B. Crude birth rate
C. Crude death rate
D. IMR
E. Expectation of life

44. **High under 5-proportionate mortality rate reflects:**
A. High birth rates
B. High child mortality rates
C. Shorter life expectancy
D. Both B and C above
E. All of the above

45. **Following indicates the magnitude of preventable mortality:**
A. IMR
B. Proportional mortality rate
C. MMR
D. Disease specific mortality
E. Under-5 mortality rate

46. **Following is not included under mortality indicator:**
A. Quality of life
B. Expectation of life at 1 year
C. Child mortality rate
D. Disease specific mortality

47. **Following are recognised morbidity indicators:**
I. Incidence and prevalence
II. Notification rates
III. Duration of stay in hospital
IV. Disability rates

Select the true answer from the code given below:
A. I, II and IV
B. I, II and III
C. II, III and IV
D. I, III and IV
E. III and IV

48. **Following are the two types of disability rates:**
I. Incidence type
II. Place type
III. Period type
IV. Person type
V. Event type

Select the correct answer from the code given below:
A. I and II only
B. II and III only
C. III and IV only
D. IV and V only

49. **Expectation for life, free of disability is known as:**
A. Park's index
B. Broca's index
C. Sullivan's index
D. Smith's index
E. None of the above

50. Following three nutritional status indicators are considered important as indicators of health status, *except* for one:

A. Measurements of weight, height, mid arm circumference (MAC) of preschool children

B. Hts. of children (wt. sometimes) at school entry

C. Prevalence of low birth wt. (< 2.5 kg)

D. None of these

51. Following are frequently used indicators of health care delivery system:

I. Doctor-population ratio

II. Doctor-nurse ratio

III. Population-bed ratio

IV. Population per health/subcentre

V. Population per traditional birth attendant

Select the true answer from the code given below:

A. I, II, III, IV and V All

B. I, III and V only

C. II, IV and V only

D. I, II, III and V only

52. Following are recognised indicators of social and mental health:

I. Suicide, homicide, other acts of violence and crime

II. Road traffic accidents

III. Juvenile delinquency

IV. Smoking, alcohol, drug abuse, consumption of tranquillizers and obesity

V. Family violence, battered baby and battered wife syndromes and neglected and abandoned youth in the neighbourhood

Select the true answer from the code given below:

A. I, III and V

B. I, II and III

C. I, II, III and IV

D. I, II, III, IV and V All

53. Amongst the following environmental indicators the most useful indicators are the following:

A. Air pollution

B. Access to safe water and sanitation facilities

C. Radiation and noise pollution

D. Exposure to toxic substances in food or drink

E. All of the above

54. Following are the recognised examples of utilization rates:

I. Proportion of infants who are "fully immunized against the six (6) EPI diseases

II. Proportion of pregnant women who receive antenatal care, or have their deliveries supervised by trained birth attendant

III. Percentage of the population using the various methods of family planning

IV. Bed-occupancy rate

V. Average length of stay in hospital

Select the true response from the code given below:

A. I, III and V

B. I, II and III

C. I, II, III, IV and V All

D. I, IV and V

E. I, II, III and IV only

55. Following are recognised socio-economic indicators of health, *except* for one:

A. Per capita GNP

B. Per capita "caloric" availability

C. Expendency ratio

D. Male literacy rates

56. The single most important indicator of political commitment is:

A. Allocation of adequate resources

B. Proportion of GNP spent on health services

C. Proportion of GNP spent on health related activities

D. Proportion of total health resources devoted to primary health care
E. All of the above

57. **Social indicators, as defined by the United Nations statistical office, have divided it into how many categories?**
A. Only 6
B. 12
C. 14
D. 16
E. None of the above

58. **Which of the following international agency uses the "BASIC NEEDS INDICATORS"?**
A. WHO
B. UNICEF
C. ILO
D. UNESCO
E. IRC

59. **Following are true about India: Demographic profile:**
I. Total population (estimated 1991 census)-844 million
II. Population doubling time (at current growth rate)-30 years
III. Population below 15 years (1992)-35.7%
IV. Sex ratio (females per 1000 males)-939 (1991)
V. Literacy rate (1991 census)-52.11%
Select the false answer from the code given below:
A. I and II only
B. I, II and III only
C. I and III only
D. IV only
E. I, II, III, IV and V All

60. **Infant mortality rate (IMR) in the whole world by 2000 AD is:**
A. 50/1000 live birth
B. 66.6/1000 live birth
C. 16/1000 live birth
D. 80/1000 live birth

61. **In India, which state has got highest death rate?**
A. Orissa
B. Bihar
C. UP
D. MP
E. Rajasthan

62. **In India, which of the following state has recorded the highest infant mortality rate in 1998?**
A. M.P.
B. Bihar
C. U.P.
D. Orissa
E. Rajasthan

63. **The death rate in Uttar Pradesh in 1998 is:**
A. 9 B. 10
C. 11 D. 11.5
E. 12

64. **If the IMR in Orissa is 122, then what is the IMR in Kerala state?**
A. 122 B. 77
C. 17 D. 80
E. None of these

65. **In India, which of the following health structure provide the secondary health care?**
A. PHC
B. Additional PHC
C. Community health centre
D. District hospitals
E. Both C and D above

66. **By the end of March 1992, how many PHC's are existing in India?**
A. 10,000
B. 15,000
C. 20,000
D. 22,441
E. 51,200

67. At present, if 80% of urban population has safe water availability, then what % of rural people has been benefited by such water availability?

A. Only 1% **B.** 10%
C. 25% **D.** 37%
E. 47%

68. Which of the following statements is/are true?

A. Tertiary health care is provided by the teaching hospital and institution and other apex hospitals
B. The adequate sanitation facilities are available to only 30% in the urban and only 1% of the rural population
C. Village health guides and trained dais are selected by the local community and trained to deliver primary health care
D. All of the above
E. Both A and C but not 'B' above

69. Almost half of the reported dentist, in the world are in which continent?

A. Asia
B. Europe
C. Australia
D. Latin America

70. The four states in India has been described cynically as the "waterloo" of India's health and family welfare programmes:

I. Himachal Pradesh
II. Uttar Pradesh
III. Madhya Pradesh
IV. Bihar
V. Rajasthan

Select the false answer from the code given below:

A. I only
B. I and II only
C. I, II and III only
D. II, III, IV and V

71. If the annual population growth rate in India is 2.03%, then what is the estimated annual global rate of population?

A. 1.0% **B.** 1.12%
C. 1.23% **D.** 1.36%
E. 1.63%

72. Following nations has already achieved zero-population growth rate:

I. UK
II. USA
III. Austria
IV. Belgium
V. FRG

Select the false answer from the code given below:

A. I and II only
B. II and III only
C. II only
D. IV and V only

73. Following countries have shown population growth > 3% per annum, *except* for one:

A. South Africa
B. Libya
C. Congo
D. Nigeria
E. Zambia

74. Following Muslim nations have more than 3 (> 3) population growth per annum currently, *save* for one:

A. Iraq
B. Turkey
C. Saudi Arabia
D. UAE
E. Libya only

75. "Multitude of services rendered to individual families or communities by the agents of the health services or professions, for the purpose of promoting, maintaining, monitoring or restoring health. This is the definition of:

A. Health care
B. Medical care
C. Health system
D. All of the above
E. Both A and B but not C above

76. Following are the recognised characteristics of health care:

I. Appropriateness
II. Comprehensiveness
III. Adequacy
IV. Availability
V. Accessibility
VI. Affordability
VII. Feasibility

Select the true answer from the code given below:

A. I, II, III, V and VI
B. II, IV and VI only
C. III, IV, V and VI only
D. IV, VI and VII only
E. I, II, III, IV, V, VI and VII All

77. Statement (S): "Health system" is intended to deliver health services.
Reason (R): Because it constitutes the management sector and involves organizational matters.

A. Both (S) and (R) are true but unrelated to cause and effect
B. Both (S) and (R) are true and related to cause and effect
C. (S) is true but (R) is false
D. (R) is true, (S) is false
E. Both (S) and (R) are false

78. Following are the recognised components of the health system:

I. Concepts (e.g. health and disease)
II. Ideas (e.g. equity, coverage, effectiveness, efficiency, impact)
III. Objects (e.g. hospitals, health centres health programmes)
IV. Persons (e.g. provides and consumers)

Select the true answer from the code given below:

A. I and II only
B. II and III only
C. I, II, III and IV All
D. II, III and IV

79. In India, the 1st referral level in the health system is:

A. PHC and subcentres
B. District hospital only
C. Community health centres
D. Both B and C above
E. All of the above

80. "Who has less than full professional qualifications in a particular field and is supervised by a professional worker." This is the definition of:

A. Auxiliary worker
B. Barefoot doctors
C. Paramedicals
D. All of the above
E. None of the above

81. Health for all by 2000 AD means what?

A. Complete leprosy cure
B. Total tuberculosis eradication
C. Equity in health
D. Preparation of AIDS vaccine

82. The concept of primary health care came into limelight in .... following an international conference in "ALMA ATA", USSR.

A. 1978 **B.** 1981
C. 1983 **D.** 1985
E. 1990

83. "Essential health care based on practical, scientifically sound and socially acceptable methods and technology made universally accessible, to individuals and families in the community through their full participation and at a costs that the community and the country can afford to maintain at every stage of their development in the spirit of self-determination." This is the definition of:

A. Integrated health care
B. Primary health care
C. Comprehensive health care
D. Basic health services

84. The declaration of Alma Ata stated that primary health care includes at least the following:

I. Health education about existing health problems and methods of preventing and controlling them
II. Promotion of food supply and proper nutrition
III. An adequate supply of safe water and basic sanitation
IV. MCH care including family planning
V. Immunization against infectious disease
VI. Prevention and control of endemic disease
VII. Appropriate treatment of common disease and injuries
VIII. Provision of essential drugs

Select the true answer from the code given below:

A. I, III, V and VII only
B. II, IV, VI and VIII only
C. I, III, V and VIII
D. I, II, III, IV, V, VI and VII only
E. I, II, III, IV, V, VI, VII and VIII All

85. It is true about "HFA by 2000 AD" is that it is mainly concerned with the following:

A. Health services being provided by government with active participation of community
B. Hospital based services
C. Community health services
D. Health services being provided by government with passive participation of community

86. The Ministry of Health and Family Welfare, Government of India evolved a "National Health Policy" in 1982, keeping in view the national commitment to attain the goal of "HFA by 2000 AD". This policy has approved by Parliament in which year?

A. 1985
B. 1982
C. 1983
D. 1986
E. 1990

87. "State of social dysfunction" is otherwise known as:

A. Illness
B. Sickness
C. Disease
D. Both A and B above
E. None of the above

88. The concept of HSR (health services research) was developed during:

A. 1980-81
B. 1981-82
C. 1982-83
D. 1983-84

89. "Health services research" (HSR) or health practice research is now called as:

A. Health systems research
B. Biomedical research
C. Intersectoral research
D. Both B and C but not A
E. All of the above

90. "The systematic study of the means by which biomedical and other relevant knowledge is brought to bear on the health of individuals and communities under a given set of conditions." This statement defines:

A. Intersectoral research
B. Biomedical research
C. HSR
D. Both A and B but not 'C' above
E. All of the above

91. Following is/are the true definition of disease as defined by WHO:

A. A condition in which body health is impaired, a departure from a state of health, an alteration of the human body interrupting the performance of vital functions

B. A condition of the body or some part or organ of the body in which its functions are disrupted or deranged
C. A maladjustment of the human organisms to environment
D. Any deviation from normal functioning or state of complete physical or mental well-being
E. None of the above

92. **"A subjective state of the person who feels aware of not being well." This statement defines what?**
A. Sickness only
B. Disease only
C. Illness only
D. All of the above
E. Both A and B but not C above

93. **"Epidemiological triad" includes:**
I. Agent
II. Vector
III. Host
IV. Carrier
V. Environment
Select the correct answer from the code given below:
A. I, II and III only
B. I, III and IV only
C. I, II and V only
D. I, III and V only
E. I, II, III, IV and V All

94. **Which of the following is aptly called the "modern diseases of civilization"?**
A. Lung cancer
B. Coronary heart disease
C. Chronic bronchitis
D. Mental illness
E. All of the above

95. **Following factors are involved in the pathogenesis of coronary heart disease:**
I. Excess of fat intake
II. Lack of physical exercise
III. Smoking only
IV. Obesity only
Select the true answer from the following code given below:
A. I, II and III only
B. I, II, III and IV only
C. I and III only
D. II and III only
E. I, II, III, IV and V All

96. **The "web of causation" model of disease causation was suggested by whom?**
A. Mac Mahon and Pugh
B. Pattenkofer
C. John Ryle
D. Ketchy

97. **The "web of causation" model of disease causation is ideally suited in cases of:**
A. Acute disease
B. Subacute cases
C. Chronic cases
D. All of these

98. **The natural history of disease is best established by:**
A. Agent
B. Host
C. Environment
D. Cohort studies
E. All of the above

99. **"Agent, host and environment" are collectively referred as:**
A. Secular triad
B. Epidemiological triad
C. Ecological triad
D. Pathogenetic triad
E. All of the above

100. **The final outcome of any disease may be:**
A. Recovery
B. Disability
C. Death
D. All of these
E. Both A and C

101. **Which is the one way of measuring the virulence?**
A. Case fatality rate
B. Infectivity

C. Pathogenecity only
D. Sequelae only
E. All of the above

102. **Following endogenously produced chemical agents are produced in human body in diseased state, *except* for:**
A. Urea (ureamia)
B. Calcium carbonate (kidney stones)
C. Uric acid (podagra)
D. Serum bilirubin (icterus)
E. None of these

103. **Following social agents are involved in disease causation:**
I. Poverty
II. Smoking, abuse of drugs and alcohol
III. Unhealthy life styles
IV. Social isolation
V. Maternal deprivation
Select the true answer as per code given below:
A. I and II only
B. I, II and III only
C. I, II, III, VI and V All
D. I, II, III and V only

104. **In epidemiological terminology, which of the following is referred to as "SOIL"?**
A. Human host
B. Agent
C. Environment only
D. All of the above
E. Both B and C above

105. **Recognised risks factors for STROKE causation includes the following, *save* for one:**
A. High blood pressure
B. Elevated cholesterol
C. Smoking
D. Type A personality only
E. None of these

106. **Consider the following statement about spectrum of disease:**
I. The term "spectrum of disease" is a graphic representation of variations in the manifestations of disease
II. At one end of the disease spectrum are subclinical infections which are not ordinarily identified and at the other end are total illnesses
III. In the middle of the spectrum lie illnesses ranging in severity from mild to severe
IV. This above different C/M are simply reflections of individuals different states of immunity and receptivity
Choose the true answer as per code given below:
A. I, II and IV only
B. I, II, III and IV All
C. II and IV
D. II, III and IV

107. **Which is an excellent example of the "spectral concept of disease"?**
A. Malnutrition
B. Tuberculosis
C. Hansen's disease
D. Diabetes mellitus
E. Coronary artery disease

108. **The "floating tip of the iceberg" represents what?**
A. Spectrum of disease
B. Clinical cases
C. Latent cases
D. Presymptomatic and undiagnosed cases
E. Carriers

109. **The concept of which prevention is comparatively less relevant to control efforts?**
A. Primary prevention
B. Secondary prevention
C. Tertiary only
D. All of the above
E. Both A and B above

110. **The "all or none phenomenon" has been exhibited by:**
A. Disease eradication
B. Disease control
C. Disease elimination

D. Monitoring
E. Disease surveillance

111. In the modern day, the concept of prevention has been grouped into how many levels?
A. Only one B. Two
C. Three D. Four
E. Seven

112. Regarding primordial prevention, which is false?
A. Prevention of chronic diseases
B. It is secondary prevention in its purest sense
C. Here efforts are directed towards discouraging children from adopting harmful lifestyles
D. The main intervention in primordial prevention is through individual and mass education

113. Following is an example of primordial prevention:
A. Low salt diet to prevent hypertension
B. Chlorination of water
C. Inculcating healthy life-styles in children
D. All of the above
E. Both A and B above

114. All the following are good example of secondary prevention *save* for one:
A. Use of calipers
B. Mammography
C. Treatment of hypertension
D. Mass trachoma treatment
E. None of these

115. Which is regarded as the tertiary prevention?
A. Health promotion
B. Specific protection
C. Early diagnosis treatment
D. Disability limitation and rehabilitation
E. None of the above

116. Which is an imperfect tool in the control of transmission of disease?
A. Primordial prevention
B. Primary prevention
C. Secondary prevention
D. Tertiary prevention

117. One of the most cost-effective interventions among the health promotion is:
A. Health education
B. Environmental modifications
C. Nutritional interventions
D. Lifestyle and behavioural changes

118. A mass treatment approach is used in the control of following disease, *but* one:
A. Leprosy
B. Yaws, pinta and bejel
C. Trachoma
D. Malaria only
E. None of these

119. When a patient report late in the pathogenesis phase, the mode of intervention is:
A. Health promotion
B. Disability limitation
C. Specific protection
D. Early diagnosis treatment

120. The sequence of events leading to disability and handicap are as follows:
I. Disease
II. Disability
III. Impairment
IV. Handicap
Select the correct sequence as per following code:
A. I, III, II and IV
B. III, I, II and IV
C. II, I, III and IV
D. I, II, III and IV

121. The most effective way of dealing with the disability problem in developing countries is:
A. Primordial prevention
B. Primary prevention
C. Secondary prevention
D. Tertiary prevention
E. None of these

122. The leading cause of death in USA is:
A. Pneumonia
B. Accidents
C. Heart disease
D. Cancers
E. Both B and D above

123. Which is described as the "silent epidemic" of the century is an important cause of morbidity and mortality?
A. Alzheimer's disease
B. Suicide
C. Cancer
D. Tuberculosis

124. Which disease best exemplify the basic science, clinical science and population medicine altogether?
A. Heart disease
B. Tuberculosis
C. Cancer
D. Diphtheria

125. In Greek mythology, the serpent testifies what?
A. Disease
B. Hygeia
C. Art of healing
D. Drug

126. The term "Social medicine" was 1st introduced by whom?
A. CEA Winslow
B. Maxy-Rosenau
C. Alfred Grotjhan
D. Jules Guerin
E. Emil Fisher

127. Who was 1st appointed as Professor of social medicine at Oxford?
A. Alfred Grotjahn
B. John Ryle
C. Crew
D. Jules guerin

128. "An ivory tower of disease" is the name given to:
A. Hospital
B. Social medicine
C. Community medicine
D. Public health
E. All of the above

129. Recognised functions of a Physician include:
A. The care of the individual
B. The care of the community
C. The Physician as a teacher
D. All of these
E. Both A and B above

130. Who 1st classify the disease in the 17th century?
A. John Ryle
B. John Graunt
C. Crew
D. Alfred Grotjhan

131. The International classification of disease (ICD) produced by WHO and accepted for national and international use, has been received once every:
A. 3 years
B. 5 years
C. 7 years
D. 10 years
E. 12 years

132. The latest version of ICD, has come into effect on January 1, 1993, which is the:
A. Fifth one
B. Sixth one
C. Seventh one
D. Eight one
E. Tenth one

133. How many volumes are found in ICD-10?
A. Single
B. Two
C. Three
D. Four
E. Five

134. Human Development Index (HDI) is measured by all, *except:*
A. Under five mortality
B. Life expectancy at birth
C. Literacy
D. Per capita income

135. Human Development Index (HDI) includes:
- **A.** Life expectancy, GDP and per capita income
- **B.** Education, life expectancy and purchasing power
- **C.** Education, social status and life expectancy
- **D.** All of these

136. Provision of carotene rich diet in order to prevent Xero-ophthalmia is:
- **A.** Health promotion
- **B.** Rehabilitation
- **C.** Specific protection
- **D.** Early diagnosis and treatment

137. The measure used to express the global burden of disease i.e., how a healthy life is affected by disease is:
- **A.** Age specific incidence rate
- **B.** Case fatality rate
- **C.** Life expectancy
- **D.** Disability-adjusted life year

138. Most important component of level of living is:
- **A.** Health
- **B.** Education
- **C.** Occupation
- **D.** Housing

139. The value of HDI in India is:
- **A.** 0.500
- **B.** 0.545
- **C.** 0.505
- **D.** 0.540

140. Optimal healthy life includes all, *but* one:
- **A.** Moderate physical exercise
- **B.** Mental peace
- **C.** Athletic involvement
- **D.** Sufficient nutrition

141. Following is *not* true of ICD:
- **A.** It is revised once in every 10 years
- **B.** It was devised by UNICEF
- **C.** The 10th revision consists of 21 major chapters
- **D.** It is accepted for national and international use

Answers

1 A	2 C	3 D	4 C	5 B	6 A	7 D	8 B	9 E	10 B
11 C	12 A	13 C	14 C	15 A	16 B	17 E	18 A	19 B	20 E
21 D	22 E	23 C	24 D	25 B	26 A	27 D	28 C	29 A	30 B
31 A	32 C	33 B	34 D	35 E	36 A	37 B	38 C	39 A	40 B
41 A	42 B	43 D	44 E	45 B	46 A	47 B	48 D	49 C	50 D
51 A	52 D	53 B	54 C	55 D	56 A	57 B	58 C	59 D	60 A
61 C	62 D	63 E	64 C	65 E	66 B	67 E	68 D	69 B	70 A
71 E	72 C	73 A	74 B	75 A	76 E	77 B	78 C	79 B	80 A
81 C	82 A	83 B	84 E	85 A	86 C	87 B	88 B	89 A	90 C
91 E	92 C	93 D	94 E	95 B	96 A	97 C	98 D	99 B	100 D
101 A	102 E	103 C	104 A	105 D	106 B	107 C	108 B	109 C	110 A
111 D	112 B	113 C	114 A	115 D	116 C	117 A	118 A	119 B	120 A
121 B	122 C	123 A	124 B	125 C	126 D	127 B	128 A	129 D	130 B
131 D	132 E	133 C	134 A	135 B	136 C	137 D	138 A	139 B	140 C
141 B									

C·H·A·P·T·E·R **THREE**

Nutrition and Health

DIRECTION: Following MCQ's are provided with a few suggestive answers/completions. Only one answer is correct. You have to identify the *BEST* one in each case.

1. Following statements/facts are true about nutrition:

I. Nutrition may be defined as the science of food and its relationship to health

II. Nutrition is concerned primarily with the part played by nutrients in body growth, development and maintenance

III. The word nutrients or "food-factor" is used for specific dietary constituents such as proteins, vitamins and minerals

IV. Good nutrition means "maintaining a nutritional status that enables us to grow well and enjoy good health

Select the true response from the code given below:

A. I, II and IV
B. I and IV only
C. III and IV only
D. I, II and IV only
E. II, III and IV only

2. Statements (S): Dietetics is the practical application of the principles of nutrition; Reason (R): Because it includes the planning of meals for the well and the sick:

A. Both (S) and (R) are true, but do not explain each other
B. Both (S) and (R) are true, and correctly explain each other
C. (S) is true, (R) is false
D. Both (S) and (R) are false

3. Following statements are true regarding nutrition:

I. Protein, CHO (carbohydrate) and fat has been recognized early in the 19th century as energy-yielding foods

II. The discovery of vitamins at the turn of the present century has "rediscovered" the science of nutrition

III. Between the two world wars, research on protein gained momentum

IV. Nutrition gained recognition as a scientific discipline, with roots in physiology and biochemistry

Select the true response from the following code:

A. I and II only
B. I and III only
C. II and III only
D. I, II, III and IV only
E. I and IV only

4. **All vitamins and essential amino acids has been discovered by about:**
   A. 1920
   B. 1930
   C. 1940
   D. 1950
   E. 1970

5. **Statement (S): The science of nutrition was extending its influences into other fields .... agriculture, animal husbandary, economics and sociology.**
   Reason (R): Because this led to "green revolution" and "white revolution" in the country and increased food production.
   A. Both (S) and (R) are true and correctly explains each other
   B. Both (S) and (R) are true but not related to each other
   C. (S) is true, (R) is false
   D. (R) is true, (S) is false
   E. Both are false

6. **Which agency has initiated the international activities in the field of nutrition?**
   A. FAO only
   B. League of Nations
   C. WHO
   D. UNICEF

7. **Dietary factors have got specific role in the pathogenesis of following noncommunicable disease; *except*:**
   A. Coronary heart disease only
   B. Diabetes mellitus only
   C. Cancer only
   D. Diabetes insipidus only

8. **Epidemiological methods are now increasingly used not only in the elucidation of disease aetiology and identification of risk factors of disease, but also in the planning and evaluation of nutritional programmes.**
   A. True
   B. False

9. **In the global campaign of Health for All (HFA), promotion of proper nutrition is one of the eight elements of primary health care.**
   A. True
   B. False

10. **Following foods are regarded as body-building foods:**
    I. Milk only
    II. Meat, poultry, fish and eggs
    III. Pulses only
    IV. Groundnut only
    Select the true answer from the following:
    A. Only I and III
    B. I and IV
    C. I, II, III and IV All
    D. I and II only
    E. I, II and III'only

11. **Classification of foods on the basis of chemical composition include the following:**
    A. Protein, CHO and fats
    B. Protein, CHO, fats and vitamins
    C. Protein, CHO, fats, vitamins and mineral only
    D. Protein, CHO, fats, vitamins, minerals and water

12. **Following are regarded as body building food *but* one of the following:**
    A. Milk
    B. Fats
    C. Meat and fish
    D. Pulses only

13. **Following food are regarded as energy yielding:**
    I. Cereals and sugars
    II. Roots and tubers
    III. Fats and oils
    IV. Milk and poultry
    Select the correct answer from the following code:

A. I, II and III only
B. III and IV only
C. I and II only
D. I, II, III and IV All

14. All the following are regarded as protective food, *save* for one:
A. Vegetables only
B. Fruits only
C. Milk
D. Oils

15. How many nutrients which are normally supplied through the foods we eat?
A. 25 only
B. 50 only
C. 60 only
D. 75
E. 80

16. Most natural food contain more than one nutrient.
A. True
B. False

17. Statement (S): Protein, fats and carbohydrates are often called "proximate principles".

Reason (R): Because they form the main bulk of food.
A. Both (S) and (R) are true but donot explain each other
B. Both (S) and (R) are true and truly explain each other
C. Only (S) is true, (R) is false
D. Both (S) and (R) are false

18. Following foods are included under macronutrients, *but* one:
A. Proteins
B. Fats only
C. Carbohydrate
D. Vitamins

19. Statement (S): Vitamins and minerals are called micronutrients.

Reason (R): Because its absence does not affect the health.
A. Both (S) and (R) are true and related to each other
B. Both (S) and (R) are true but not related to each other
C. (S) is true, (R) is false
D. (S) is false, but (R) is true

20. In the Indian dietary system, "proximate principle" (macronutrients) contribute to the total energy intake in the following proportions:
I. Protein—(7 to 15%)
II. Fats—(10 to 30%)
III. Carbohydrates—(65 to 80%)
IV. Protein—(15 to 30%)

Select the true answer from the code given below:
A. I, II and III only
B. I and II only
C. II and IV only
D. II, III and IV

21. Which of the following statements regarding protein is/are true?
A. They are complex organic nitrogenous compounds
B. They consists of C, H, O, N and S in varying amounts
C. They also contain P and Fe plus other elements
D. Both A and B but not 'C' above
E. All of the above

22. Protein differ from carbohydrates and fats in that they contain:
A. Phosphorous
B. Nitrogen
C. Sulphur
D. Iron only

23. What % of nitrogen is found in protein?
A. 4% only
B. 8%
C. 16%
D. 20%

24. Protein constitute about how much % of the body weight in an adult?
A. 5% only
B. 10% only
C. 16% only
D. 20% only

25. Statement (S): Out of 24 amino acids that are stated to be needed by the human body only I are essential amino acids.
Reason (R): Because they are not synthesized by body in adequate amounts.
A. Both (S) and (R) are true and correctly explains each other
B. Both (S) and (R) are true but do not explain each other
C. (S) is true, (R) is false
D. (R) is true, (S) is false

26. Following are recognized essential amino acids *but* one:
A. Tryptophan
B. Tyrosine
C. Methionine
D. Threonine only
E. Phenylalanine only

27. Following are non-essential amino acids:
I. Glycine only
II. Lysine only
III. Serine and proline
IV. Glutamic acid
Select the correct answer from the code given below:
A. I and II only
B. I, III and IV only
C. III and IV only
D. II and III only
E. II, III and IV only

28. Statement (S): Both essential and non-essential amino acids are needed for synthesis of tissue proteins.
Reasons (R): Because absence of a single essential amino acid will lead to negative nitrogen balance.
A. Both (S) and (R) are true and (R) is the true explanation of (S)
B. Both (S) and (R) are true but (R) is not the true explanation of (S)
C. (S) is true but (R) is false
D. Both (S) and (R) are false

29. Following are recognized important biological functions exhibited by essential amino acids:
A. Formation of niacin from tryptophan
B. Methyl group from methionine for choline synthesis
C. Methionine provides methyl group for folates and nucleic acid synthesis
D. All of the above
E. Both A and B but not 'C' above

30. Cystine and tyrosine are esential for premature babies.
A. True
B. False

31. Proteins are needed by the body for the following:
I. Body building
II. Repair and maintenance of body tissues
III. Maintenance of osmotic pressure
IV. Formation of plasma protein, enzyme, hormones etc.
Select the correct response from the following code:
A. I and III only
B. I, II, III and IV
C. I, III and IV
D. I and IV only

32. Following proteins are regarded as biologically complete, *save* for one:
A. Meat
B. Milk
C. Soyabean only
D. Fish
E. Egg only

33. The reference proteins are obtained from:
A. Fish
B. Meat
C. Soyabean only
D. Egg
E. Any of these

34. New tissues cannot be formed unless all the essential amino acids are present in the diet.
A. True
B. False

35. A protein is said to be "biologically complete" if it contains all the essential amino acids in amounts corresponding to human needs.
A. True
B. False

36. From the nutritional standpoint, animal proteins are rated superior to vegetable proteins because they are "biologically complete".
A. True
B. False

37. Statement (S): Egg proteins are considered to be the best among food proteins. Reason (R): Because of their high biological value and digestibility.
A. Both (S) and (R) are true and correctly explain each other
B. Both (S) and (R) are true explain each other
C. (S) is true but (R) is false
D. (S) is false but (R) is true

38. The CM1 response and the bactericidal activity of leucocytes have been found to be lowered in severe form of protein energy malnutrition.
A. True
B. False

39. The "limiting" amino acids is cereals protein include:
I. Methionine
II. Lysine
III. Threonine
IV. Valine
V. Tryptophan
Select the correct answer from the code given below:
A. I and II only
B. II and III only (IV and V only)
C. I, II and IV only
D. I, II, III, IV and V only
E. I, II, III, IV and V All

40. Lysine in cereals and methionine in pulses are good example of:
A. Essential amino acid
B. Supplementary action
C. First limiting amino acid
D. Non essential amino acid

41. "Vegetable proteins" are found in the following *except*:
A. Pulses
B. Beans
C. Cereals only
D. Oil-seed cakes
E. None of these

42. Statement (S): In India cereals and pulses are the main sources of dietary protein. Reason (R): Because they are cheap, easily available and consumed in bulk.
A. Both (S) and (R) are true and truly explained each other
B. Both (S) and (R) are true but does not explained each other
C. (S) is true, (R) is false
D. (S) is false but (R) is true
E. Both false

43. The most practical method of evaluation of protein quality is:
A. Biological value
B. Net protein utilization
C. Protein efficiency ratio
D. Digestibility coefficient

44. The reutilization of amino acids is a major contributary factor to the economy of protein metabolism.

A. True

B. False

45. Statement (S): The net protein utilization (NAU) is considered of more practical value.

Reasons (R): Because it is the product of biological value and digestibility coefficient divided by 100.

A. Both (S) and (R) are true and correctly explains each other

B. Both (S) and (R) are true but does not explain each other

C. (S) is true but (R) is false

D. Both (S) and (R) are false

46. The overall rate of turn-over in adult man is equivalent to replacement between 1 to 2% of body protein each day.

A. True

B. False

47. Following battery of tests have been suggested to assess the state of protein nutrition:

I. Arm-muscle circumference

II. Total body nitrogen

III. The creatinine-height index

IV. Serum albumin and transferrin

Select the true response from the code given below:

A. I and II only

B. II and III only

C. II, III and IV only

D. I. II, III and IV

48. At the present moment the best measure of the state of protein nutrition is probably:

A. Arm-muscle circumference

B. Serum albumin

C. The creatinine-height index

D. Serum transferrin

E. Total body nitrogen only

49. A level of 3.0 gm/dL of serum albumin indicates:

A. Mild degree of malnutrition

B. Moderate degree of malnutrition

C. Severe degree of malnutrition

D. A normal level

50. Serum albumin and transferrin assess the ability of the liver to synthesize proteins.

A. True

B. False

51. The ICMR (1981) recommended 1.0 gm protein/kg body weight for an adult assuming an NPU of 65 for the dietary proteins.

A. True

B. False

52. What amount of body fat in the adipose tissue is in the form of triglycerides?

A. 25%

B. 45%

C. 69%

D. 89%

E. 99%

53. In the normal human subjects, adipose tissue constitute what percent of body weight?

A. 5 to 9%

B. 10 to 15%

C. 16 to 25%

D. 26 to 41 %

E. > 50%

54. The accumulation of one kg of adipose tissue corresponds to how much quantity of energy?

A. 770 Kcals

B. 6600 Kcals

C. 7700 Kcals

D. 9000 Kcals

55. Following are recognized members of saturated fatty acids, *save* for one:

A. Oleic acid

B. Lauric acid

C. Palmitic acid

D. Stearic acid only

E. None of these

56. Statement (S): The most important essential fatty acid is linoleic acid.
Reason (R): Because linolenic and arachidonic acids are synthesized from it.
A. Both (S) and (R) are true but not related to each other
B. Both (S) and (R) are true and explained each other
C. (S) is true and (R) is false
D. Both (S) and (R) are false

57. Which of the following is not a polyunsaturated fatty acids?
A. Linolenic acid
B. Linoleic acid only
C. Oleic acid only
D. Arachidonic acid

58. The polyunsaturated fatty acids are mostly found in vegetable oils, and the saturated fatty acids mainly in animal fats.
A. True
B. False

59. Which of the following oils contains greatest contents of saturated fatty acids?
A. Palm oil
B. Butter only
C. Coconut oil
D. Cottonseed oil
E. Margarine only

60. Least quantity of saturated fatty acid are seen in the following oils/fats:
A. Soyabean oil
B. Safflower oil
C. Corn oil
D. Sunflower seed oil
E. Both C and D above

61. Least amount of monounsaturated fatty acids are found in following oils/fats:
A. Groundnut oil
B. Butter only
C. Coconut oil
D. Palm oil only
E. Soyabean oil only

62. Which of the following fats/oil contains greatest quantity of monounsaturated fatty acids?
A. Margarine only
B. Groundnut oil
C. Cottonseed oil
D. Sunflower oil

63. Not all polyunsaturated fatty acids are essential.
A. True
B. False

64. The least amount of polyunsaturated fatty acids are found in which oils/fats?
A. Palm oil
B. Butter
C. Coconut oil
D. Corn oil

65. The highest amount of polyunsaturated fatty acids are found in which oils/fats?
A. Sunflower oil
B. Safflower oil
C. Corn oil only
D. Soyabean oil only
E. Cottonseed oil only

66. The greatest percentage of linoleic acid is found in:
A. Soyabean oil
B. Seasame oil
C. Groundnut oil
D. Safflower oil
E. Corn oil only

67. Arachidonic acid is exclusively found in the following food materials, *but* one:
A. Fish oil only
B. Milk fat only
C. Meat only
D. Eggs only
E. None

68. "Fish oil" contains the following essential fatty acid:
I. Arachidonic acid
II. Linoleic acid

III. Eichosapentaenoic acid
IV. Linolenic acid

Select the true answer from the code given below:

A. I and II only
B. III only
C. I, II and IV
D. I, II, III and IV

69. The percentage of linoleic acid in the following foodstuffs is less than 50% *except*:

A. Palm oil only
B. Mustard oil
C. Coconut oil
D. Sesame oil only
E. Soyabean oil only

70. The percentage of linoleic acid in the following foodstuffs is more than 50%, *except*:

A. Safflower oil
B. Sunflower oil
C. Corn oil
D. Groundnut
E. Soyabean oil

71. Statement (S): Coconut and palm oils have an extremely high percentage of saturated fatty acids.
Reason (R): Because they belong to the category of vegetable oils.

A. Both (S) and (R) are true and truly explains each other
B. Both (S) and (R) are true but not related to each other
C. (S) is true and (R) is false
D. (R) is true and (S) is false
E. Both (S) and (R) are false

72. Animal fats are mostly saturated fats *except* cod liver oil and sardine oil.

A. True
B. False

73. "INVISIBLE FATS" (small quantities of fat) are found in the following food materials:

I. Cereals
II. Pulses
III. Nuts
IV. Vegetables

Select the true answer from the code given below:

A. I and II only
B. I and III only
C. II and III only
D. I, II, III and IV

74. Among the following foodstuffs, which of the following contains greatest percentage of invisible fats?

A. Rice only
B. Bajra only
C. Wheat
D. Jowar

75. "PROSTAGLANDINS" (Local hormones) play a major role in controlling following physiological function:

I. Vascular homeostasis
II. Kidney function
III. Acid secretion in stomach
IV. GIT motility
V. Lung physiology
VI. Reproduction

Select the correct response from the code:

A. I, II and III only
B. II, III and V only
C. I, II, III and V only
D. I, II, III, IV and V only
E. I, II, III, IV, V and VI All

76. Statement (S): "VANASPATI or DALDA" is prepared from the hydrogenation of vegetable oils.
Reason (R): Because of that it contains highest percentage of polyunsaturated fatty acids.

A. Both (S) and (R) are true and truly explains each other
B. Both (S) and (R) are true but unrelated cause and effect

C. (S) is true but (R) is false
D. Both (S) and (R) are false

77. During the process of hydrogenation of vegetable oils, its high polyunsaturated fats get converted into saturated fatty acids hence their essential fatty acid content is drastically reduced.
A. True
B. False

78. Statement (S): Refining only improves the quality and taste of oils.
Reason (R): Because it removes the free fatty acid and rancid materials.
A. Both (S) and (R) are true and explain each other
B. Both (S) and (R) are true but not related to each other
C. (S) is true but (R) is false
D. Both (S) and (R) are false

79. Statement (S): Vanaspati or Dalda is fortified with Vitamin A 2500 IU and Vitamin D 175 IU per 100 gms.
Reason (R): Because it lacks fat soluble vitamins.
A. Both (S) and (R) are true but do not explain each other
B. Both (S) and (R) are true and explains each other fully
C. (S) is true but (R) is false
D. Both (S) and (R) are false

80. Following are relevant about fats and disease:
I. Obesity only
II. Phrenoderma only
III. Coronary heart disease
IV. Cancer
Select the true response from the code given below:
A. I and II only
B. I, II and III only
C. I, II, III and IV
D. III and IV only

81. Deficiency of essential fatty acids in the diet is associated with rough and dry skin, known as:
A. Phrenoderma
B. Toad skin
C. Both of the above
D. Neither

82. "Phrenoderma" is reported from following states in India, *save* for one:
A. Kerala
B. Bihar
C. Gujarat only
D. Karnataka

83. "Phrenoderma" is characterized by horny papular eruptions on the posterior and lateral aspects of limbs and on the back and buttocks:
A. True
B. False

84. "Phrenoderma" can be cured rapidly by administration of:
A. Linseed oil only
B. Vitamin B complex
C. Safflower oil only
D. All of the above
E. Both B and C above

85. Diets high in fat increase the risk of following cancer:
I. Adrenal cancer
II. Breast cancer
III. Colon cancer
IV. Endometrial cancer
Select the true response from the following code:
A. I and IV only
B. I and II only
C. II and III only
D. I, II, III and IV

86. The WHO expert committee on prevention of coronary heart disease has recommended how much percent of total dietary energy to be provided by fats?
A. 5%

B. 10%
C. 20 to 30%
D. 40%
E. > 40% but < 50%

87. The ICMR (1981) has recommended a daily intake of not more than .... of total energy intake through fats:
A. 10%
B. 20%
C. 30%
D. 40%
E. 50%

88. Which of the following statements are true about carbohydrates?
A. CHO is the main source of energy providing 4 Kcals per one gram
B. CHO is essential for the oxidation of fats
C. CHO is necessary for the synthesis of certain non-essential amino acids
D. All of the above
E. Both A and B but not C above

89. Following are main sources of carbohydrates:
I. **Margarine**
II. **Starches**
III. **Sugar**
IV. **Cellulose**

Select the true response from the following code:
A. I and III only
B. I, II and III only
C. II and IV only
D. I, II, III and IV only
E. II, III and IV only

90. Statement (S): Starch is basic to the human diet.

Reason (R): Because it is found in abundance in cereals, roots and tubers.
A. Both (S) and (R) are true and correctly explains each other
B. Both (S) and (R) are true but not related to cause and effect
C. (S) is true, (R) is false
D. Both (S) and (R) are false

91. The carbohydrate reserve (Glycogen) of a human adult is about:
A. 250 gm
B. 500 gm
C. 750 gm
D. 1000 gm
E. 1250 gm

92. When the dietary carbohydrates do not meet the energy needs of the body, protein and glycerol from dietary and endogenous sources are used by the body to maintain glucose homeostasis?
A. True
B. False

93. Following are recognized examples of sugars:
I. **Glucose**
II. **Fructose**
III. **Galactose**
IV. **Sucrose**
V. **Lactose**
VI. **Maltose**

Select the true response from the code given below:
A. I, II and IV only
B. II, IV and V only
C. I, II, IV and V only
D. I, II, III, IV and V only
E. I, II, III, IV, V and VI All

94. Statement (S): Dietary fibre which is mainly non-starch polysaccharide is a physiologically important component of the diet.

Reason (R): Because it is found in vegetables, fruits and grains.
A. Both (S) and (R) are true but not related to each other
B. Both (S) and (R) are true and related to each other
C. (S) is true but (R) is false
D. Both (S) and (R) are false

95. Following statements are true regarding dietary fibres:

A. These all are degraded to a greater or lesser extent by the microflora in the human colon

B. Fibre may also have a role in weight reduction

C. Fibre helps reduce the tendency to constipation by encouraging bowel movements

D. All of the above

E. Both B and C true but not A

96. The conversion of Vitamin A can be done in the following way to retinol equivalent (RE):

I. 1 mcg of retinol = 1 mcg of RE

II. 1 mcg of β-carotene = 0.167 mcg of RE

III. 1 mcg of other carotenoids = 0.084 mcg of RE

Select the correct response from the code given below:

A. I only

B. I, II and III only

C. I and II only

D. II and III only

97. In which year the term "retinol" was introduced for Vitamin A-1 alcohol?

A. 1935

B. 1950

C. 1960

D. 1970

E. 1980

98. The international unit of Vitamin A is equivalent to:

A. 0.3 mcg of retinol

B. 0.55 mcg of retinol palmitate

C. Both of the above

D. None of these

99. Recognised functions of Vitamin 'A' includes:

I. It is indispensable for normal vision

II. It supports growth especially skeletal growth

III. It is anti infective

IV. It may protect against some epithelial cancer (Bronchial CA)

Select the true answer from the code given below:

A. I and II only

B. II and III only

C. I and III only

D. I, II, III and IV

E. I, II and III

100. Statement (S): Vitamin A (retinol) occurs in animal foods as preformed.
Reason (R): Because Vitamin A is widely distributed in animal and plant foods.

A. Both (S) and (R) are true and (R) is the true explanation of (S)

B. Both (S) and (R) are true but (R) is not the true explanation of (S)

C. (S) is true but (R) is false

D. Both (S) and (R) are false

101. Which of the following statement regarding Vitamin A is/are true?

A. Animal foods contains preformed Vitamin A called retinol

B. Plant foods contains provitamins as carotenes

C. Carotenes are converted to Vitamin A in the small intestine

D. The darker the green leaves the higher its carotene content

E. All of the above

102. Following foods are fortified with Vitamin A:

I. Vanaspati only

II. Margarine only

III. Milk

Select the true answer from the code given below:

A. I, II and III All

B. I and III only

C. I and II only

D. II and III only

103. The most important CAROTENOID is beta carotene which has the highest Vitamin A activity.
A. True
B. False

104. The richest natural sources of retinal is/ are:
A. OX, liver only
B. Fish liver oil
C. Cheese only
D. Fish only
E. All of the above

105. The retinol equivalent (mcg/100 gm) of following vegetable foodstuffs is greatest?
A. Mango
B. Papaya
C. Carrot
D. Spinach
E. Amaranth

106. The retinol equivalent (mcg/100 gm) of following animal foods is greatest?
A. Margarine
B. Butter only
C. Liver, Ox only
D. Cod liver oil only
E. Halibut liver oil only

107. The retinol equivalent (mcg/100 gm) of following vegetable foodstuffs is lowest?
A. Amaranth
B. Green leaves
C. Tomato only
D. Orange only
E. Both A and D above

108. The retinol equivalent (mcg/ 100 gm) of following animal food is lowest?
A. Fish
B. Butter
C. Cheese
D. Margarine
E. Egg

109. Statement (S): Liver stores Vitamin A mostly in the form of retinol palmitate.
Reason (R): Because the liver has an enormous capacity to store Vitamin A.
A. Both (S) and (R) are true but not related to cause and effect
B. Both (S) and (R) are true and C related to each other
C. (S) is true but (R) is false
D. Both (S) and (R) are true

110. The "Xerophthalmia" (dry eye) comprise, the following ocular manifestations of Vitamin 'A' deficiency:
I. Nightblindness
II. Conjunctival xerosis
III. Bitot's spots
IV. Corneal xerosis
V. Keratomalacia
Select the correct response from the code given below:
A. I and II only
B. I, III and IV only
C. II, III and V only
D. I, II, III, IV and V All
E. II, III, IV and V only

111. The 1st symptoms of Vitamin 'A' deficiency is:
A. Nightblindness
B. Bitot's spot
C. Conjunctival xerosis
D. Inability to see in dimlight
E. Both A and D above

112. The 1st clinical sign of Vitamin 'A' deficiency is:
A. Nightblindness
B. Bitot's spot
C. Conjunctival xerosis
D. Corneal xerosis
E. Both B and C above

113. Which of the following eye condition is regarded as a grave medical emergency?
A. Conjunctival xerosis
B. Bitot's spot
C. Corneal xerosis
D. Keratomalacia only
E. Any of the above

114. Following statements are true regarding the Bitot's spot, *except* for one:

A. They are triangular, pearly-white or yellowish, foamy spots on the bulbar conjunctiva on either side of cornea
B. They are frequently unilateral
C. Bitot's spots in young children usually indicate Vitamin 'A' deficiency
D. In older persons, these spots are often inactive sequelae of earlier disease
E. Non of these

115. A deficiency of Vitamin 'A' causes an increase in morbidity and mortality due to respiratory and intestinal infection.

A. True
B. False

116. Statement (S): Keratomalacia is one of the major causes of blindness in India. Reason (R): Because it is frequently associated with protein calorie malnutrition (PCM).

A. Both (S) and (R) are true but are unrelated to each other
B. Both (S) and (R) are true and are related to each other
C. (S) is false but (R) is true
D. Both (S) and (R) are false

117. The extraocular manifestations of Vitamin A deficiency include all the following, *but* one:

A. Anorexia
B. Follicular hyperkeratosis
C. Growth retardation
D. None of these

118. Nearly all of the early stages of xerophthalmia can be reversed by giving:

A. 2 lakh IU of Vitamin A orally
B. 110 mg of retinol palmitate orally
C. 2 lakh IU of Vitamin A and 110 mg retinol palmitate orally on two consecutive days
D. 2 lakh IU of Vitamin A IM
E. 110 mg retinol palmitate IM

119. Vitamin A deficiency can be prevented by reducing the frequency and severity of following contributory factors:

A. PCM
B. Respiratory tract infections
C. Measles
D. Diarrhoea
E. All of the above

120. The recommended daily intake of Vitamin A (retinol) is:

A. 750 mcg in adult males
B. 750 mcg in adult women
C. 750 mcg in pregnant ladies
D. All of the above

121. The daily intake of Vitamin A recommended by ICMR in 0 to 6 months of infants is:

A. 250 mcg
B. 300 mg
C. 400 mcg
D. 1000 mcg
E. 750 mcg

122. If the daily intake of Vitamin A recommended by ICMR in 13 to 15 years adolescents is 750 mcg then what should be the amount needed for 16 to 19 years adolescents?

A. 1000 mcg
B. 750 mcg
C. 500 mcg
D. 300 mcg
E. 250 mcg

123. If the daily intake of vitamin A recommended by ICMR in 6 to 12 months infants is 300 mcg, then what will be the amount for 4 to 6 years children?

A. 300 mcg
B. 400 mcg
C. 500 mcg
D. 750 mcg
E. 1000 mcg

124. The amount of vitamin A as recommended by ICMR during lactation in females is:
- **A.** 750 mcg
- **B.** 500 mcg
- **C.** 300 mcg
- **D.** 750 and 400 mcg

125. Following are the recognized toxicity of Vitamin A and its congeners, *except* for one:
- **A.** Nausea and vomiting
- **B.** Splenomegaly only
- **C.** Anorexia and sleep disorders
- **D.** Teratogenic effects
- **E.** Enlarged liver and papillary oedema

126. Regarding Vitamin D, which of the following statement is false?
- **A.** The nutritionally important Vitamin D in man are calciferol (Vitamin D2) and cholecalciferol (D3)
- **B.** Calciferol may not be derived from irradiation of ergosterol (a plant sterol)
- **C.** Cholecalciferol is the naturally occurring (preformed) Vitamin D which is found in animal fats and fish liver oils
- **D.** It is also derived from exposure to UV rays (Sunlight) which convert the cholesterol in the skin to Vitamin D
- **E.** Vitamin D is stored mainly in the fat depots

127. Following Vitamin is regarded as a kidney hormone:
- **A.** Vitamin A only
- **B.** Thiamine
- **C.** Vitamin D
- **D.** Vitamin K only
- **E.** All the above

128. The richest source of Vitamin D is:
- **A.** Shark liver oil
- **B.** Halibut liver oil
- **C.** Cod liver oil
- **D.** Fish fat only

129. Statement (S): Vitamin D is unique among other vitamins.
Reason (R): Because it is derived from both sunlight and food materials.
- **A.** Both (S) and (R) are true but not related to each other
- **B.** (S) is true but (R) is false
- **C.** (S) is false but (R) is true
- **D.** Both (S) and (R) are true and related to each other
- **E.** Both (S) and (R) are false

130. Vitamin D is synthesized by the body by the action of UV rays of sunlight on:
- **A.** Calceferol
- **B.** Ergosterol
- **C.** 7-dehydrocholesterol
- **D.** 25 OH cholecalciferol
- **E.** 1, 25 dihydroxy cholecalciferol

131. The poor dietary sources of Vitamin D is:
- **A.** Fish fat
- **B.** Butter
- **C.** Eggs only
- **D.** Whole milk only

132. Which of the following statement regarding the Vitamin D deficiency is/are correct?
- **A.** In young children, Vitamin D deficiency causes rickets
- **B.** In adults, Vitamin D deficiency causes osteomalacia
- **C.** Osteomalacia occurs mainly in women especially during pregnancy and lactation
- **D.** Both A and B above but not C
- **E.** All of the above

133. Statement (S): Muslim women are more frequently suffer from Vitamin 'D' deficiency.
Reason (R): Because of purdah system.
- **A.** Both (S) and (R) are true and (R) is the true explanation of (S)
- **B.** Both (S) and (R) are true but does not explain each other

C. (S) is true but (R) is false
D. Both (S) and (R) are false

134. Following are the recognised functions of Vitamin D and its metabolites, *except* for one:
A. Promotes intestinal absorption of calcium and phosphorus
B. Decreases tubular reabsorption of phosphate
C. Stimulates normal mineralization
D. Affects collagen maturation
E. Enhances bone resorption

135. "Rickets" is observed in following age groups:
A. < 6 months
B. > 6 months < 1 year
C. > 1 year but < 2 years
D. 6 months to 2 years
E. 5 to 15 years

136. The bony lesions of rickets include the following:
I. Curved legs
II. Deformed pelvis
III. Pigeon chest
IV. Harrison's sulcus
V. Rickety rosary
VI. Kyphoscoliosis
Select the true response from the following code:
A. I, II and IV
B. II, III and V
C. I, II, III and V
C. I, II, III, IV and V
E. I, II, III, IV, V and VI All

137. In adults Vitamin D deficiency may result in osteomalacia which occurs mainly in women, especially during pregnancy and lactation when requirements of Vitamin D are increased.
A. True
B. False

138. Statement (S): Fraser urges caution regarding Oral supplementation of Vitamin D.
Reason (R): Because orally administered Vitamin D appears to bypass the protective mechanism that prevents excessive 25(OH) D3 formation.
A. Both (S) and (R) are true but are not related to each other
B. Both (S) and (R) are true and correctly explains each other
C. (S) is true but (R) is false
D. Both (S) and (R) are false

139. The most practical approaches in developing countries to prevent Vitamin D deficiency include:
I. Educating parents to expose their children regularly to sunshine
II. Periodic dosing of young children with Vitamin D
III. Vitamin D fortification of food especially milk
IV. Education about Vitamin D uses
Select the correct answer from the following code given:
A. I and III only
B. II and IV only
C. I and II only
D. I, II, III and IV only

140. One I.U. of Vitamin D is equivalent to:
A. 0.1 µg of calciferol
B. 0.01 µg of calciferol
C. 0.25 µg of calciferol
D. 0.025 µg of calciferol

141. The following are true regarding the daily requirement of Vitamin D in following:
I. Adults–2.5 mcg (100 IU)
II. Infants and children–5.0 mcg (200 IU)
III. Pregnant ladies–10.0 mcg (400 IU)
IV. Lactating ladies–10.0 mcg (400 IU)

Select the true answer from the code given below:
A. I and III only
B. I and II only
C. II and IV only
D. I, II and III only
E. I, II, III and IV all ture

142. "TOCOPHEROLS" is the generic name for which of the following vitamins?
A. Vitamin 'E' only
B. Vitamin 'B' only
C. Vitamin 'A' only
D. Vitamin 'C' only
E. Thiamine of Vitamin 'B' complex family

143. Biologically the most potent tochopherol is:
A. Alpha-tocopherol
B. Beta-tocopherol
C. Gamma-tocopherol
D. Delta-tocopherol
E. Epsilon-tocopherol only

144. Strike the false statement regarding Vitamin 'E':
A. By far the richest sources are vegetable oils, cottonseed, sunflower seed, egg yolk and butter
B. Foods rich in polyunsaturated fatty acids are also rich in Vitamin 'E'
C. The usual plama level of Vitamin 'E' in adults is between 0.8 and 1.4 mg per 100 ml
D. The current estimate of Vitamin E requirement is about 25 mg per day per adult

145. Following, *but* one, statements are true regarding Vitamin 'K':
A. It occurs in two major forms—Vitamin K_1 and Vitamin K_2
B. Human milk is richer source of Vitamin K than cow's milk
C. Vitamin K_1 is found mainly in fresh green vegetables particulary dark green ones, and in some fruits
D. Vitamin K_2 is synthesized by the intestinal bacteria, which is quite sufficient for human

146. Statement (S): Administration of oral antibiotic may cause a deficiency of Vitamin 'K'.
Reason (R): Because antibiotic causes suppression of normal intestinal flora that synthesize vitamin K_2.
A. Both (S) and (R) are true and (R) is the true explanation of (S)
B. Both (S) and (R) are true but (R) is not the true explanation of (S)
C. (S) is true but (R) is false
D. Both (S) and (R) are false

147. Which organ stores Vitamin K in human being?
A. Pancreas
B. Gall bladder
C. Liver only
D. Large intestine
E. Kidneys only

148. Which of the following statement is/are true?
A. The role of Vitamin K is to stimulate the production and/or the release of certain coagulation factors
B. In Vitamin K deficiency, the prothrombin content of blood is markedly decreased
C. In Vitamin K deficiency the blood clotting time is considerably prolonged
D. All of the above
E. Both B and C but not A above

149. The daily Vitamin K requirement for adult man is:
A. 0.03 mg/kg
B. 0.06 mg/kg
C. 0.15 mg/kg
D. 1 mg/kg
E. None of the above

150. Statement (S): Newborn infants tend to be deficient in Vitamin 'K'.

Reason (R): Because of minimal stores of prothrombin at birth and lack of an established intestinal flora.

A. Both (S) and (R) are true but are not related to each other
B. Both (S) and (R) are true and are related to each other
C. (S) is true but (R) is false
D. (R) is true but (S) is false
E. Both (S) and (R) are false

151. All infants or those at increased risk should receive a single intramuscular dose of a Vitamin K preparation (0.1-0.2 mg of menadione sodium bisulphite or 0.5 mg of Vitamin K_1) by way of prophylaxis soon after birth.

A. True
B. False

152. Following statements are true regarding Thiamine (Vitamin B_1), but one:

A. It is essential for the utilization of carbohydrates
B. Thiamine pyrophosphate (TPP), the coenzyme of cocarboxylase plays a part in activating transketolase, and enzyme involved in the direct oxidative pathway for glucose
C. In thiamine deficiency, there is accumulation of pyruvic and lactic acids in the tissues and body fluids
D. The main source of thiamine in the diet of Indian people is cow's milk

153. The richest dietary sources of thiamine mg/100 gm:

A. Whole wheat
B. Gingelly seeds
C. Mutton only
D. Almonds only
E. None of the above

154. The main source of thiamine in the diet of Indian people is cereals (rice and wheat) which contribute from 60 to 85% of the total supply.

A. True
B. False

155. Daily requirements of thiamine is .... of energy intake.

A. 0.1 mg/1000 Kcals
B. 0.5 mg/100 Kcals
C. 0.5 mg/1000 Kcals
D. 1.5 mg/1000 Kcals

156. Following statements are true regarding thiamine (Vitamin B_1), *save* for one:

A. Thiamine is readily lost from rice during the process of milling
B. Much of the thiamine in fruits and vegetables is generally lost during prolonged storage
C. Thiamine is also destroyed in toast and in cereals cooked with baking soda
D. None of these

157. "Beri-Beri" is a deficiency disease due to lack of:

A. Biotin
B. Thiamine
C. Pyridoxine
D. Selenium

158. "Beri-Beri" may occur in following forms:

A. The dry form characterised by nerve involvement
B. The wet form characterised by heart involvement
C. Infantile beri-beri seen in infants between 2 and 4 months of life
D. Both A and B above
E. All of the above

159. Wernicke's encephalopathy (seen often in alcoholics) may be characterised by following:

I. Ophthalmoplegia
II. Polyneuritis
III. Ataxia
IV. Mental deterioration

Select the true answer from the code given below:
A. I and II only
B. II and III
C. III and IV only
D. I, II and III
E. I, II, III and IV all true

160. A patient presents with loss of appetite, absence of ankle and knee jerks and presence of calf tenderness. Most likely he is suffering from:
A. Motor neurone disease
B. Pyridoxine deficiency
C. Thiamine deficiency
D. Neurosyphilis
E. None

161. In the Western countries, "BERI-BERI" is most commonly due to excessive alcohol consumption.
A. True
B. False

162. Thiamine should also be given prophylactically to people with:
A. Persistent vomiting
B. Prolongd gastric aspiration
C. Prolonged fasting
D. All the above
E. A and C only

163. The body content of thiamine is placed at 30 mg and if more than this is given it is only lost in the urine.
A. True
B. False

164. Deficiency of riboflavin is widespread in India particularly in populations where .... is the staple died.
A. Rice
B. Wheat
C. Jowar
D. Bajra
E. Pulses

165. The most common lesion associated with riboflavin deficiency is:
A. Glossitis
B. Angular stomatitis
C. Cheilosis
D. Nasolabial dyssebacia
E. All of the above

166. The "erythrocyte glutathione reductase activation test" was carried by NIN Hyderabad to demonstrate which of the following?
A. Vitamin 'A'
B. Vitamine 'K'
C. Riboflavin
D. Pyridoxine only
E. None of the above

167. "Hyporiboflavinosis" may have subtle functional effects such as:
I. Impaired neuromotor function
II. Wound healing
III. Increased susceptibility to cataract

Select the true response from the following code:
A. I only
B. I and II
C. III only
D. I, II and III only

168. Riboflavine deficiency almost always occurs in association with deficiencies of other Vitamin B complex like pyridoxine (Vitamin B_6).
A. True
B. False

169. Richest natural sources of riboflavin includes all the following, *except* for one:
A. Milk
B. Liver
C. Kidney
D. Fish
E. Eggs

170. Daily requirement of riboflavin is .... of energy intake.
A. 0.2 mg/1000 Kcal
B. 0.6 mg/1000 Kcal
C. 0.3 mg/1000 Kcal
D. 1.0 mg/1000 Kcal

171. Following statements are true regarding NIACIN or NICOTINIC ACID *except* for one:
- **A.** It is necessary for the metabolism of carbohydrate fat and protein
- **B.** It is excreted in urine as such
- **C.** It is needed for the normal functioning of the skin, intestinal and nervous systems
- **D.** In maize it occurs in bound form hence unavailable to the consumer

172. Niacin differs from the other vitamins of the B Complex group in that an essential amino acid .... serves as its precursor:
- **A.** Glycine
- **B.** Threonine
- **C.** Tryptophan only
- **D.** Methionine only
- **E.** Any of the above

173. Niacin is excreted in urine in which form?
- **A.** Nicotinic acid only
- **B.** N-methyl pyridones
- **C.** N-methyl-nicotinamide
- **D.** Both B and C above
- **E.** All of the above

174. The recommended daily allowance of Niacin is .... of energy intake.
- **A.** 6.6 mg/1000 Kcal
- **B.** 0.6 mg/1000 Kcal
- **C.** 1.6 mg/1000 Kcal
- **D.** 3.6 mg/1000 Kcal

175. To produce 8 mg of niacin, how much quantity of tryptophan is needed?
- **A.** 60 mg
- **B.** 480 mg
- **C.** 240 mg
- **D.** 580 mg
- **E.** 880 mg

176. Niacin deficiency results in pellagra, which is characterised by the following:

I. Glossitis and stomatitis
II. Diarrhoea
III. Dermatitis
IV. Dementia

Select the true answer from the following code:
- **A.** I and II only
- **B.** II and III only
- **C.** II, III and IV only
- **D.** I, III and IV only
- **E.** I, II, III and IV All

177. Recognised mental changes of Pellagra includes which of the following?

I. Euphoria
II. Depression
III. Irritability
IV. Delirium

Select the true answer from the following code:
- **A.** I and II only
- **B.** I, II and IV
- **C.** II and IV
- **D.** II, III and IV only

178. In India, pellagra is prevalent in:
- **A.** Andhra Pradesh
- **B.** Bihar
- **C.** Karnataka
- **D.** Maharashtra
- **E.** Madhya Pradesh only

179. Excess of which amino acid appears to interfere in the conversion of tryptophan to niacin?
- **A.** Valine
- **B.** Leucine only
- **C.** Lysine only
- **D.** Methionine
- **E.** Phenylalanine only

180. Gopalan and others are of the opinion that amino acid imbalance caused by an excess of leucine is the cause of pellagra in:
- **A.** Rice eaters only
- **B.** Maize eaters only
- **C.** Jowar eaters only

D. Both B and C above
E. All of the above

181. Pyridoxin (Vitamin B_6) exists in following forms:
I. Pyridoxine
II. Pyridoxal
III. Pyridoxamine
IV. Pyrimethamine
Select the true response from the code given below:
A. I and II only
B. II and III only
C. I, II and III only
D. I, II, III and IV All

182. Following statements are true about pyridoxine *save* for one:
A. It does not play an important role in the metabolism of amino acids, fats and carbohydrate
B. It is widely distributed in milk, liver, meat, egg yolk, fish
C. Whole grain cereals, legumes and vegetables are good sources of Vitamin B_6
D. Its deficiency is associated with peripheral neuritis
E. Riboflavin deficiency impairs the optimal utilization of pyridoxine

183. Following are the recognized requirements of pyridoxine in the following situation, *except* for:
A. During pregnancy-2.5 mg/day
B. During lactation-2.5 mg/day
C. Young adults-2 mg/day
D. Patients receiving INH-5 mg/day

184. The amount of pantothenic acid excreted in the urine per day is about:
A. 1 mg B. 2 mg
C. 3 mg D. 4 mg
E. 5 mg only

185. The administration of following folic acid antagonists in early gestations may produce abortions or congenital malformations, *except* for one:
A. Alcohol only
B. Pyrimethamine
C. Cotrimoxazole only
D. Penicillin only
E. None of these

186. If the daily recommended intake of folic acid in healthy adult is 100 mcg, then what should be the intake in children?
A. 100 mcg B. 150 mcg
C. 200 mcg D. 300 mcg
E. 400 mcg

187. The chief storage site for Vitamin B_{12} is:
A. Spleen
B. Liver
C. Bone marrow
D. Lymphnodes

188. The amount of Vitamin B_{12} stored in the liver is:
A. 1 mg B. 1 gm
C. 2 mg D. 3 mg
E. 5 mg only

189. Following species require Ascorbic acid (Vitamin C) in their diet:
A. Man only
B. Monkey only
C. Guinea pig only
D. All of the above
E. Both A and B above

190. Statement (S): In Vitamin 'C' deficiency local haemorrhages occur and the bones get fracture easily.
Reason (R): Because lack of vitamin 'C' impairs collagen synthesis.
Select the true answer from the code given below:
A. Both (S) and (R) are true and are related to cause and effect
B. Both (S) and (R) are untrue and are not related to cause and effect
C. (S) is true, but (R) is false
D. (R) is true, (S) is false
E. Both (S) and (R) are false

191. Which of the following vitamin inhibits NITROSAMINE formation by the intestinal mucosa?
A. Vitamin 'A' only
B. Vitamin 'C'
C. Riboflavin
D. Folic acid

192. Which is regarded as one of the richest sources of Vitamin 'C' both in the fresh as well as in the dry condition?
A. Indian gooseberry (Amla)
B. Guava
C. Orange
D. Lime

193. Among the following vegetables which contains the least amount of ascorbic acid?
A. Brinjal
B. Radish
C. Amaranth
D. Cabbage
E. Potatoes

194. Which of the following vegetables (per 100 gm) contains the greatest amount of Vitamin 'C' (ascorbic acid)?
A. Amaranth
B. Spinach
C. Cabbage
D. Cauliflower

195. Statement (S): The bioavailability of minerals like iron and zinc may be low in a vegetarian diet.

Reason (R): Because of the presence of phytic acid.

Choose the correct answer as per code given below:
A. Both (S) and (R) are true, but not related to cause and effect
B. Both (S) and (R) are true and are related to cause and effect
C. (S) is true, (R) is false
D. (R) is true, (S) is false
E. Both (S) and (R) false

196. If a litre of cow's milk provides 1200 mg of calcium, then 1 litre of human milk provides how much quantity of calcium?
A. 1200 mg
B. 900 mg
C. 300 mg
D. 600 mg
E. 1000 mg

197. The average adult body contains about 1200 mg of calcium then the amount of phosphorous in adult human is:
A. 200 gm
B. 400 gm
C. 300 gm
D. 400 to 700 gm
E. 100 gm

198. If the amount of sodium in adult human body is 100 gm, then the amount of potassium would be:
A. 50 gm
B. 100 gm
C. 250 mg
D. 100 mg
E. 250 gm

199. Magnesium is essential for the normal metabolism of:
A. Na^+ only
B. K^+ only
C. Ca^{++} only
D. Both B and C above
E. All of the above

200. Iron is essential for many functions in the body including:
I. Hb formation
II. Brain development and function
III. Regulation of body temperature and muscle activity
IV. Catecholamine metabolism

Select the true answer as per code given below:
A. I only
B. I and IV only
C. I, II, III and IV All
D. I, II and III only

201. Regarding IRON, following statements are true, *except*:
A. Each gm of Hb. contains about 3.34 mg of iron
B. Iron is mostly absorbed from duodenum and upper small intestine in the ferrous state (Fe^{++})
C. The total daily iron loss in adult male is 1 mg and menstruating women is 2 mg
D. The adult human contains about 3 to 4 gm of iron

202. The absorbed iron is transported as plasma ferritin and stored in the following organs *save* for one:
A. Lymph nodes
B. Bone marrow
C. Liver
D. Spleen
E. Kidney

203. Following substances in Indian diet inhibits iron absorption:
I. Phytates in bran
II. Phosphates in egg yolk
III. Tannin in tea
IV. Oxalates in vegetables

Choose the true answer as per following code:
A. I and II only
B. I, II and III
C. I, II, III and IV All
D. I, III and IV only

204. "Latent iron deficiency" is the most widely prevalent stage of iron deficiency seen in India has the following features:
A. Iron stores are exhausted but anaemia has not occurred as yet
B. Its recognition depends upon measurement of serum ferritin
C. The % saturation of transferrin falls from a normal value of 30% to less than 15%
D. All of these
E. Both B and C above

205. At all ages the normal MCHC should be:
A. 15%
B. 20%
C. 25%
D. 30%
E. 34%

206. Following statements are true regarding the evaluation of iron status, *save* for one:
A. Haemoglobin concentration is a relatively sensitive index of nutrient depletion
B. Serum iron concentration is a more useful index than Hb concentration
C. Serum transferin saturation should be above 16% (normal value 30%)
D. None of these

207. To test the efficiency of pasteuization the following tests are done, *except*:
A. Phosphatase test
B. Standard plate count
C. Milk ring test
D. Coliform count

208. Consider the following facts about serum ferritin:
I. The single most sensitive tool for evaluating the iron status is by measurement of serum ferritin
II. It reflects the size of iron stores in the body
III. It is the most useful indicator of iron status in a population where the prevalence of iron deficiency is not high
IV. Values below 10 mcg/L probably indicate an absence of stored iron

Choose the correct answer as per following code:
A. I and II only
B. I, II, III and IV All
C. II, III and IV only
D. I, II and III only

209. The adult human body contains about how much quantity of iodine?
A. 25 mg

B. 36 mg
C. 50 mg
D. 75 mg
E. 100 mg

210. The best sources of iodine is:
A. Sea fish only
B. Sea salt
C. Cod liver oil
D. All of the above
E. Both A and B above

211. Consider the following statements:
I. The blood level of iodine is about 8 to 12 mcg/dl
II. About 50% of iodine comes from foods eaten
III. Cabbage, cauliflower and other members of Brassica group contains goitrogens that produce goitre
IV. Most important among the dietary goitrogens are probably cyano-glycosides and the thiocyanates

Choose the correct answer as per code given below:
A. I only
B. I and II only
C. I, II and III only
D. II and IV only
E. I, III and IV only

212. The most abundant element in nature is:
A. Na^+
B. K^+
C. Fluorine (Fl)
D. Iron (Fe)
E. Mg^{++}

213. About what % of fluoride in the body is found in bones and teeth?
A. 12%
B. 20%
C. 50%
D. 75%
E. 96%

214. Regarding zinc, all are correct, *save* for one:
A. Zinc is active in the metabolism of glucides and proteins
B. It is required for the synthesis of insulin
C. The average adult contains 1.2 to 2.3 mg of zinc
D. Animal foods such as meat, milk and fish are dependable sources
E. Its deficiency results in growth failure, sexual infantilism, delayed wound healing

215. Low circulating zinc levels may cause following clinical conditions:
I. Liver disease
II. Pernicious anaemia
III. Thalassaemia
IV. Myocardial infarction

Choose the correct answer as per following code:
A. I, II, III and IV All
B. I and II only
C. I, II and III only
D. II and IV only

216. "Hypocupremia" (low serum Cu^{++}) occurs in patients with:
A. Nephrosis
B. Wilson's disease
C. Protein energy malnutrition
D. Infants fed for prolonged period exclusively on cow's milk
E. All of the above

217. The best documented abnormality of copper deficiency is:
A. Lymphocytosis
B. Neutrophilia
C. Neutropenia only
D. Monocytosis
E. Eosinophilia

218. Hypercuperemia (high serum Cu^{++}) is seen in the following:
I. Leukaemia
II. Hodgkin's disease
III. Hyperthyroidism
IV. Severe anaemia
V. Haemochromatosis
VI. Myocardial infarction

Choose the true answer as per following code:

A. I, II, III and IV
B. I, II, III, IV, V and VI All
C. II, III and V
D. I, III and V

219. The occurrence of unusual glucose tolerance curves are responsive to:

A. Cobalt
B. Selenium
C. Chromium
D. Molybdenum
E. All of the above

220. Deficiency of which trace elements is associated with mouth and oesophageal cancer?

A. Zinc
B. Cobalt
C. Chromium
D. Molybdenum
E. Selenium

221. People subsisting mainly on white or polished rice are prone to develop:

A. Anaemia
B. Beri-beri
C. Pellagra
D. Diabetes mellitus

222. The incorporation of opaque-2 gene into which cereal has greatly improved the quality of its protein content?

A. Maize
B. Wheat
C. Rice only
D. All of these
E. Both B and C above

223. Regarding jowar (sorghum), which is NOT true?

A. It is also known as kaffir corn or milo
B. It is a major crop grown in India next only to wheat and rice
C. Its protein is limiting in lysine and threonine
D. Its excessive consumption may cause pellagra
E. It is the cheapest among millets

224. Which of the following PULSES contain Vitamin 'C'?

A. Soyabean
B. Bengal gram
C. Black gram
D. Red grain

225. Presence of high amounts of OLIGOSACCHARIDES is known to be associated with flatulence in the following:

A. Rice
B. Bajra
C. Pulses only
D. Ragi

226. Which nuts is regarded as the richest source of iron?

A. Groundnut
B. Pistachio
C. Almonds
D. Cashewnut

227. Which nuts contain greatest quantity of proteins?

A. Groundnuts
B. Walnuts
C. Cashewnuts
D. Almonds only

228. "Carotene" is almost NIL in the following fruits, *except* for one:

A. Grapes
B. Guava
C. Orange only
D. Sitaphal only

229. "Lactose" content of which of the following species of milk is highest?

A. Human
B. Buffalo
C. Cow
D. Goat only

230. The term "toned" milk is an Indian coinage. It has a composition nearly equivalent's to following milk:
A. Human
B. Cows
C. Buffalo
D. Goat
E. Ass only

231. Following vitamins are contained in egg, *but* one:
A. Vitamin A
B. Vitamin D
C. Vitamin C only
D. Vitamin E
E. Vitamin K only

232. Which of the following animal foods contain all the nine essential amino acids needed by the body in right proportion?
A. Meat
B. Liver
C. Fish
D. Egg
E. Any of the above

233. A cup of which of the following beverages provides maximum calories per cup of 150 ml?
A. Cocoa
B. Coffee
C. Tea
D. Both A and B above
E. All of these

234. One million joules is equivalent to how much kilocalories?
A. 4184 Kcal
B. 0.239 Kcal
C. 239 Kcal
D. 1000 Kcal

235. If the Indian reference man (60 kg. wt.) needs 45 Kcal/kg/24 hrs energy, then the Indian reference woman (50 kg) needs how much?
A. 30 Kcal/kg/day
B. 35 Kcal/kg/day
C. 40 Kcal/kg/day
D. 45 Kcal/kg/day
E. 50 Kcal/kg/day

236. In infants the total EAA 42 mg/kg per day is required then adults should require how much of EAA per day?
A. 742 mg/kg/day
B. 352 mg/kg/day
C. 261 mg/kg/day
D. 216 mg/kg/day
E. 84 mg/kg/day

237. In India, what % of pregnancy culminates in LBW babies?
A. 15%
B. 20%
C. 25%
D. 30%
E. 50% only

238. The incidence of PEM in India in preschool age children is:
A. 1%
B. 1 to 2%
C. 3%
D. 4%
E. 5.5%

239. NOT seen in the MARASMUS child is:
A. Irritable
B. No oedema
C. Severe loss of subcutaneous fat
D. Good appetite
E. No hepatomegaly

240. Which is NOT an usual findings in KWASHIORKOR?
A. Oedema
B. Apathetic
C. Plasmal amino acid ratio elevated
D. Poor appetite
E. Flaky paint dermatosis

241. Xerophthalmia refers to all the ocular manifestations of Vitamin A deficiency

in man. It is most common in children aged:

A. 1 year
B. 2 years
C. 1 to 3 years
D. 1 to 5 years
E. > 5 years

242. The states badly affected by xerophthalmia includes (upto 1998):

I. Andhra Pradesh
II. Tamil Nadu
III. Karnataka
IV. Bihar
V. West Bengal

Choose the true answer as per code given below:

A. I, II and III
B. I, II, III and IV
C. II, III and IV
D. I, II, III, IV and V All
E. I, III and V

243. The Government of India started its national Vitamin A prophylaxis programme for the prevention of blindness in children in 1970 based on periodic massive dosing of .... retinol palmitate in oil every 6 months.

A. 2 lakhs IU
B. 110 mg
C. Both of the above
D. Neither

244. By far the most frequent cause of nutritional anaemia is:

A. Iron deficiency
B. Vitamin B_{12} only
C. Folate
D. All of these
E. Both B and C above

245. The world's biggest goitre belt is:

A. Africa
B. Himalaya goitre belt
C. Australian goitre belt
D. European goitre belt
E. None of the above

246. In 1960s, it was estimated that about 9 million persons were affected by goitre, currently in India how much population in sub-Himalayan goitre belt of India has been suffering of goitre?

A. 9 million
B. 18 million
C. 55 million
D. 140 million

247. "Two-in-one" salt contains:

A. Salt and Iron
B. Salt and Iodine
C. Salt and Iodine and T4
D. Salt and Iron and Iodine
E. None of the above

248. Under the national IDD control activities, the Government of India proposed to completely replace common salt with iodized salt in a phased manner by:

A. 1992
B. 1993
C. 1995
D. 1998
E. 2001

249. One 1M injection of iodized oil (poppy seed oil) of 1 ml would provide protection for about:

A. 1 year
B. 2 years
C. 3 years
D. 4 years
E. 5 years

250. In dental fluorosis, mottling is best seen on the:

A. Molar of upper jaw
B. Incisors of upper jaw
C. Molar of lower jaw
D. Incisors of lower jaw

251. The toxic C/M of fluorosis includes the following *save* for:

A. Dental fluorosis

B. Skeletal fluorosis
C. Genu valgum
D. Muscular fluorosis
E. None of these

252. "Crippling fluorosis" may ensue, when the concentration of fluoride in body exceeds:
A. 3 mg/L
B. 5 mg/L
C. 7 mg/L
D. 10 mg/L

253. NEERI, Nagpur has developed a technique for defluoridation of water called as:
A. Gondwana technique
B. Nalgonda technique
C. Peston technique
D. Sulabh International technique

254. Neurolathyrism results when diets containing more than 30% of this Khesari dhal if taken over a period of:
A. 1 month
B. 2 months
C. 2 to 6 months
D. 6 to 12 months

255. Neurolathyrism is nowadays prevalent in:
A. M.P. only
B. U.P.
C. Bihar
D. Orissa
E. All of the above

256. Which of the following vitamin helps to control in cases of neurolathyrism?
A. Vitamin A
B. Vitamin C
C. Vitamin B_6
D. Vitamin D
E. Vitamin E

257. The body's best bulwark against CHD is:
A. Linoleic acid
B. LDL
C. Thromboxanes
D. Prostacycline

258. Coronary heart disease rates are lowest in populations eating high:
A. Protein diet
B. Fatty diet
C. Carbohydrate diet
D. Salty diet
E. Both A and D above

259. The highest incidence of hypertension is found in:
A. USA
B. U.K.
C. Canada
D. North Japan
E. East European nations

260. Excessive consumption of alcohol can increase the risk of diabetes mellitus (DM) by:
A. Damaging liver
B. Damaging pancreas only
C. Promoting obesity
D. All of these
E. Both B and C above

261. DIABETICS ate an average .... per day more than nondiabetics:
A. 250 Kcal
B. 1000 Kcal
C. 500 Kcal
D. 750 Kcal
E. 1500 Kcal

262. Consider the following statements:
I. The high fat intake accounts for the high incidence of colon cancer in western communities
II. The risk of stomach CA has been related to a deficiency of Ascorbic acid (Vitamin C)
III. The risk of colon CA is inversely related to the consumption of dietary fibre
IV. Heavy drinking (alcohol) increases the risk of liver CA

Choose the correct answer as per code given below:
A. I and II only
B. I, II and III
C. I, II, III and IV All
D. II and IV only
E. I and III only

263. Regarding assessment of nutritional status, the most important lab. test carried out in nutritional surveys includes:
A. Serum protein estimation
B. Hb estimation
C. Serum retinol
D. Serum albumin only
E. Prothrombin time

264. Indicator of maternal nutrition includes:
A. Birth weight
B. Height for age
C. Weight for age
D. All of these
E. Both B and C above

265. Malnutrition comprises following forms:
A. Undernutrition only
B. Overnutrition
C. Imbalance
D. Specific deficiency
E. All of the above

266. Following international agencies are working in close collaboration helping the national governments in different parts of the world in their battle against malnutrition:
I. FAO
II. UNICEF
III. WHO
IV. World Bank
V. UNDP
VI. CARE

Choose the true answer as per code given below:
A. I, II and III only
B. I, II, IV and V only
C. I, II, III and VI only
D. I, II, III, IV and V only
E. I, II, III, IV, V and VI All

267. Following animal infections that may be transmitted to man through animal milk has got primary importance, *except* for one:
A. Tuberculosis
B. Staphylococcal enterotoxin poisoning
C. Q fever only
D. Cowpox only
E. Brucellosis only

268. Following infections primary to man that can be transmitted through milk includes all, *but* one:
A. Typhoid and paratyphoid fever
B. Viral hepatitis
C. Diphtheria
D. Enteropathogenic E.coli only
E. None of these

269. Regarding methylene blue reduction test, which is false?
A. It is an indirect method for detection of microbes in milk
B. The test is carried out on the milk accepted for pasteurization
C. It is based on the observation that bacteria growing in milk bring about a decrease in the colour imparted to milk
D. The milk which remains blue the shortest is considered to be the best quality
E. In conducting the test, definite quantities of methylene blue are added to 10 ml of milk and the sample is held at a uniform temperature of 37°C until the blue colour has disappeared

270. Which of the following method of Pasteurisation of milk has been the recommended method for small and rural communities?
A. Holder method
B. HTST method
C. Vat method

D. UHT method
E. Both A and C above

271. Which test is widely used to check the efficiency of Pasteurization?
A. Phosphatase test
B. Standard plate count
C. Coliform count
D. Both B and C above
E. All of the above

272. Ingestion of contaminated meat may produce all, *except*:
A. Actinomycosis
B. Helminthiasis
C. Tuberculosis only
D. Fasciola hepatica
E. T. solium/T. saginata

273. Following diseases can be transmitted by fish:
A. Vibrio parahaemolyticus
B. Salmonella species
C. Clostridium botulinum type E
D. All of these
E. Both A and C above

274. Following infections are likely to be transmitted by food handlers:
I. Diarrhoea, dysenteries, typhoid and paratyphoid fevers
II. Enteroviruses and viral hepatitis
III. Protozoal cysts and eggs of helminths
IV. Streptococcal and staphylococcal infections
Choose the true answer as per code given below:
A. I only
B. I and II only
C. I, II, III and IV All
D. I, II and IV
E. I, II and III only

275. Persons having the following conditions should not be permitted to handle food or utensils?
A. Wounds
B. Otitis media
C. Skin infections
D. All of the above
E. Both A and C above

276. Following may cause food intoxications, *but* one:
A. Lathyrism
B. Botulism
C. Ergot
D. Staphylococcal
E. Streptococcal infections

277. Following foodborne intoxications are due to FUNGI *save* for one:
A. Endemic ascites
B. Aflatoxin
C. Ergot
D. Fusarium toxin

278. In CANNED FOOD, chemical poisoning ensues due to:
A. Mercury
B. Lead
C. Cadmium
D. Iron
E. TCP only

279. Following PARASITES have been recognised as foodborne infections:
I. Taeniasis and hydatidosis
II. Trichinosis
III. Oxyuriasis
IV. Amoebiasis
V. Ascariasis
Select the true answer as per following code:
A. I and IV only
B. IV and V only
C. I, II, III, IV and V All
D. I, III, IV and V only

280. "Neurolathyrism" is due to toxin called BOAA which stands for:
A. β–oxalyl amino alanine
B. β–oxalo acetic acid

C. β–oxalo amino acid
D. β–oxalyl ammonium alurete

281. "BOAA" is a food toxin found in:
A. Aflatoxins
B. Groundnut
C. Khesari dhal
D. Sorghum

282. To prevent aflatoxicosis, it is desirable that moisture content in the storage of foodgrains should be kept below:
A. 1%
B. 10%
C. 5%
D. 16%
E. 20%

283. Following foodgrains have a tendency to get infested during flowering stages by the ERGOT, *but* one:
A. Groundnut
B. Bajra
C. Rye
D. Sorghum
E. Wheat

284. "Aflatoxin" is produced by the following:
A. Aspergillus flavus
B. Aspergillus parasiticus
C. Aspergillus niger
D. Both A and B above
E. All of these

285. "Claviceps fusiformis" causes what?
A. Aflatoxicosis
B. Ergotism
C. Fusarium toxins
D. Epidemic dropsy
E. Endemic ascites

286. The upper safe limit for the ergot alkaloids has been estimated to be .... per 100 grams of the food material.
A. 0.05 mg
B. 0.1 mg
C. 0.5 mg
D. 1 mg
E. 5 mg

287. Who among the following isolated "SANGUINARINE" from argemone oil and found out its chemical formula as well?
A. Sarkar *et al.* (1926)
B. Lal and Roy (1937)
C. Mukherji *et al.* (1941)
D. Chopra *et al.* (1939)

288. "Sanguinarine" interferes with the oxidation of .... which gets accumulated in the blood?
A. Lactic acid
B. Pyruvic acid
C. Alginic acid
D. Acetic acid

289. "Sanguinarine" is obtained from:
A. Argemone mexicana
B. Brassica rapa
C. Claviceps purpura
D. Jhunjhunia seeds
E. Fusarium incamatum

290. "Epidemic dropsy" is NOT seen in following age groups:
A. Adolescents
B. Breast fed infants
C. Children
D. Adults

291. Which is the most sensitive test for detecting argemone oil yet devised?
A. Phosphatase test
B. Nitric acid test
C. Paper chromatography test
D. All of the above
E. Both B and C above

292. "Epidemic dropsy" results due to consumption of:
A. Argemone oil
B. Khesari dhal
C. Mustard oil
D. Ergot

293. Most of the cases of "Endemic Ascites" in India has been reported from which state?
A. Assam
B. Bihar
C. M.P.
D. U.P.
E. Orissa

294. "Jhunjhunia poisoning" is caused by:
A. Aflatoxin
B. Argemone mexicana
C. Aspergillus
D. Crotolaria
E. Fusarium incamatum

295. NOT true about Endemic Ascites is:
A. An outbreak of rapidly developing ascites and jaundice
B. Affects both sexes of all age groups except infants
C. Caused by fusarium (Pyrrolizidina alkaloids) hepatotoxins
D. The overall mortality is about 40%

296. In India, which govern the rules and regulations of food additives?
A. The Prevention of Food Adulteration Act
B. The fruit products order
C. Both of the above
D. Neither A nor B

297. Recognised examples of food fortification includes all the following, *but* one:
A. Addition of vanilla essence in icecream
B. Fluoridation of water
C. Iodization of salt
D. In vanaspati or milk
E. Addition of Vitamin A

298. In India, common adulterants used for asafoetida includes the following, *save* for one:
A. Sand
B. Grit
C. Resins
D. Date husk
E. Gums

299. In India, common adulterants used for coffee powder is:
A. Date bush
B. Tamarind husk
C. Chicory
D. Both A and C above
E. All of the above

300. "Lead chromate" powder is used as adulterant for:
A. Dhania powder
B. Haldi powder
C. Chilli powder
D. Coffee powder
E. All of the above

301. Prevention of Food Adulteration Act was enacted by the Indian Parliament in which year?
A. 1947
B. 1952
C. 1954
D. 1960
E. 1964

302. Statement (S): The voluntary agencies and consumer guidance societies can play a vital role in curbing food adulteration.
Reason (R): Because the general public, traders and food inspectors are all responsible for perpetuating this evil.
Choose the true answers as per code given below:
A. Both (S) and (R) are true, and are related to cause and effect
B. Both (S) and (R) are true but are unrelated to cause and effect
C. (S) is true, (R) is false
D. (R) is false, (S) is false
E. (R) is true, (S) false

303. Adulteration of edible oils with which of the following results in paralysis and death?
A. Argemone oil
B. Trycresyn phosphate (TCP)
C. BOM only

D. All of the above
E. Both A and C above

304. The Prevention of Food Adulteration Act was amended in the following years, *save* for one:
A. 1964
B. 1976
C. 1986
D. 1996
E. 1954

305. Who organises in service training programme for different functionaries responsible for implementation of the PFA Act?
A. UNICEF
B. WHO
C. DGHS
D. Ministry of Food, Government of India

306. Which is the principal organ of the joint FAO/WHO food standards programme formulates food standards for international market?
A. The Agmark standard
B. Codex alimentarius
C. PFA standards
D. Bureau of International Standards

307. To obtain a minimum level of quality of foodstuffs attainable under Indian conditions, which of the following is usually applicable?
A. The Agmark standards
B. ISI mark
C. Codex alimentarius
D. PFA standards

308. Following nutrition programme is operated by Ministry of Education:
A. Mid-day meal programme
B. ICDS
C. SNP only
D. Balwadi nutrition programme

309. Ministry of Health and Family Welfare organises the following nutrition programme in India, *but* one:
A. Vitamin A prophylaxis programme
B. SNP only
C. Prophylaxis against nutritional anaemia
D. Iodide deficiency disorders control programme

310. Which of the following nutrition programme has NOT been organised by Ministry of Social Welfare?
A. SNP
B. Balwadi nutrition programme only
C. Mid-day meal programme
D. ICDS programme

311. The National Goitre Control Programme was launched in which year in India?
A. 1952
B. 1962
C. 1972
D. 1982
E. 1992

312. A National Programme for the Prevention of Nutritional Anaemia was launched by the Government of India during the:
A. 1st five-year plan
B. 3rd five-year plan
C. 4th five-year plan
D. 5th five-year plan
E. 7th five-year plan

313. Following Government agencies are involved in implementing the nutritional anaemia prevention in urban areas?
A. ICDS
B. MCH only
C. PHC only
D. All of the above
E. Both A and B above

314. "SNP" was started in which year?
A. 1970
B. 1973
C. 1975
D. 1980
E. 1990

315. Consider the following statements about SNP:

I. The nutritional benefit of children below 6 years of age, pregnant and nursing mothers and is in operation in urban slums, tribal areas and backward rural areas

II. The supplementary food supplies about 300 Kcal and 10 to 12 gms. of protein per child per day

III. The beneficiary mothers receive daily 500 Kcal and 25 gm of protein

IV. Such supplements provided to the target groups throughout the year

Choose the true answer as per code given below:

A. I and II only
B. I, II and IV only
C. I and IV only
D. I, II and III only
E. I, II, III and IV All

316. Each Anganwadi unit covers a population of about:

A. 100
B. 300
C. 500
D. 750
E. 1000

317. Under ICDS programme, field supervision is done by:

A. CDPO
B. Mahila mandals
C. Mukhyasevikas
D. All of the above

318. The Midday Meal Programme (MDMP) because part of the Minimum Needs Programme in the:

A. 1st five-year plan
B. 3rd five-year plan
C. 5th five-year Plan
D. 7th five-year plan
E. 8th five-year plan

319. Under MDMP, according to NIN the minimum number of feeding days in a year should be .... to have the desired impact on the children.

A. 180 days
B. 230 days
C. 300 days
D. 250 days
E. 360 days

320. If a person is NOT using any types of PULSES in his/her diet, then which of the following mould be the best supplementation?

A. Two eggs
B. 50 gm of meat
C. 50 gm of fish
D. One egg and 30 gm of meat
E. Any of the above

321. Following additional allowances (food items) during pregnancy are recommended over and above the daily needs, *save* for one:

A. Fat 7 gm
B. Cereal 35 gm
C. Pulses 15 gm
D. Milk 100 gm
E. Sugar 10 gm

322. Total calories from additional foods during pregnancy amounts to how much?

A. 100 Kcal
B. 200 Kcal
C. 293 Kcal
D. 400 Kcal

323. Nutritional calories from additional foods during lactation .... amounts to how much?

A. 100 Kcal
B. 200 Kcal
C. 400 Kcal
D. 550 Kcal

324. Following pulses has highest content of iron:

A. Bengal gram

B. Soyabean
C. Red gram
D. Black gram

325. The recommended daily energy intake of an adult woman with heavy work is:
A. 1800 Kcal
B. 2100 Kcal
C. 2300 Kcal
D. 2900 Kcal

326. The best indicator for monitoring the impact of iodine deficiency disorder control programme is:
A. Iodine level in soil
B. Neonatal hypothyroidism
C. Prevalence of goitre among school children
D. Urinary I_2 levels among pregnant women

327. Dates are rich source of:
A. Calcium
B. Iron
C. Carotene
D. Vitamin C

328. The nodal ministry for ICDS programme centre is:
A. Ministry for rural development
B. Ministry for human resource development
C. Ministry for health and family welfare
D. Social justice

329. ICDS scheme is sponsored by:
A. Ministry of Health and Family Welfare
B. Ministry of Social Welfare
C. Ministry of Education
D. All of the above

330. Soyabean is deficient in:
A. Tryptophan
B. Lysine
C. Methionine
D. Threonine

331. Soyabean is rich in:
A. Alanine
B. Glycine
C. Aspartic acid
D. Lysine

332. Community health guide measures malnutrition by:
A. MAC
B. Height and weight
C. Skin fold thickness
D. All of the above

333. Severe wasting is:
A. < 50%
B. < 60%
C. < 70%
D. < 80%

334. Classification of grades of PEM given by Indian academy of paediatrics as adopted:
A. ICMR standards
B. Standards adopted by NIN, Hyderabad
C. Local standards
D. NCHS standards

335. The 1st and the most common C/M of epidemic dropsy is:
A. Bilateral leg swelling
B. GIT upsets
C. Sarcoid
D. Cardiac decompensation

336. The Hb cut off level for determining prevalence of anemia among pregnant women in India is:
A. < 15 gm/dL
B. 13 gm/dL
C. < 11gm/dL
D. < 7gm/dL

337. Fat content is highest in:
A. Beef
B. Mutton
C. Chicken
D. Fish

338. Additional calorie requirement during lactation is:
A. 450 Kcal

B. 550 Kcal
C. 650 Kcal
D. 750 Kcal

339. The edible oil yields highest quantity of polyunsaturated fatty acid is:
A. Corn oil
B. Coconut oil
C. Sunflower oil
D. Groundnut oil

340. Maximum amount of PUFA is in:
A. Palmitic acid
B. Stearic acid
C. Oleic acid
D. Linoleic acid

341. Highest % of EFA is found in:
A. Corn oil
B. Butter fat (ghee)
C. Sunflower seed oil
D. Groundnut oil

342. Highest amount of linoleic acid is in:
A. Sunflower oil
B. Safflower oil
C. Corn oil
D. Coconut oil

343. All are of vegetable origin, *except*:
A. Vitamin A
B. Vitamin B
C. Vitamin C
D. Vitamin B_{12}

344. On exposure to sunlight which vitamin get lost?
A. Vitamin C
B. Vitamin A
C. Vitamin B_1
D. Vitamin B_6

345. The WHO criterion for evidence of a xerophthalmia problem in the community is:
A. Corneal ulcers in > 0.5% of population of 6 months to years age
B. Night blindness prevalence of >1% in 6 months to 6 years age group
C. Prevalence of bitot spots >2% in 6 months to 6 years age group
D. None of these

346. Protein content highest per 100 gm is:
A. Groundnut B. Milk
C. Egg D. Meat

Answers

1 A	2 B	3 D	4 B	5 A	6 B	7 D	8 A	9 A	10 C
11 C	12 B	13 A	14 D	15 B	16 A	17 B	18 D	19 C	20 A
21 E	22 B	23 C	24 D	25 A	26 B	27 B	28 A	29 D	30 A
31 B	32 C	33 D	34 A	35 A	36 A	37 B	38 A	39 B	40 C
41 E	42 A	43 B	44 A	45 A	46 A	47 B	48 B	49 C	50 A
51 A	52 E	53 B	54 C	55 A	56 B	57 C	58 A	59 C	60 E
61 C	62 B	63 A	64 C	65 B	66 D	67 A	68 B	69 E	70 D
71 A	72 A	73 D	74 B	75 E	76 C	77 A	78 A	79 B	80 C
81 C	82 B	83 A	84 B	85 C	86 C	87 B	88 D	89 E	90 A
91 B	92 A	93 E	94 B	95 B	96 B	97 C	98 C	99 D	100 A
101 E	102 A	103 A	104 B	105 C	106 E	107 D	108 A	109 B	110 D
111 E	112 C	113 D	114 B	115 A	116 B	117 B	118 C	119 E	120 D
121 C	122 B	123 A	124 D	125 B	126 B	127 C	128 B	129 D	130 C
131 D	132 E	133 A	134 B	135 D	136 E	137 A	138 B	139 C	140 D
141 E	142 A	143 A	144 D	145 B	146 A	147 C	148 B	149 A	150 B
151 A	152 D	153 B	154 A	155 C	156 D	157 B	158 E	159 E	160 C
161 A	162 D	163 A	164 A	165 B	166 C	167 D	168 A	169 D	170 B
171 B	172 C	173 D	174 A	175 B	176 E	177 D	178 A	179 8	180 D
181 C	182 A	183 D	184 C	185 D	186 A	187 B	188 C	189 D	190 A
191 B	192 A	193 A	194 C	195 D	196 C	197 D	198 E	199 D	200 C
201 B	202 A	203 C	204 D	205 E	206 C	207 C	208 B	209 C	210 D
211 E	212 C	213 E	214 C	215 A	216 E	217 C	218 B	219 C	220 D
221 B	222 A	223 E	224 B	225 C	226 B	227 A	228 C	229 A	230 B

231 C	232 D	233 A	234 C	235 C	236 E	237 D	238 B	239 A	240 B
241 C	242 D	243 C	244 A	245 B	246 C	247 D	248 A	249 D	250 B
251 D	252 D	253 B	254 C	255 E	256 B	257 A	258 C	259 D	260 D
261 B	262 C	263 B	264 A	265 E	266 E	267 D	268 E	269 D	270 E
271 A	272 B	273 D	274 C	275 D	276 E	277 A	278 B	279 C	280 A
281 C	282 B	283 A	284 D	285 B	286 A	287 C	288 B	289 A	290 B
291 C	292 A	293 C	294 D	295 C	296 C	297 A	298 D	299 E	300 B
301 C	302 A	303 B	304 D	305 C	306 B	307 D	308 A	309 B	310 C
311 B	312 C	313 B	314 A	315 B	316 E	317 A	318 C	319 D	320 E
321 A	322 C	323 D	324 B	325 D	326 B	327 A	328 B	329 B	330 C
331 D	332 B	333 C	334 D	335 A	336 C	337 B	338 B	339 C	340 D
341 A	342 B	343 D	344 A	345 B	346 D				

C•H•A•P•T•E•R **FOUR**

Social Sciences and Medicine

DIRECTION: Following MCQ's are provided with a few suggestive answers/completions. Only one answer is correct. You have to identify the *BEST* one in each case.

1. **Following factors predisposes to ill health, *except:***
   A. Poverty and poor sanitation
   B. Inadequate housing
   C. Malnutrition
   D. Lack of education
   E. None of these
2. **"Psychophysiological stress reactions" are involved in following disease, *but* one:**
   A. Huntington's chorea
   B. Rheumatoid arthritis and obesity
   C. Intestinal ulceration constipation
   D. Diarrhoea
   E. Epilepsy
3. **Following disciplines are included under the behavioural sciences, *save* for one:**
   A. Sociology
   B. Economics
   C. Social psychology
   D. Social anthropology
   E. None of these
4. **The study of the physical, social and cultural history of man is known as:**
   A. Sociology
   B. Political science
   C. Anthropology
   D. Economics
   E. None of these
5. **The concept of medical sociology was first proposed by whom and when?**
   A. Lamuhar Kalakki (1902)
   B. Barbara Jones (1901)
   C. Charles Mcintire (1894)
   D. McIver (1903)
6. **Who said, "A man who can live without society is either a beast or God"?**
   A. Anderson
   B. Babes Earnest
   C. Charles Darwin
   D. Aristotle
   E. Sir Issac Newton
7. **Learned behaviour which has been socially "acquired" is the definition of:**
   A. Culture
   B. Acculturation
   C. Socialism
   D. Customs
   E. Anthropology
8. **"Acculturation" means what?**
   A. Standard of living
   B. Culture contact
   C. Social control mechanisms
   D. Culture

9. **Acculturation can be acquired by the following:**
   I. **Trade and commerce**
   II. **Industrialization**
   III. **Propagation of religion**
   IV. **Conquest**
   V. **Education**

   Select the true answer as per code given below:
   A. I, II and III only
   B. I, II, III and IV only
   C. I, II, III, IV and V All
   D. I, III and V only
   E. II, III and IV only

10. **The seat of primary emotions e.g. anger, joy and hunger lies in the:**
    A. Thalamus
    B. Hypothalamus
    C. Cerebral cortex
    D. Cerebellum
    E. Internal capsule

11. **Following are recognised organic response *save* for one:**
    A. Emotions
    B. Skills
    C. Feelings
    D. Tension

12. **Intellectual responses include the following:**
    I. **Perceptions**
    II. **Thinking**
    III. **Reasoning**
    IV. **Skills**
    V. **Habits**

    Choose the false answer as per code given:
    A. I, II and III
    B. I, III and V
    C. IV and V
    D. I, IV and V

13. **The most common emotion of man is:**
    A. Anger B. Fear
    C. Jealousy D. Sympathy

14. **The most important factor in the NFPP for eligible couples to adopt a small family norm is:**
    A. Incentives
    B. Lust
    C. Legislation
    D. Motivation
    E. All of the above

15. **Statement (S): Doctor should cultivate the habit of correct observation.**
    Reason (R): Because correct observation leads to correct thinking, reasoning and learning.

    Select the true answer as per code given below:
    A. Both (S) and (R) are true and are related to each other
    B. Both (S) and (R) are true and are unrelated to each other
    C. (S) is true, (R) is false
    D. (R) is true, (S) is false
    E. Both (S) and (R) are false

16. **Following biophysical phenomenon occurring in the universe has been attributable to observation, *save* for one:**
    A. Hippocrates foundation of modern medicine
    B. Newton—theory of Gravitation
    C. Fleming—discovery of Penicillin
    D. James Watt—discovery of Diesel engine

17. **The disorders of perception includes the following:**
    A. Imperception
    B. Illusion
    C. Hallucinations
    D. Both B and C above
    E. All of these

18. **A gross error of perception is called as:**
    A. Hallucination
    B. Imperception
    C. Both A and B above
    D. None of these

19. Mistaking a rope for a snake is a:
A. Imperception
B. Illusion
C. Hallucination
D. All of these
E. None of these

20. Seeing objects that donot exist hearing sounds that are false, seeking objects moving in a room are called as:
A. Imperception
B. Illusion
C. Hallucination
D. All of these
E. None of these

21. Which is NOT included under the 3 components of attitudes?
A. Observation
B. A cognitive element or knowledge
C. An affective or feeling
D. A tendency to action

22. The responsibility to develop healthy attitudes devolves upon:
A. Parents only
B. Teachers
C. Religious leaders
D. Elders only
E. All of the above

23. Which is NOT included under the most significant interest?
A. Security
B. Beliefs
C. Pleasure
D. Self-esteem

24. The powerful motives that stimulate learning is:
A. Encouragement
B. Praise
C. Reward
D. Success
E. All of these

25. The curve of learning reaches its peak between years of age:
A. 5 years
B. 5 to 10 years
C. 10 to 20 years
D. 22 to 25 years
E. After 30 years

26. Following are ways of measuring student's learning:
A. MCQ's
B. Essay writing
C. Project work
D. Oral and practical examiantions
E. All of the above

27. Following are recognised external sources of frustration, *save* for one:
A. Lack of intellectual ability
B. Failures
C. Unemployment
D. Defeats

28. When a person, instead of accepting failure and correcting himself tries to make excuses and justifies his behaviour. It is called:
A. Escape mechanism
B. Rationalization
C. Compensation
D. Projection

29. Sometimes the individual blames others for his mistakes or failures. Then it is called as:
A. Projection
B. Rationalization
C. Escape mechanism
D. Displacement
E. None of these

30. When the student who is not good in his studies may distinguish himself in sports or dramatics, music etc. It is known as:
A. Regression
B. Projection
C. Compensation
D. Displacements
E. Escape mechanism

31. Some students pretend illness and do not appear for examinations is known as:
A. Rationalization
B. Escape mechanism
C. Projection
D. Displacement
E. Regression

32. Some people resort to weeping when something goes wrong is called:
A. Regression
B. Projection
C. Compensation
D. Displacement
E. Escape mechanism

33. The basic personality traits are established by the ages of ....
A. 2 years
B. 4 years
C. 6 years
D. 8 years
E. 18 years

34. The personality traits we look for in a doctor includes:
I. Kindness and honesty
II. Patience and tolerance
III. Perseverance and consciousness
IV. Thoroughness and initiative
Choose the correct answer as per code given:
A. I, II and III
B. I, II, III and IV
C. II and IV
D. III and IV

35. To a layman, which of the 4 components of human personality considered as most important?
A. Intelligence
B. Behaviour
C. Physical
D. Emotional
E. All of these

36. The 1st intelligence test was devised by whom?
A. Terman
B. Binet and Simon
C. Binet and Coleman
D. Gessel
E. All are involved

37. The 4 sectors of intellectual development like motor ability, adoptive behaviour, language development and personal-social behaviour has been developed by whom?
A. Terman
B. Binet and Simon
C. Gessel
D. All of the above

38. The concept of mental age has been given by:
A. Binet and Simon
B. Gessel
C. Terman
D. All of the above
E. Both B and C above

39. When the mental age is the same as chronological age, the I.Q. is:
A. 50
B. 60
C. 80
D. 100
E. 120

40. When a 10 years old child exhibit a mental age of 5 years. The I.Q. would be:
A. 50
B. 60
C. 70
D. 80
E. 100

41. If the I.Q. range is 0 to 24, then the individual is said to be:
A. Moron
B. Idiot
C. Imbecile
D. Border line

42. I.Q. near 140 and above has been called as:
A. Normal
B. Imbecile
C. Near genius
D. Very superior
E. Catamite

43. The chief values of discovering a child's I.Q. is:
A. As an aid in determining the right time to enter school
B. The selection of applicants for college and professional school
C. Educational guidance
D. The use of intelligent test to the therapist
E. All of the above

44. The "Universal Declaration of Human Rights" (1948) consists of how many articles?
A. 10
B. 20
C. 30
D. 40
E. 50 articles

45. The 1st country to give its citizens a constitutional right to all health services is:
A. India
B. Russia
C. Germany
D. Britain

46. Which of the following lacks leadership?
A. Crowd
B. Mob
C. Herd
D. All of the above
E. B and C above

47. Following is a recognised temporary social group, *save* for one:
A. Mob
B. Herd
C. Crowd
D. Band
E. None of the above

48. "Democracy" is seen in:
A. India
B. USA
C. China
D. All of the above
E. Both A and B above

49. "Oligarchy" system of Government is seen in all, *but* one:
A. UK
B. Saudi Arabia
C. Cambodia
D. Thailand
E. None of the above

50. "Monarchy" is seen in:
A. UK
B. Nepal
C. Both of the above
D. None of the above

51. "Socialistic" system is seen in:
A. Poland
B. Germany
C. China
D. Both A and C above
E. All of the above

52. "Autocracy" is not seen in:
A. Jordan
B. Ethiopia
C. Thailand
D. All of the above
E. Both A and B above

53. The phase of nuclear family cycle ends with:
A. Death of survivor
B. Birth of 1st child
C. Birth of last child
D. 1st spouse died

54. "Union is strength" is the motto of:
A. Nuclear family
B. Three generation family
C. Extended family
D. All of these

55. **POLYANDRY (marriage of several men with one women) is found in India in:**
A. Todas of Nilgiri hills
B. Nayars in Malabar coasts
C. Inhabitants of Jaunsar Bawar in UP
D. All of the above

56. **Kuppuswamy socioeconomic criteria for urban people does not include:**
A. Residential address
B. Education
C. Income
D. Occupation

57. **Hollingshed in USA, socioeconomic status, utilizes 3 variables, *but* one:**
A. Residential address
B. Income
C. Education
D. Occupation

58. **"Almoner" was a medical social worker appointed in:**
A. India
B. USA
C. UK (England)
D. Denmark

59. **According to consumer protection act (CPA-1986) following are relevant facts about medicare:**
A. The decision should be taken within 3 to 6 months
B. No court fee payment
C. Person can plead his own case
D. All of these
E. Both A and B above

60. **The Immoral Traffic (prevention) Act" was promulgated in which year?**
A. 1956
B. 1966
C. 1976
D. 1986
E. 1996.

61. **"Panchayat samiti" is located at the:**
A. Village level
B. Block level
C. district level
D. Commissionary level

62. **The current literacy rate in India is:**
A. 40%
B. 45%
C. 50%
D. 52%
E. 65%

63. **In India, Agriculture accounts for nearly .... of the national income.**
A. 33%
B. 44%
C. 55%
D. 66%
E. 77%

64. **The lowest per capita GNP (1994) is seen in:**
A. India
B. Pakistan
C. Thailand
D. Japan
E. Switzerland

65. **In India the life expectancy at birth is 62, then in 1996, IMR is how much?**
A. 62
B. 74
C. 80
D. 84
E. 90

66. **Acquisition of skills is known as:**
A. Psychomotor learning by skill
B. Affective learning by attitudes
C. Cognitive learning by knowledge
D. Learning by conditioned reflex

67. **The poverty line limit for rural areas in the purchasing capacity for a daily intake of 2400 Kcal per person. What calorie limit if for urban areas?**
A. 2400 Kcal
B. 2100 Kcal
C. 1900 Kcal
D. 2600 Kcal

68. **An environmental factor associated with mental illness is:**
   A. Anxiety
   B. Emotional stress
   C. Broken home
   D. Frustration

69. **Which is needed for daily living according to WHO?**
   A. Emotional skill
   B. Interpersonal skill
   C. Social skill
   D. Academic skill

70. **Which science is most used in community medicine?**
   A. Anthropology
   B. Politics
   C. Psychology
   D. Economics

Answers

1 E	2 A	3 B	4 C	5 C	6 D	7 A	8 B	9 C	10 A
11 B	12 C	13 B	14 D	15 A	16 D	17 E	18 A	19 B	20 C
21 A	22 E	23 B	24 E	25 D	26 E	27 A	28 B	29 A	30 C
31 B	32 A	33 C	34 B	35 C	36 B	37 C	38 A	39 D	40 A
41 B	42 C	43 E	44 C	45 B	46 A	47 D	48 E	49 A	50 C
51 D	52 C	53 B	54 C	55 D	56 A	57 B	58 C	59 D	60 D
61 B	62 D	63 B	64 A	65 B	66 A	67 B	68 C	69 D	70 A

CHAPTER FIVE

Epidemiology of Communicable Diseases

DIRECTION: Following MCQ's are provided with a few suggestive answers/completions. Only one answer is correct. You have to identify the *BEST* one in each case.

1. RESPIRATORY INFECTIONS

1. Consider the following statement(s):

I. Smallpox was once a major killer throughout the world has been totally eradicated

II. The last indigenous case in India occurred on 17th May 1975 in Bihar

III. India's last known case of smallpox, an importation from Bangladesh occurred on 24th May 1975

IV. India was proclaimed to be no longer a smallpox-endemic country on 5th July 1975

V. India was declared smallpox-free by an international commission for assessment of smallpox eradication in April 1977

Select the true answer as per code given below:

A. I, II and V
B. I, II, III and IV
C. I, II, III and V
D. I, II, III, IV and V All
E. I, III and IV only

2. The world's last case of smallpox, apart from lab. accident occurred in:

A. Somalia
B. Bangladesh
C. China
D. Indonesia
E. Europe

3. The WHO declared on which date that smallpox had totally been eradicated from world arena?

A. 26th October 1977
B. 1st April 1977
C. 8th May 1980
D. 24th May 1978

4. A resolution from WHO's executive board to the World Health Assembly in May 1996 recommended that the stocks of smallpox virus kept at Government research centers in Russia and USA be destroyed in which year?

A. 2000 **B.** 1999
C. 1998 **D.** 1997
E. 2010

5. **Most cases of human monkeypox has occurred in which country?**
   A. South Africa
   B. Latin America
   C. Zaire
   D. China
   E. Spain

6. **Which is NOT true about human monkeypox infection?**
   A. Have been recognised in 7 nations of western and central Africa
   B. Most victims are young children
   C. Belong to the genus orthopox virus
   D. The presumed I.P. is 30 days
   E. Localised lymphadenopathy

7. **All are true about human monkeypox infection, *save* for one:**
   A. The secondary attack rate is 15%
   B. Smallpox vaccination is protective
   C. Extensive rash causes significant mortality in children
   D. It is a rare disease
   E. The reservoir host is monkey

8. **Following are true about tanapox, *except* for one:**
   A. Clinically disease is heralded by fever and 1 to 2 pustular lesions lasting upto 6 weeks
   B. It is reported in East and Central Africa
   C. The reservoir of infection is Tanafish
   D. It is a zoonotic disease, spread by mosquitos
   E. Smallpox vaccination is not protective against it

9. **The causative agent for chickenpox is:**
   A. Varicella
   B. V-Z virus
   C. Human (α) herpes virus '3'
   D. All of the above
   E. Both A and B but not C above

10. **Characteristics F/O rash of varicella virus (chickenpox) includes all, *except:***
    A. Superficial
    B. Unilocular dew drop like appearance
    C. Pleomorphic
    D. An area of inflammation around vesicles
    E. Evolution of rash is slow

11. **Herpes zoster virus is closely related to the virus of:**
    A. Varicella
    B. Herpes simplex
    C. Rubella
    D. Rubeola
    E. Variola

12. **Chickenpox rash is commonly seen in the:**
    A. Legs
    B. Behind the ear
    C. Axilla (armpit)
    D. Face
    E. Upper limbs

13. **In chickenpox scabs begin to form how many days after the rash appears?**
    A. 1 to 2 days
    B. 4 to 7 days
    C. 4 to 5 days
    D. 7 to 14 days
    E. 10 to 14 days

14. **A 8-year-old unvaccinated boy appears with a history of mild fever for a day followed by superficial, pleomorphic, unilocular rash mainly over trunk and axilla. There is an irregular rise and fall of temperature. The most likely diagnosis is:**
    A. Smallpox
    B. Rubella
    C. Chickenpox
    D. Rubeola (Measles)
    E. Drug rash

15. **Following *but* one, are true regarding varicella:**
    A. The secondary attack rate in household contacts approaches 90%
    B. Occurs primarily among children under 10 years of age

C. The virus tends to present in abundance during pustular stage
D. The portal of entry of virus is the respiratory tract

16. Which is NOT true about varicella or chickenpox?
A. It shows a seasonal trend in India
B. Pleomorphism is a characteristic
C. Most patients are infected by face to face contact
D. Congenital varicella
E. Temperature does not rise with each fresh crops of rash

17. Recognised characteristics of smallpox rash includes all, *but* one:
A. Axilla affected
B. Palms and soles frequently involved
C. Centrifugal
D. Rash predominately on extensor surfaces

18. Following are recognised complications of varicella, *save* for:
A. Hemorrhages
B. Pneumonia
C. Acute cerebellar ataxia and Reye's syndrome
D. Encephalitis only
E. None of these

19. "OKA strain" of virus is used to prepare a live attenuated vaccine against:
A. Smallpox
B. Rubeola
C. Chickenpox
D. Rubela
E. Herpes simplex

20. Maternal varicella during pregnancy may cause fetal wastage and birth defects like:
A. Cutaneous scars
B. Atrophied limbs
C. Microcephaly
D. LBW
E. All of these

21. The word "RUBEOLA" means what?
A. Red spots
B. Blue spots
C. Black spots
D. Yellow spots

22. Which of the following historical facts about measles is NOT true?
A. The earliest description of measles was given by the noted Arab physician—Abu Bacr
B. Panum (1946) did classical studies on the epidemiology of measles
C. Enders and his colleagues (1954) in USA isolated the measles virus
D. Measles vaccine was 1st used in a clinical trial in 1958
E. A live measles vaccine was licensed for use in 1963

23. Measles tend to become epidemic when the proportion of susceptible children reaches about how much?
A. 10%
B. 15%
C. 20%
D. 30%
E. 40%

24. Today, out of 30 million affected children worldwide, how many succumb, to measles?
A. 1 million
B. 2 million
C. 3 million
D. 4 million
E. 5 million

25. In developing nations, case fatality rate due to measles range from:
A. 0.2 to 3%
B. 2 to 15%
C. 3 to 20%
D. 4 to 25%
E. 5 to 50%

26. The case fatality rate for measles in India is:
A. 1%
B. 2%
C. 1.8% to 7.6%
D. 2.1 to 16.0%
E. 4.0 to 20.0%

27. Measles is caused by:
A. Rubeola
B. Rubella
C. Variola
D. RNA paramyxoviruses
E. Varicella

28. The secondary attack rate for measles among susceptible household contacts is:
A. 30%
B. 40%
C. 50%
D. 60 to 70%
E. > 80%

29. Regarding measles, which is incorrect?
A. The virus can survive outside the human body for any length of time
B. The virus has been grown in cell cultures
C. The only source of infection is cases
D. Infective material is secretions of nose, throat and respiratory tract of a case during prodromes and early stages of eruption

30. Which is NOT correct about measles?
A. One attack of measles generally confers life-long immunity
B. Infants are protected by maternal antibodies upto 6 months of age
C. Measles tends to be very severe in the malnourished child
D. Recipients of measles vaccine are contagious to others

31. The pathognomonic lesion of measles is:
A. Forscheimmer spots
B. Koplik's spots
C. Enders spots
D. All of these

32. In measles Koplik's spot is seen during:
A. Prodromal stage
B. Eruptive phase
C. Postmeasles stage
D. All of the above

33. Diagnosis of measles is based on:
A. Typical rash
B. Koplik's spot
C. Both of the above
D. None of the above

34. The most serious complications of measles include all, *but* one:
A. Febrile convulsions
B. Encephalitis
C. SSPE
D. Pneumonitis

35. Encephalitis in measles occurs in about .... cases.
A. 1 in 100
B. 1 in 250
C. 1 in 500
D. 1 in 750
E. 1 in 1000

36. All cases of severe measles and all cases of measles in areas with high case fatality rates should be treated with:
A. Vitamin 'A'
B. Vitamin 'B_6'
C. Vitamin 'C'
D. Vitamin 'D' only
E. Vitamin 'E'

37. Following measles outbreak in locality, vaccine to be given at what age?
A. At birth
B. 3 months
C. 6 months
D. 9 months
E. 12 months

38. In most developing countries, 9 months is the optional age for measles vaccination.
A. True
B. False

39. If the I.P. and naturally occurring measles is 10 days, then what should be the I.P. of vaccine induced measles?
A. 1 day
B. 3 days
C. 5 days
D. 7 days
E. 10 days

40. Toxic shock syndrome (TSS) occurs when measles vaccine is contaminated or the same vial is used for more than one session on the same day or next day.
A. True
B. False

41. Which is NOT true about German measles (Rubella)?
A. Rubella virus (RNA) Togavirus was discovered in 1962
B. Infectivity is minimum when the rash is erupting
C. Vaccine made in 1967
D. Transmitted by droplets or droplet nuclei
E. J.P.—18 days

42. For diagnosis of Rubella the most widely used serological tests is:
A. Virus culture
B. ELISA
C. HAI
D. Radio-immunoassay

43. Following complications may be seen in Rubella infection:
A. Arthralgia
B. Encephalitis
C. Thrombocytopenic purpura
D. All of the above

44. In Rubella, the most common congenital defect includes all, *but* one:
A. IUGR
B. Cardiac malformation
C. Cataract
D. Deafness
E. None of the above

45. Congenital Rubella infection during 1st trimester may result in all, *except:*
A. PDA
B. Cataract
C. Glaucoma
D. Deafness
E. None of the above

46. Congenital rubella is a .... infection.
A. Acute
B. Chronic
C. Subclinical
D. Both B and C above
E. All of the above

47. The % of foetuses infected is minimum during what stage of gestation?
A. < 11 weeks
B. 11 to 16 weeks
C. 17 to 26 weeks
D. 27 to 36 weeks

48. Among various rubella vaccine RA 27/3 vaccine prepared in 1979 is given as a single dose of 0.5 ml subcutaneously.
A. True
B. False

49. The most characteristic feature of rubella is:
A. Fever and rhinorrhoea
B. Enlargement of cervical lymph glands
C. Fever and rhinorrhoea
D. All of these
E. Both A and C above

50. Regarding vaccination strategy against rubella, which is true?
A. To protect women of child-bearing age
B. Children aged 1 to 14 years
C. All children at one year of age
D. All of the above
E. Both A and B above

51. NOT true about mumps is:
A. The disease tends to be more severe in adults
B. There are several serotypes

C. Single attack confers almost life-long immunity
D. Largely an endemic disease
E. Peak incidence is in winter and spring

52. The most common complications of mumps is:
A. Arthritis
B. Parotitis
C. Orchitis
D. Pancreatitis
E. All of the above

53. In mumps secondary attack rate is estimated to be about:
A. 56%
B. 66%
C. 76%
D. 86%
E. 96%

54. The control of mumps is difficult because the disease is infectious before a diagnosis can be made.
A. True
B. False

55. The 1st influenza pandemic during the present century occurred in:
A. 1818-19
B. 1860-61
C. 1918-19
D. 1932-33
E. 1957-58

56. The virus of 1st influenza pandemics is known swine influenza virus.
A. True
B. False

57. Consider the following statements:
I. There are 3 types of influenza virus (A, B, C) of which A and B are responsible for epidemics of disease throughout the world
II. Influenza A and B viruses have two distinct surface antigens-H and N
III. The haemaglutinin (H) antigen initiates infection following attachment of the virus to susceptible cells
IV. The neuraminidase (N) antigen is responsible for release of the virus from the infected cell

Select the true answer as per code given below:
A. I and II only
B. I, II and III only
C. I, II, III and IV All
D. I and III only
E. III and IV only

58. The influenza A virus is unique among the viruses because it is frequently subject to antigenic variation, both major and minor.
A. True
B. False

59. In influenza A virus, when the antigenic change is gradual over a period of time, it is called as a:
A. Antigenic shift
B. Antigenic drift
C. Both of the above
D. Neither A nor B

60. The influenza 'A' strains occurring between 1946 and 1957 have been called:
A. H_1N_2
B. H_2N_2
C. H_1N_2
D. H_3N_2
E. All of these

61. At present following *but* one type of influenza virus are circulating in the world:
A. A (H_1N_1)
B. Influenza 'B'
C. Influenza 'C'
D. A (H_3N_2)
E. None of the above

62. Following influenza infection secretory antibodies develop in respiratory tract and consists predominantly of:

A. IgA_1
B. IgA_2
C. IgG
D. IgM only

63. Following influenza infection antibodies appear in about 7 days after the antibody level drops to pre-infection levels.

A. True
B. False

64. In India influenza epidemics have been occurred during:

A. Winter
B. Rainy season
C. Summer
D. All of the above

65. The I.P. of influenza is:

A. 6 to 12 hours
B. 18 to 72 hours
C. 4 to 6 days
D. 7 to 10 days

66. In influenza, for virus isolation, naso-pharyngeal secretions are the best specimens for obtaining large amounts of virus-infected cells.

A. True
B. False

67. Which of the following influenza vaccine is recommended for children?

A. Killed vaccine
B. Live attenuated
C. Split virus
D. Neuraminidase specific

68. "Guillain-Barre syndrome" may occur following which influenza vaccination?

A. Live attenuated
B. Split virus
C. Neuraminidase
D. Killed
E. Recombinant

69. Which drug is useful against influenza 'A' virus?

A. Amantadine
B. Rimantidine
C. Cyclosporin
D. Tetracycline
E. Both A and B

70. Regarding Diphtheria, which is false?

A. I.P. –2 to 6 days
B. Its causative agent has high invasive power
C. It produces a powerful exotoxins
D. Affects usually children aged 1 to 5 years
E. The source of infection may be a case or carrier

71. NOT true regarding diphtheria is:

A. In diphtheria, the -phage (bacteriophage) carrying the gene for toxin production
B. Females are only affected
C. Cases of diphtheria occur in all seasons
D. Commonly the portal of entry is the respiratory tract

72. The nasal carriers are particularly dangerous as a source of infection because of frequent shedding of the organism into the environment, than do throat carriers.

A. True
B. False

73. A case or carrier may be considered non-communicable, when atleast 2 culture properly obtained from nose and throat, ... apart, are negative for diphtheria bacilli.

A. 10 days
B. 7 days
C. 24 hours
D. 48 hours
E. 5 days

74. Schick test surveys in India reveal that 70% of children over 3 years and 9% over the age of 5 years are already immune to diphtheria.

A. True
B. False

75. Diphtheria may be transmitted by:
A. Cups
B. Thermometers
C. Toys
D. Pencils
E. All of these

76. Recognised C/F of diphtheria includes all, *save* for one:
A. Sore throat
B. Bullnecked appearance
C. Ulcer
D. Hoarseness
E. None

77. The mildest form of respiratory diphtheria is:
A. Faucial
B. Laryngeal
C. Nasal
D. Pharyngotonsillar
E. Laryngotracheal

78. When Schick test is positive, the person is:
A. Susceptible to diphtheria
B. Immune to diphtheria
C. Carriers
D. None

79. In diphtheria, carriers should be treated with 10 days course of oral:
A. Ampicillin
B. Bacitracin
C. Rifampicin
D. Doxycycline
E. Erythromycin

80. The pertussis component in DPT vaccine enhances the potency of the:
A. Tetanus
B. Pertussis
C. Diphtheria toxoid
D. All of the above
E. Both A and B

81. A person who shows diphtheria bacillus in his throat swab and shows positive reaction to Schick test is most likely to be:
A. Incubatory carrier
B. Healthy
C. Convalescent
D. Temporary carriers

82. The recommended prophylaxis for non-immunized contacts of a diphtheria case is:
A. ADS only
B. ADS and Diphtheria toxoid
C. Chemotherapy and diphthcria toxoid
D. ADS and chemotherapy

83. If a child who has received DPT vaccine has severe reaction like convulsion the decision about immunization would be:
A. Donot give any immunization
B. Give DT only
C. Give diphtheria toxoid only
D. Give DPT after one month of reaction

84. D.P.T. vaccine is not recommended in children above the age of 5 years because:
A. Pertussis is not common after the age of 5 years
B. Vaccine is likely to cause severe reaction in that age group
C. Diphtheria is not common after the age of 5 years
D. Both A and B
E. All of the above

85. The therapeutic dose of diphtheria antitoxin by IM route is:
A. 500 to 5000 IU
B. 1000 to 10,000 IU
C. 10,000 to 30,000 IU
D. 40,000 to 1 lakh

86. A "Hundred day cough" is the name given to which diseases by Chinese?
A. Whooping cough
B. Pneumonia
C. T.B.
D. Diphtheria

87. Clinical disease of pertussis is associated with:
A. Noncapsulated phage I strain
B. Encapsulated phase I strain
C. Phase II strain
D. Phage III strain

88. Which is NOT true regarding pertussis or whooping cough?
A. B. pertussis infects not only man but animal as well
B. The source of infection is the case of pertussis
C. It is most infective during catarrhal stage
D. Secondary attack rate averages 90% in unimmunized household contacts

89. The chief complications of pertussis includes:
A. Bronchitis
B. Bronchopneumonia
C. Bronchiectasis
D. All of the above
E. Both A and B

90. The clinical illness of pertussis generally lasts for about:
A. 1 to 2 weeks
B. 2 to 3 weeks
C. 3 to 4 weeks
D. 4 to 5 weeks
E. 6 to 8 weeks

91. In which disease maternal antibody does not appear to give protection to infant?
A. Measles
B. Pertussis
C. Rubella
D. All of the above
E. Both B and C above

92. The DOIC against pertussis is:
A. Ampicillin
B. Bacitracin
C. Cyclosporin
D. Doxicycline
E. Erythromycin

93. In whooping cough antibiotics are given:
A. To reduce the frequency of spasm
B. To reduce the severity of spasm
C. To control secondary bacterial infections
D. To shorten illness
E. All of these

94. An infant was immunized against DPT and within 24 hours of vaccination he developed mild/moderately high fever, moderate pain and occasional convulsion. It is most likely due to which component of DPT?
A. Diphtheria
B. Pertussis
C. Tetanus
D. Due to all of these

95. The control of pertussis would never be 100% even if immunization coverage is 100% because whooping cough vaccines have never been claimed to be more than .... effective.
A. 50%
B. 60%
C. 70%
D. 80%
E. 90%

96. The fatality of typical untreated cases of meningococcal meningitis is about:
A. 50%
B. 60%
C. 70%
D. 80%
E. 100%

97. In meningococcal meningitis, with early diagnosis and treatment, case fatality rates have declined to less than how much?
A. 10%
B. 15%
C. 20%
D. 25%
E. 33%

98. "Meningitic belt" is the name given to those areas or zone that are lying:
A. Between 1 and 5 degree S of equator in tropical Africa
B. Between 5 and 15 degree S of the equator in tropical Africa
C. Between 5 and 15 degree S of the equator in tropical Africa
D. Between 1 and 5 degree N of the equator in tropical Africa

99. Meningococci is found in:
A. Nasopharynx of carriers and other body fluids and secretions of cases
B. Only nasopharynx of carriers
C. Nasopharynx of cases and carriers
D. All of these

100. Regarding meningococcal meningitis, which is false?
A. Carriers are the most important source of infection
B. The disease spreads mainly by droplet infection
C. The portal of entry is the nasopharynx
D. The I.P. is 18 days

101. The DOIC for meningococcal meningitis is:
A. Penicillin
B. Tetracycline
C. Cotrimoxazole
D. Rifampicin

102. The carrier state of meningococcal meningitis must be treated with:
A. Penicillin
B. Rifampicin
C. Tetracycline
D. Erythromycin

103. In meningococcal meningitis cases rapidly lose their infectiousness within .... of specific treatment.
A. 6 hours
B. 12 hours
C. 24 hours
D. 36 hours
E. 48 hours

104. Meningococcal meningitis vaccine gives protection for:
A. 6 months
B. 1 year
C. 2 years
D. 3 years
E. Life long

105. Meningococcal vaccine is NOT recommended for use in:
A. Infants
B. Children under 2 years
C. Pregnant women
D. All of the above

106. Infection of the respiratory tract are perhaps the most common human ailment.
A. True
B. False

107. The upper respiratory tract infections include all, *but* one:
A. Otitis media
B. Pharyngitis
C. Epiglottitis
D. Common cold

108. "Croup syndrome" is associated with:
A. Adenovirus
B. Bordetella pertussis
C. Influenza 'A'
D. Parainfluenza 1 and 2

109. Bronchiolitis is caused by:
A. RSV
B. Adenovirus
C. Parainfluenza
D. Influenza

110. "Acute epiglottitis" is caused by:
A. Staph. aureus
B. H. influenzae type 'b'
C. Klebsiella
D. Adenoviruses

111. Epidemiologically a Schick positive person with throat swab positive for diphtheria bacilli is termed as:
A. Incubatory carrier
B. Case
C. Convalescent carrier
D. Immune
E. Susceptible

112. The influenza virus strain not responsible for pandemics and antigenic variation is:
A. Type 'A'
B. Type 'B'
C. Type 'C'
D. Both A and B
E. All of the above

113. The interepidemic survival of influenza virus is because of:
A. Mild sporadic cases
B. Animal reservoir
C. Carriers
D. Avian reservoir
E. All of the above

114. Epidemiologically a Schick +ve person swab negative (–ve) for diphtheria bacilli is termed as:
A. Incubatory carrier
B. Immune convalescent
C. Susceptible
D. Immune non carrier

115. Epidemiologically a Schick negative person with throat swab +ve for diphtheria bacillus is termed as:
A. Incubatory carrier
B. Susceptible
C. Immune non carrier
D. Immune convalescent carrier

116. The I.P. of mumps is:
A. 1 to 10 days
B. 12 to 14 days
C. 14 to 18 days
D. 14 to 21 days

117. Epidemiologically a person with negative Schick test and throat swab negative for diphtheria bacilli is termed as:
A. Incubatory carrier
B. Susceptible
C. Immune convalescent carrier
D. Immune noncarrier
E. None of those

118. A child developed oedema of legs and feet and petechiae below knee after measles vaccination. The diagnosis will be:
A. Atypical measles
B. Reaction to vaccine
C. Haemorrhagic measles
D. Purpuric measles incipient
E. None of these

119. "The best policy for prevention and control is to allow free exposure to the risk of infection in a defined age group." The disease is:
A. Measles
B. Mumps
C. Chickenpox
D. German measles
E. Influenza

120. If a child after infection with bacillus parapertussis develops infection with bacillus pertussis, then the attack will:
A. Be mild
B. Escape clinical attack
C. Be severe
D. Give modified picture
E. Not show any effect

121. The pertussis infection mainly spreads by:
A. Fomite
B. Infected dust
C. Droplets
D. Droplet nuclei
E. All of the above

122. Fast breathing is present when the respiratory rate is:
A. 60 breaths per minute or more in a child less than 1 month of age

B. 50 breaths per minute or more in a child aged 2 months upto 12 months
C. 40 breaths per minute or more in a child aged 12 months upto 5 years
D. All of these
E. Both A and B above

123. In severely malnourished children with pneumonia, fast breathing and chest indrawing may not be as evident as in other children:
A. True
B. False

124. Cyanosis is a sign of hypoxia:
A. True
B. False

125. A child having severe pneumonia has the following signs:
A. Chest indrawing
B. Nasal flaring
C. Grunting
D. Cyanosis
E. All of these

126. Young infants are those who are less than:
A. 1 month of age
B. 1 week of age
C. 2 months of age
D. 6 months of age
E. 1 year of age

127. Recognised sign of very severe disease includes:
I. Not able to drink
II. Convulsions
III. Abnormally sleepy of difficult to wake
IV. Strider in calm child
V. Severe malnutrition

Select the true answer as per following code given below:
A. I, II, III and IV
B. I, II, III, IV and V All
C. I, III and V
D. II and V
E. II, III and V

128. Statement (S): Mild chest indrawing is normal in young infants.
Reason (R): Because their chest wall bones are soft.
A. Both (S) and (R) are true and are related to one another fully
B. Both (S) and (R) are true but are unrelated to cause and effect
C. (S) true, (R) false
D. (R) true, (S) false
E. Both (S) and (R) false

129. The DOIC for the treatment of pneumonia in children aged 2 months upto 5 years is:
A. Ampicillin
B. Chloramphenicol
C. Cotrimoxazole
D. Doxicycline

130. Cotrimoxazole should not be given to premature babies and cases of neonatal jaundice.
A. True
B. False

131. Statement (S): Antibiotics are not recommended for coughs and colds.
Reasons (R): Because majority of cases are caused by viruses and antibiotics are not effective.
A. Both (S) and (R) are true but are unrelated to cause and effect
B. (S) and (R) are true and are related to cause and effect
C. (S) true, (R) false
D. (R) true, (S) false
E. Both (S) and (R) are false

132. The DOIC in children with sign of very severe disease is:
A. Ampicillin
B. Benzyl penicillin
C. Chloramphenicol
D. Cotrimoxazole

133. Treatment with chloramphenicol in very severe disease (Pneumonia) should not be given more than:
A. 24 hours
B. 48 hours
C. 72 hours
D. 96 hours
E. 5 days

134. A child who has tender, enlarged lymph nodes in the front of the neck and a white exudate on the throat is classified as having:
A. A viral sore throat
B. Staphylococcal sore throat
C. Streptococcal sore throat
D. Diphtheritic sore throat
E. None of these

135. To prevent rheumatic fever a single injection of benzathine penicillin is given:
A. True
B. False

136. A child with wheezing may present as a case of:
A. Wheezing without any accompanying respiratory distress
B. Recurrent wheezing
C. Wheezing accompanied with respiratory distress
D. All of these
E. Both A and C

137. Management of a case with any respiratory distress for children less than 10 kg involves:
A. Oral salbutamol 1 mg 8 hourly
B. Oral salbutamol 2 mg 8 hourly
C. Oral salbutamol 3 mg 8 hourly
D. Oral salbutamol 4 mg 8 hourly

138. ARI control programme was taken up as a pilot project in the country (INDIA) in:
A. 1985
B. 1990
C. 1991
D. 1992
E. 1995

139. Since 1992-93 the ARI programme is being implemented as part of the CSSM programme.
A. True
B. False

140. The total number of infectious case of tuberculosis in the world today is about:
A. 10 million
B. 15 to 20 million
C. 15 to 40 million
D. 50 to 100 million

141. In T.B. the prevalence of infection means proportion of persons who:
A. Are tuberculin +ve
B. Show tubercle bacilli in sputum
C. Shows sign of tuberculosis in X-ray
D. Have cough, fever, pain chest > 15 days

142. In India as per longitudinal survey of National Tuberculosis Institute, Bangalore, the prevalence of infection is:
A. 5%
B. 10%
C. 30%
D. 50%
E. Just 1% only

143. In India, prevalence of infection for T.B is minimum in which age groups?
A. 5 to 9 years
B. 10 to 14 years
C. 15 to 24 years
D. 0 to 4 years
E. 35 to 44 years

144. In India prevalence of infection for T.B. is maximum in which age group?
A. 0 to 10 years
B. 14 to 24 years
C. 25 to 34 years
D. 45 to 54 years
E. 55+ years

145. In which year WHO declared Tuberculosis as a global emergency?
A. 1990
B. 1991
C. 1992
D. 1993
E. 1994

146. In USA, the number of T.B. cases increased by:
A. 3%
B. 7%
C. 14%
D. 20%
E. 25%

147. In T.B. cure rates of upto 95% fall to 56% or less with INH + Rifampicin resistance, and among AIDS patients infected with bacilli resistant to both drugs, a case fatality rate of 91% has been reported in one study.
A. True
B. False

148. As per criterion laid down by WHO, which country in the world has succeeded in reaching the point of control in tuberculosis i.e. < 1% tuberculin +ve among children in the age group 0 to 14 years?
A. U.S.A.
B. U.K.
C. Canada
D. Australia
E. None so far

149. The National Tuberculosis Institute, Bangalore undertook three longitudinal surveys at following places, *but* one:
A. Delhi
B. Banglaore
C. Chingleput
D. Mumbai
E. None of the above

150. Currently the rate of infection (T.B.) in India is:
A. 1%
B. 1 to 2%
C. 3%
D. 5%

151. In India, at present the prevalence of sputum +ve cases of tuberculosis per thousand population is about:
A. 1
B. 2
C. 3
D. 4
E. 10

152. The incidence of new cases of T.B. (confirmed by culture) was about:
A. 1 per 1000
B. 2 per 1000
C. 3 per 1000
D. 4 per 1000
E. 5 per 1000

153. India's biggest public health problem is:
A. Kala-azar
B. Malaria
C. Tuberculosis
D. Filaria
E. Hookworm

154. Which of the following statement is not true about Tuberculosis?
A. In females the peak of tuberculous prevalence is below 35 years
B. Life span of tuberculous patients has decreased
C. Prevalence represents a cumulative experience of a population to recent and remote infection with Mycobacterium tuberculosis
D. T.B. is found more frequently in slum dwellers and low social class

155. By Ziehl-Neelsen method, T.B. bacilli (AFB) are stained:
A. Blue
B. Yellow
C. Red
D. Black
E. Green

156. One of the best indicators for evaluating the tuberculosis problem and its trend is:
A. Case rate
B. Annual infection rate
C. Tuberculin conversion index
D. Both B and C

157. Regarding Mycobacterium tuberculosis, which is wrong?
A. Indian strain are more virulent than European one
B. The disease is caused by both human and bovine type
C. Males are more affected than females
D. It is a gram +ve bacilli

158. Following *but* one, are true statements in respect of Tuberculosis:
A. The actively multiplying bacilli are found in the walls of pulmonary cavities
B. Actively mutiplying bacilli are found in the walls of macrophages
C. The persisters are usually found in the solid caseous lesion
D. Slowly multiplying forms are found inside the macrophages
E. The more rapidly a bacillary strain multiplies the more susceptible it is to the bactericidal action of chemotherapeutic drugs

159. Regarding atypical mycobacterias, which is the wrong pair?
A. Photochromogen—M. Kansasi
B. Scotochromogens—M. Scrofulaceum
C. Non-photochromogens—M. Intercellulare
D. Rapid growers—M. fortuitum
E. None of these

160. Who has classified Atypical Mycobacteria?
A. Robert Koch
B. Runyon
C. Louis Pasteur
D. William Boyd

161. In T.B. patients are infective as long as they remain untreated. Effective antimicrobial treatment reduces infectivity by 90% within:
A. 48 hours
B. 7 days
C. 21 days
D. 1 month
E. 3 months

162. Which disease is described as a barometer of social welfare?
A. Measles
B. Tetanus
C. T.B.
D. Diphtheria
E. Any of these

163. The best method to differentiate in between an atypical mycobacteria and mycobacterium tuberculosis is:
A. By animal inoculation
B. By Grams staining
C. By C/M only
D. By culture only
E. All of the above

164. Who discovered the Tuberculin test?
A. Von Pirquet
B. Robert Koch
C. Runyon
D. Louis Pasteur

165. Currently Tuberculin test is done by following methodology, *except:*
A. Mantoux test
B. Dick test
C. Heaf test
D. Tine test

166. Statement (S): The heaf test is usually preferred for testing large groups of people.
Reason (R): Because it is quick and easy to perform, reliable and cheap.
A. Both (S) and (R) are true, and are related to cause and effect

B. (S) and (R) are true, but are unrelated to cause and effect
C. (S) true, (R) false
D. (R) true, (S) false
E. Both (S) and (R) are false

167. The standard PPD as acclaimed by W.H.O. contains how much of tuberculin unit?
A. 5000 TU/mg
B. 50,000 TU/mg
C. 5 lakhs TU/mg
D. 15,000 TU/mg

168. In India, how much quantity of tuberculin is used as a test dose?
A. 0.1 TU
B. 0.5 TU
C. 1 TU
D. 5 TU
E. 10 TU

169. For routine tuberculin testing the dose of PPD given in India is:
A. 1 TU
B. 2 TU
C. 3 TU
D. 4 TU
E. 5 TU

170. Which test is employed to measure the prevalence of T.B. in a community?
A. BCG test
B. Tuberculin test
C. Both of the above
D. None of the above

171. For Mantoux testing the PPD advocated by WHO is:
A. PPD-B
B. PPD-Y
C. PPD-RT-23
D. PPD (PPD-5)

172. Tuberculin test shows that the following persons have more risk of developing tuberculosis:
A. Those with induration less than 5 mm
B. Those with 6 to 9 mm induration
C. Those with induration 20 mm or more
D. Both A and C above
E. All of the above

173. A repeat tuberculin test shows that the person had positive reaction initially and now shows negative reaction. This means:
A. Elimination of viable tubercle bacilli
B. Booster effect of previous test
C. Patient is given injection streptomycin
D. Both A and B above
E. All of the above

174. In an area if the frequency distribution of tuberculin test revealed bimodal distribution for the size of reaction the conclusion will be:
A. Variation incidence in different age groups
B. Prevalence of atypical mycobateria
C. Doubtful sensitivity to tuberculin
D. All of the above
E. Both A and C above

175. A person with fulminant tuberculous infection will have the following tuberculin reaction.
A. Mild
B. Moderate
C. Negative
D. Severe with sloughing
E. Normal

176. If a child below 2 years is found to be tuberculin +ve, it is an indirect evidence of an active tuberculous lesion in the body even if it is not manifest.
A. True
B. False

177. The WHO defines that tuberculosis control "is said to be achieved when the prevalence of natural infection in the age group 0 to 14 years is of the order of 1 percent. This is about .... in India?
A. 10%
B. 20%

C. 30%
D. 40%
E. 50%

178. The time from receipt of infection to the development of a positive tuberculin test ranges from:
A. 1 to 3 weeks
B. 3 to 6 weeks
C. 6 to 9 weeks
D. 9 to 12 weeks

179. Tuberculosis is transmitted mainly by the following:
A. Fomites
B. Droplet
C. Droplet nuclei
D. All of the above
E. Both B and C

180. Safe and practicable disposal of AFB +ve sputum in the house with no sanitary facilities can be done by:
A. Burning
B. Boiling
C. Disinfectants
D. All of the above
E. Both A and C

181. A sputum +ve case of T.B. is declared as cured when the:
A. Sputum becomes AFB negative
B. Two smears taken one month apart are AFB negative
C. Two smears three months apart are AFB negative
D. All of the above

182. A patient on anti-Koch's treatment complains of red coloured urine. It is due to:
A. INH
B. PAS
C. Thiacetazone
D. Rifampicin
E. Pyrazinamide

183. Which anti-Koch's drug produce an influenza like illness?
A. Rifampicin
B. INH
C. PAS
D. Thiacetazone
E. Pyrazinamide

184. Concurrent administration of PAS should be avoided with:
A. INH
B. Rifampicin
C. Thiacetazone
D. Pyrazinamide

185. If Rifampicin is stopped for some reasons, it should not be restarted within .... weeks to avoid hypersensitivity:
A. 1 week
B. 2 weeks
C. 3 weeks
D. 6 weeks
E. 12 weeks

186. Sputum is taken on 3 mm wire loop and seven of size 10 × 20 mm is made what is the minimum number of acid fast bacilli that should be seen to label the case as open case?
A. One
B. Two
C. Three
D. Four
E. Five

187. Transmission of T.B. is more dangerous in the case of:
A. Culture the cases
B. Smear the cases
C. Both of the above
D. Neither A nor B

188. In India, under district tuberculosis programme (DTP) which type of C/P in a patient should be given priority to be screened for tubeculous foci elsewhere, *except* for one:

A. Night sweating
B. Pain chest
C. Cough of about 3 weeks duration
D. Continuous fever
E. Haemoptysis

189. Which is the most powerful anti-Koch's drug?
A. PAS
B. RMP
C. INH
D. Streptomycin
E. Pyrazinamide

190. Which anti-Koch's should preferably be given on empty stomach before breakfast?
A. INH
B. Thiacetazone
C. PAS
D. RMP
E. P-zide

191. Which antituberculous is active against persisters or dormant bacilli present is solid caseous lesions?
A. PAS
B. INH
C. Ethambutol
D. Pyrazinamide
E. RMP

192. Regarding INH, all are true, *save* for one:
A. It is active against both intracellular and extracellular bacilli
B. It should be given preferably in divided doses
C. Its action is most marked on rapidly multiplying bacilli
D. It is less active against slow multipliers

193. The most common toxicity of INH in slow inactivators is:
A. Peripheral neuropathy
B. Jaundice
C. Hyperglycemia
D. Blood dyscrasia

194. Recognised toxcicity of streptomycin includes all, *but* one:
A. Vestibular damage
B. Nystagmus
C. Renal damage
D. Deafness

195. Which anti-Koch's is most active against slow multiplying bacilli found inside macrophages, and affected by other drugs?
A. INH
B. PAS
C. Streptomycin
D. Ethambutol
E. Pyrazinamide

196. The sterilizing ability of rifampicin has been enhanced by:
A. PAS
B. INH
C. Pyrazinamide
D. All of the above
E. Both A and B

197. Following antituberculous drugs are bactericidal, *except:*
A. INH
B. RMP
C. Streptomycin
D. Pyrazinamide
E. Ethambutol

198. In adults T.B. patients, PAS has been replaced by which drug?
A. INH
B. RMP
C. Ethambutol
D. Streptomycin
E. Thiacetazone

199. "Retrobulbar neuritis" occurs due to:
A. RMP
B. Thiacetazone
C. P. zide
D. Streptomycin
E. Ethambutol

200. Which anti-Koch's causes GIT disturbances, blurring of vision, haemolytic anaemia and urticaria?
A. INH
B. Pyrazinamide
C. Thiacetazone
D. Streptomycin
E. PAS

201. The main role of the bacteriostatic drugs as to prevent the emergence of INH resistant strains.
A. True
B. False

202. The most frequently used combination under daily regimen in India is:
A. INH + RMP
B. INH + Thiacetazone
C. INH + PAS
D. INH + Streptomycin

203. The standard by weekly regimen used in India is:
A. Streptomycin
B. INH
C. Pyridoxine
D. All of the above
E. Both A and B

204. An antituberculous drug regime in named 2RHSZ-4HR. Here 2 and 4 indicate:
A. Code number of the regime
B. The number of drugs given are in two phases
C. The number of months these drugs are given
D. All of the above
E. None of these

205. An anti-Koch's regime is named 2RHSZ-4H_2R_2. The suffix 2 to Hand R here means:
A. The number of drugs given are in two phases
B. The number of months these drugs are given
C. Code number of regime
D. Frequency of administration in a week

206. The 1st human was vaccinated against BCG by intradermal technique in:
A. 1927
B. 1906
C. 1921
D. 1915

207. BCG vaccine was considered as a safe preventive measure against T.B. in:
A. 1927
B. 1936
C. 1948
D. 1951
E. 1961

208. Calmette and Guerin-two French scientist, prepared BCG vaccine after 230 subcultures over 13 years.
A. True
B. False

209. The WHO has recommended "Danish 1331" strain for BCG vaccine production.
A. True
B. False

210. Following successful BCG vaccination a tuberculin negative individual becomes tuberculin positive in:
A. 1 to 5 weeks
B. 5 to 10 weeks
C. 6 to 12 weeks
D. 8 to 14 weeks

211. BCG vaccine can be given along with:
A. OPV
B. DPT
C. Both
D. Neither

212. Contraindications to BCG vaccine include all, *except:*
A. Infective dermatosis
B. Generalised eczema
C. Hypogammaglobulinemia
D. None of these

213. Backbone of National T.B. control programme is:
A. PHC
B. UHC
C. Developmental blocks
D. District T.B. centre
E. All of the above

214. The main strategy in National T.B. control programme is:
A. To trace contacts
B. To detect and treat as many cases of T.B. as possible
C. To give free treatment
D. To give BCG vaccination to all population

215. Principles of National T.B. control programme are following, *except:*
A. Isolation of T.B. cases
B. BCG vaccination
C. Early case detection
D. Domiciliary chemotherapy

216. Following is a peripheral health institution under National T.B. control programme:
A. Subcentre
B. PHC
C. Referral hospital
D. District hospital

217. Out of 460 districts in India, District T.B. centres have been established in how many districts?
A. 100
B. 200
C. 360
D. 446
E. 460

218. The Government of India, WHO, and World Bank together reviewed the National Tuberculosis Programme (NTP) in which year?
A. 1990
B. 1991
C. 1992
D. 1993
E. 1994

219. The revised strategy for NTP includes:
A. Achievement of 85% cure rate amongst infections cases of T.B
B. Detecting 70% of estimated cases through sputum microscopy
C. Involvement of NGOs
D. DOTs
E. All of these

220. Worldwide the number of people infected with both HIV and T.B. is rising and would reach .... million by 2000 AD.
A. One
B. Two
C. Three
D. Four
E. Ten

221. T.B. appears to continue as an important communicable disease problem because of following reasons throughout world:
I. The chronic nature of disease
II. The concentration of disease in older age gr
III. The ability of T.B. bacilli to remain alive in the human body for years
IV. The high prevalence of infection and high reactivation rate
V. Emergence of drug resistant strain
VI. Association of T.B. and HIV

Select the true answer as per code given below:
A. I, III and V
B. I, II, III and IV
C. I, II, III, IV and V
D. I, II, III, IV, V and VI All

222. A resolution from WHO's executive Board to the World Health Assembly in May 1999 recommended that the stocks of smallpox virus kept at Russia and USA as vaccine be destroyed in the year:
A. 1999
B. 2000
C. 2002
D. 2006

223. In India, measles vaccine is best given at what age?
A. 6 months
B. 9 months
C. 12 months
D. 15 months

224. Currently 2nd dose of measles vaccine is used as a routine in the following countries *but* one:
A. India
B. Sweden
C. Czechoslovakia
D. Russia (USSR)

225. The HDC–Edmonston–Zagreb strain vaccine may protect children from .... months of age against measles:
A. 1 to 2
B. 2 to 3
C. 3 to 4
D. 4 to 6

226. Regarding measles vaccine, which is false?
A. The reconstituted vaccine is given in a single subcutaneous dose of 0.5 ml
B. The diluting fluid for reconstituting vaccine must be kept cold at 0°C in deep freeze
C. The reconstituted vaccine should be kept on ice and used within one hour
D. Measles vaccine has recently been adapted for aerosol administration

227. Measles vaccine should not be used after .... of opening the vial.
A. 1 hour
B. 2 hours
C. 3 hours
D. 4 hours

228. The disease is worldwide in distribution and tend to occur in epidemics, in non-immunized populations, every 6 to 8 years is:
A. Rubeola
B. Rubella
C. Chickenpox
D. Mumps

229. Norman Gregg (1941), an ophthalmologist reported an epidemic of congenital cataracts associated with other congenital defects in children born to mothers who had .... during their pregnancies.
A. Rubeola
B. Measles
C. German measles
D. Mumps

230. The following years are relevant in respect to rubella virus:
I. Teratogenic potential–1941
II. Isolation of virus–1962
III. Development of attenuated vaccine–1967

Select the wrong facts as per code given below:
A. I only
B. I and II only
C. I, II and III All
D. None of these

231. In which year WHO global surveillance activities have identified human infection with a new influenza virus called A (H_5N_1) in Hongkong?
A. 1997
B. 1998
C. 1999
D. 2000

232. Which group of influenza virus appears to be antigenically stable?
A. Group 'A'
B. Group 'B'
C. Group 'C'
D. All of these

233. In which year influenza virus involved only shift in 'H' antigen?
A. 1946
B. 1957
C. 1968
D. 1997

234. In India, facilities for isolation of influenza virus is available at:

I. Pasteur Institute, Coonoor, South India
II. Haffkine Institute, Mumbai
III. School of Tropical Medicine, Kolkata
IV. AIIMS, New Delhi
V. Vallabhbhai Patel Chest Institute, Delhi
VI. AFMC, Pune

Select the true answer as per code given below:

A. I, III and IV
B. I, II, III and IV
C. I, II, III and V
D. I, II, III, IV, V and VI All

235. Following are regarded as a newer influenza vaccines, *except:*

A. Live attenuated vaccine
B. Split virus vaccine
C. Neuraminidase specific vaccine
D. Recombinant vaccine

236. Which is called as a sub-virion vaccine?

A. Recombinant vaccine
B. Split virus vaccine
C. Killed vaccines
D. Neuraminidase specific vaccine

237. The fatality rate for diphtheria on an average is about:

A. 5%
B. 10%
C. 15%
D. 20%

238. Which bacteriophage carrying the gene for toxin production in cases of diphtheria?

A. α–phage
B. β–phage
C. γ–phage
D. δ–phage

239. The Schick test has largely been replaced by measurement of serum antitoxin level by the haemagglutination test (HAI).

A. True
B. False

240. The secondary attack rate for pertussis in unimmunized household contacts is:

A. 30%
B. 50%
C. 70%
D. 90%

241. In developing nations case fatality rates from whooping cough in infants is ranging from:

A. 1 to 3%
B. 2 to 5%
C. 4 to 15%
D. 6 to 20%

242. Which of the following SEAR nations adopting a booster dose of pertussis vaccine in the form of DPT_4?

A. India and Bhutan
B. Srilanka and Thailand
C. DPR Korea only
D. All of these

243. Defaulter in T.B. means that a patient who returns sputum smear positive, after having left treatment for atleast:

A. 1 month
B. 2 months
C. 6 months
D. 3 months

244. Severe acute respiratory syndrome (SARS) is caused by:

A. Amoeba
B. Bacteria
C. Coronavirus
D. Drug induced

245. The earliest case of SARS was detected in:

A. India
B. Bangladesh
C. China
D. Denmark

246. The I.P. of SARS is:

A. 1 to 2 days
B. 2 to 3 days
C. 3 to 4 days
D. 3 to 5 days

247. The epidemic of the coronavirus-associated illness known as SARS apparently began in Guangdong province of China in November 2002 and possibly originated from contact with semidomesticated animals like the palm civet or the dog raccoon.

A. True
B. Partially true
C. Untrue

248. The case fatality rate for SARS is:

A. 1%
B. 5%
C. 11%
D. 25%

249. The mode of transmission of SARS is:

A. Small aerosols
B. Faeco-oral route
C. Both of the above
D. Neither A nor B

250. In SARS, coronavirus particles have been found in:

A. Giant cell
B. Type I pneumocytes
C. Type II pneumocytes
D. All of these

251. In SARS, pulmonary pathology consists of:

A. Hyaline membrane formation
B. Desquamation of pneumocytes in alveolar spaces
C. Interstitial infiltrate consisting of lymphocytes and mononuclear cells
D. All of these

252. Recognised risk factors for SARS includes:

I. Age > 50 years
II. Cardiovascular disease
III. Hepatitis
IV. Diabetes mellitus

Choose the true answer as per code given below:

A. I, II and III
B. I, II, III and IV All
C. I and IV only
D. I, II and IV

253. Lab. abnormalities in SARS include:

I. Lymphopenia ~ 50% of cases
II. Affects both CD_4^+ T-cells and also CD_8^+ T-cells and NK cells
III. TLC normal or slightly low
IIV. Thrombocytopenia as the disease progresses
V. Raised levels of aminotransferases, CPK and LDH

Choose the correct answer as per code given below:

A. I, II and III
B. I, III and V
C. I, II, III, IV and V
D. I, IV and V only

254. SARS–COV can be grown from respiratory tract samples by inoculation into vero E6 tissue culture cells, in which a cytopathic effect can be seen within days:

A. True
B. Partially true
C. Untrue

255. Which of the following statement about SARS is/are false?

A. A rapid diagnosis can be made by reverse transcriptase PCR (RT-PCR) of respiratory tract samples and plasma early in illness and of urine and stool later on
B. RT-PCR appears to be less sensitive than tissue virus culture
C. Serum antibodies can be detected by ELISA or immunofluorescence, and nearly all patients develop detectable serum antibodies within 28 days after the onset of illness

D. RT-PCR appears to be more sensitive than tissue culture, but only around 1/3rd (33.3%) of cases are +ve by PCR at initial presentation

256. Coronaviruses that cause those illnesses are frequently difficult to cultivate in vitro but can be detected in clinical samples by:
A. ELISA
B. Immunofluorescence assays
C. RT-PCR for viral RNA
D. All of those

257. Regarding treatment for SARS–which is true?
A. No specific therapy available
B. Ribavirin and glucocorticoids may be used as routine practice
C. Mainstay of therapy is symptomatic and supportive care
D. All of the above

258. In an area not covered by measles immunization, the attack rate of measles is:
A. 70%
B. 80%
C. 90%
D. 100%

259. Single most important test for case detection of TB is:
A. X-ray
B. Sputum microscopy
C. Tuberculin test
D. MMR

260. Under the revised NTCP, schedule of treatment for category I patient is:
A. 2(HRZE) + 4 $(HR)_3$
B. $2(HRZE)_3$ + 4 $(HRE)_3$
C. $2(HRZES)_3$ + 1 $(HRZE)_3$ + 5 $(HRE)_3$
D. $2(HRZ)_3$ + 4 $(HR)_3$

261. In India, maximum cases of TB in AIDS patients are due to:
A. Myco. tuberculosis
B. Myco. avium intercellulare
C. Myco. akari
D. Myco. scrofulaceum

2. INTESTINAL INFECTIONS

1. Poliomyelitis is caused by:
A. Virus
B. Bacteria
C. Chlamydia
D. Protozoon
E. None of the above

2. During the year 1996, 20,000 cases of polio were reported to W.H.O., with about 7,000 deaths.
A. True
B. False

3. What % of children upto 12 months were immunized worldwide during 1995 with OPV_3 immunization?
A. 60%
B. 50%
C. 83%
D. 73%
E. 93 %

4. Poliomyelitis is eradicable because:
A. Man is the only host
B. A long-term carrier state not known
C. The half life of excreted virus in the sewage is about 48 hours and spread can only occur during this period
D. All of the above
E. Both A and B

5. Statement (S): OPV is ideally suited for polio eradication strategies.

Reason (R): Because the live vaccine virus, by multiplying in the intestine can interrupt the trasmission of the wild poliovirus.

A. Both (S) and (R) are true, but are unrelated to cause and effect
B. Both (S) and (R) are true, and are related to cause and effect
C. (S) true, (R) false
D. (R) true, (S) false
E. Both (S) and (R) are false

6. The 1st reported epidemic of polio occurred in which year in and around Bombay city?

A. 1971
B. 1982
C. 1949
D. 1959
E. 1969

7. The 1st reported outbreak of paralytic polio in india occurred in the year:

A. 1892
B. 1951
C. 1971
D. 1949
E. 1987

8. Total prevalence of residual paralysis due to poliomyelitis = prevalence of lameness due to polio in children above five years of age multiplied by:

A. 1.25
B. 1.33
C. 1.55
D. 12.5

9. Number of clinical polio cases in an area-prevalence rate of polio induced paralyis in that area multiplied by:

A. 0.33
B. 1.33
C. 1.25
D. 0.99
E. 1.63

10. India plays an important role in the global eradication of polio because of the presence of a large number of children under 5 years of age in the country.

A. True
B. False

11. Polio is due to:

A. Togavirus
B. Rotavirus
C. Picornavirus
D. Polyomavirus
E. Enterovirus

12. The causative agent of poliomyelitis was identified by whom?

A. Robert Koch
B. Landsteiner and Popper
C. Louis Pasteur
D. Von Pirquet

13. The most vulnerable age groups for polio in India is:

A. 1 to 5 years
B. 3 to 5 years
C. 6 months to 3 years
D. 5 to 10 years

14. Which clinical spectrum of polio constitute less than one percent of infection?

A. Abortive Polio
B. Paralytic Polio
C. Inapparent Polio
D. Nonparalytic

15. Neutralizing antibody is widely recognised as an important index of immunity to polio after infection.

A. True
B. False

16. Following provocative or risk factors have been found to precipitate an attack of paralytic polio in an individual already infected:

I. Fatigue
II. Trauma
III. IM injections

IV. **Operative procedures (tonsillectomy) done during polio epidemic**
V. **Giving alum containing DPT**

Select the true answer as per code given below:
A. II, III and IV only
B. I, II, III and IV
C. I, II, III, IV and V All
D. I, III, IV and V

17. **In India most cases of poliomyelitis occurs during:**
A. Winter
B. Rainy
C. Spring
D. Summer season

18. **Faeco-oral route is the main route of spread of polio in developing nations while droplet infection during acute phase of disease is the chief mode of transmission in developed nations.**
A. True
B. False

19. **Which of the following disinfectant is ineffective in controlling proliferation and viability of polio virus?**
A. Ultraviolet rays
B. 40% formaldehyde
C. 5% lysol
D. Free residual chlorine—0.3 to 0.5 mg/L
E. Exposure to 50°C heat

20. **In cold environment the polio virus can remain viable in water for:**
A. 4 weeks
B. 4 months
C. 6 months
D. 4 years
E. Just 4 days

21. **In cold environment the polio virus can remain viable in human faeces for:**
A. 4 weeks
B. 6 weeks
C. 4 months
D. 6 months
E. 1 year

22. **Before and after appearance of C/M as case of poliomyelitis is infectious (airborne) for:**
A. 1 to 3 days
B. 4 to 6 days
C. 7 to 10 days
D. One to two weeks

23. **An epidemic of poliomyelitis is defined as occurrence of two or more cases by similar type virus within time period of:**
A. 2 weeks
B. 4 weeks
C. 6 weeks
D. 8 weeks
E. 12 weeks

24. **In poliomyelitis the ratio of clinical and subclinical cases is:**
A. 1 : 10 to 1 : 50
B. 1 : 20 to 1 : 75
C. 1 : 75 to 1 : 500
D. 1 : 75 to 1 : 1000

25. **A case of poliomyelitis can transmit infection through faeces for how many weeks after clinical attack?**
A. 1 week
B. 1 to 2 weeks
C. 2 to 3 weeks
D. Upto 4 weeks

26. **What % of paralytic poliomyelitis cases are below the age of two years?**
A. 25%
B. 50%
C. 65%
D. 80%
E. 95%

27. **The I.P. of poliomyelitis is in the range of:**
A. 3 to 35 days
B. 7 to 14 days
C. 10 to 14 days
D. 14 to 23 days

28. Following *but* one are true regarding paralytic poliomyelitis:
A. The predominant sign is asymmetrical flaccid paralysis
B. Signs of meningeal irritation is not present
C. A history of fever at the time of onset of paralysis is suggestive of polio
D. Tripod sign may be found
E. Descending paralysis

29. The paralysis of poliomyelitis is:
A. UMN type
B. LMN type
C. Extrapyramidal
D. All of the above

30. A child two years of age has loose motions, cough and painful back and stiff neck for two days during an epidemic of poliomyelitis. He can be diagnosed to have:
A. Inapparent infection
B. Abortive illness
C. Nonparalytic polio
D. Paralytic polio

31. The best course of action for control of epidemic poliomyelitis in Indian conditions today is:
A. Surveillance containment measures
B. Mass OPV drive
C. Safe water supply
D. Good sanitation measures
E. All of these

32. The 1st field trial of OPV in the year 1961 was conducted in the state of:
A. Andhra Pradesh
B. Karnataka
C. Rajasthan
D. Tamil Nadu

33. A single dose of OPV amounts to how many drops or as stated by the manufacturer on the label?
A. Only one drop
B. Two drops
C. Three drops
D. Four drops

34. Regarding OPV, which is false?
A. Described by Sabin (1957)
B. Contains type 1, 2 and 3 live attenuated virus
C. 1st dose is given when a child is 6 weeks old
D. Described by salk

35. OPV contains all the 3 forms of polio virus in live attenuated form, which type is responsible for causing vaccine associated paralytic polio?
A. Type I
B. Type II
C. Type III
D. All of the above
E. Both A and B

36. It is true that in poliomyelitis:
A. Proximal muscle groups are more involved as compared to distal ones
B. Deep tendon reflexes are diminished before the onset of paralysis
C. Cranial nerve involvement is seen in bulbar and bulbospinal forms
D. There is no sensory loss
E. All of these

37. In paralytic polio, the usual cause of death is:
A. Heart failure
B. Respiratory failure
C. Kidney failure
D. Liver failure
E. Brain failure

38. IPV induces following antibodies, *but* one:
A. IgE
B. IgM
C. IgG
D. IgA
E. None

39. Recognised advantages of IPV includes all, *save* for one:
A. Can be safely given to a person having immunodeficiency
B. Persons using steroid and radiotherapy

C. During pregnancy
D. Those over 50 years receiving vaccine for the first time
E. None

40. Improved, IPV is 100% effective after the ....
A. 1st dose
B. 2nd dose
C. 3rd dose
D. 4th dose
E. 5th dose

41. "Quadruple vaccine" contains:
A. DPT + 1 PV
B. DPT + OPV
C. DPT + BCG
D. DT + OPV + BCG

42. EPI and the national immunization programme in India recommend a primary course of 3 doses of OPV at one month intervals, commencing the 1st dose when the infant is:
A. 1 day old
B. One week old
C. 5 weeks old
D. 12 weeks old
E. 16 weeks old

43. In case of polio epidemic IPV is unsuitable because:
A. Immunity is not rapidly achieved as more than one dose is needed to induce it
B. Injections are to be avoided during epidemic owing to chance of paralytic attacks
C. It is contraindicated during pregnancy
D. Both A and B
E. All of the above

44. The 1st dose of IPV is given when the infant is:
A. 1 day old
B. 1 week old
C. 3 weeks old
D. 6 months old
E. 6 weeks old

45. To maintain "herd immunity" against polio virus, it is desirable that atleast .... of community to be immunized with OPV.
A. 33%
B. 44%
C. 66%
D. 55%
E. 88%

46. Current failure rate of OPV is in order of what percentage?
A. Just 1%
B. 5%
C. 10%
D. 20%
E. 30%

47. "Zero dose" of polio vaccine is that which is given at:
A. Birth
B. 1st week
C. 2nd week
D. 4th week
E. 6th week

48. In order to overcome the OPV failure the Indian Academy of Pediatrics advocated .... doses in community campaigns.
A. 5, 5
B. 5, 3
C. 3, 5
D. 5, 4
E. 4, 5

49. NOT true about IPV is:
A. Given subcutaneously or IM
B. Killed formolised virus
C. Costlier
D. Easy to manufacture
E. Has a longer shelf-life

50. Which of the following is/are true about OPV?
A. Induces both humoral and intestinal immunity
B. Cheaper than IPV

C. Storage and transportation needs subzero temperature unless stabilized
D. Easy to manufacture
E. All of these

51. Regarding Pulse Polio Immunization (PPI), which is true?
A. The 1st round of PPI was conducted on 9th December 1995 and 6 weeks later on 20th January 1996
B. The 1st PPIs targeted all children under 3 years of age
C. The 2nd phase of PPI was conducted on 7th December 1996 and 18th January 1997 targeting children 3 years to below 5 years of age
D. All of these
E. Both A and C above

52. Hepatitis virus Non A-Non B consists of:
A. HAV
B. HBV
C. HCV
D. Both C and D above

53. In India approximately .... people suffer from acute viral hepatitis.
A. 1 million
B. 2 million
C. 3 million
D. 4 million
E. 6 million

54. In children, majority of cases of acute hepatitis is caused by:
A. HAV
B. HBV
C. NANB
D. HDV
E. HEV

55. Among adults majority of acute hepatitis is caused by:
A. HNANB
B. HBV
C. HAV
D. Both A and B
E. All of these

56. In HAV the case fatality rate of icteric cases is less than ....
A. 1%
B. 0.1%
C. 0.5%
D. 1.5%
E. 2.0%

57. Regarding HAV, which is false?
A. The causative agent is an enterovirus (type 72)
B. It multiplies only in hepatocytes.
C. There are several serotypes
D. Faecal shedding of virus is at its highest during the later part of I.P. and early acute phase of illness
E. The virus is fairly resistant to heat and chemicals

58. In well water, HAV may survive to about:
A. 1 week
B. 5 weeks
C. 10 weeks
D. 20 weeks
E. 30 weeks

59. HAV is not affected by the following:
A. Chlorine in doses usually employed for chlorination
B. Formaline
C. Ultraviolet rays
D. Boiling for 5 mts
E. Autoclaving only

60. Which of the following is/are false regarding HAV?
A. The only reservoir of infection is human
B. Evidence of carrier state
C. Asymptomatic infections especially common in children
D. Infectivity falls rapidly with the onset of jaundice
E. HAV is excreted in the faeces for about 2 weeks before the onset of jaundice and for upto one week thereafter

61. In India, by the age of 10 years, what % of healthy persons have serological evidence of HAV infection?
- **A.** 50%
- **B.** 60%
- **C.** 70%
- **D.** 80%
- **E.** 90%

62. Regarding immune status in persons having HAV during/after attacks includes all the following, *save* for one:
- **A.** 2nd attack reported in 50% of cases
- **B.** Most people in endemic areas acquire immunity through subclinical infection
- **C.** The IgM antibody appears early in the illness and persists for over 90 days
- **D.** IgG appears more slowly and persists for many years
- **E.** Immunity after attack probably lasts for life

63. The major route of transmission of HAV is:
- **A.** Parenteral
- **B.** Faeco-oral
- **C.** Sexual
- **D.** All of the above
- **E.** Both A and B

64. The I.P. of HAV is:
- **A.** 9 to 90 days
- **B.** 10 to 30 days
- **C.** 15 to 45 days
- **D.** 25 to 30 days

65. Demonstration of which indicates past infection and immunity in HAV?
- **A.** HAV particles only
- **B.** Specific viral antigen in faeces
- **C.** Rise in anti-HAV titre
- **D.** IgG antibody
- **E.** IgM antibody

66. In HAV, control of reservoir is difficult because of following reasons:
- **A.** Faecal shedding of virus is at its peak during the I.P. and early phase
- **B.** The occurrence of large number of subclinical cases
- **C.** Absence of specific treatment
- **D.** Low social class of population are usually involved
- **E.** All of the above

67. Effective disinfectant for faeces of HAV patient is:
- **A.** 0.5% sodium hypochlorite
- **B.** 2% cresol
- **C.** 2% savlon
- **D.** All of the above

68. It has been seen that HAV gets destroyed by 1 mg/L of free residual Cl_2 in 30 mts at pH value of 8.5 or less.
- **A.** True
- **B.** False

69. Normal human Ig against HAV is recommended for:
- **A.** Susceptible persons travelling to highly endemic areas
- **B.** Close personal contacts of patients with HAV
- **C.** For the control of outbreak in institutions
- **D.** All of the above
- **E.** Both A and B

70. W.H.O. deprecated the widespread use of Ig against HAV, because:
- **A.** The individual with sub-clinical infection may still disseminate the virus in the general community
- **B.** The practice appears to be wasteful
- **C.** Repeated injection of Ig may be undesirable in healthy children
- **D.** All of the above
- **E.** Both A and B above

71. In which year, the largest epidemic of HAV was recorded in Delhi?
- **A.** 1955-56
- **B.** 1965-66
- **C.** 1975-76
- **D.** 1985-86
- **E.** 1995-96

72. Persistent HBV infection may cause progressive liver disease like:
A. Chronic active hepatitis
B. Hepatocellular C_A
C. Both of the above
D. Neither A nor B

73. Highest incidence of HBV infection is seen in all, *except:*
A. Australia
B. China
C. South East Asia
D. South America

74. In most industrialized countries, the carrier rate is less than how much for HBV?
A. < 1% B. < 2%
C. < 3% D. < 4%
E. < 5%

75. Hepatoma (primary liver C_A) is the leading cause of death in males from HBV in most of sub-Saharan Africa and much of East and South-East Asia and the Pacific region.
A. True
B. False

76. The presence of HBV infection is designated as "high" in those areas where carrier rate of more than:
A. > 1 % B. > 2%
C. > 3% D. > 4%
E. > 5%

77. By the year 2000, applying the current prevalence of carriers, it is estimated that there will be 400 million HBV carriers in the entire world if HB vaccine is not widely used.
A. True
B. False

78. HBV has implicated in major epidemic outbreak in Ahmedabad in:
A. 1783
B. 1984
C. 1994
D. 1990
E. 1996

79. HBV was discovered by whom?
A. Louis Pasteur
B. Von Pirquet
C. Blumberg
D. Dogmak

80. All are the extrahepatic C/M of HBV *except:*
A. Amyloidosis
B. Serum sickness like syndrome
C. Aplastic anaemia
D. Periarteritis nodosa
E. Glomerulonephritis

81. An increased frequency of the carrier state with HBV has been described in patients with:
A. Down's syndrome
B. Mongolism
C. Chronic renal disease
D. Lepromatous leprosy
E. All of these

82. The antigen detectable 1st in HB infection is:
A. HBe Ag
B. HBs Ag
C. HBc Ag
D. All of the above
E. Both A and C

83. The antigen indirectly detectable after other antigens in HBV infection is:
A. HBs Ag
B. HBe Ag
C. HBc Ag
D. All of the above

84. Appearance of following in the serum of HBV case indicates infectivity:
A. HBs Ag
B. HBc Ag
C. HBs Ab
D. HBe Ag
E. HBe Ab

85. Appearance of antibody to the following in the serum of viral Hepatitis B patient is considered to be of good prognostic value:
A. HBe Ag
B. HBs Ag
C. HBc Ag
D. HBe Ab
E. HBc Ab

86. Presence of HBs Ag in the serum is an indicator of:
A. Acute infection
B. Carrier state
C. Both of the above
D. Neither A nor B

87. High infection rates with HBV have been found in:
A. Percutaneous drug abusers
B. Prostitutes and homosexual population
C. Immunization, acupuncture, circumcision, scarification
D. Shared razors and tooth brushes
E. All of these

88. In HBV infection, the persistent carrier state has been defined as the presence of HBs Ag for more than:
A. 1 month
B. 3 months
C. 6 months
D. 9 months
E. 12 months

89. "Horizontal transmission" in HBV infection means transmission from:
A. Mother to child
B. Mother to father
C. Child to child
D. Father to child

90. How long case of HBV infection is regarded to be unfit for blood transfusion?
A. 20 weeks
B. 28 weeks
C. 30 weeks
D. 36 weeks
E. 40 weeks

91. Main source for transmission of HBV is:
A. Contaminated blood
B. Saliva
C. Sweat
D. Semen
E. Vaginal fluid

92. Which is false regarding hepatitis B vaccine (plasma derived)?
A. Based on HBs Ag from the plasma of human carriers of HBV
B. Vaccine is a formalin inactivated sub-unit viral vaccine for IM injection
C. 1 ml dose of vaccine is given in 3 doses at 0, 1 and 6 months provide 95% antibody response
D. Protective level of antibody lasts for 1 year

93. Hepatitis 'B' Ig is used for those acutely exposed to HBs Ag- +ve blood like:
A. Surgeons, nurses or laboratory workers
B. Newborn infants of carrier mothers
C. Sexual contacts of acute HBV infected patients
D. All of the above

94. HB Ig would provide passive protection for about:
A. 1 month
B. 2 months
C. 3 months
D. 4 months
E. 6 months

95. Regarding RDNA-yeast derived vaccine against HBV, all true, *but* one:
A. Licensed for use for the 1st time in USA (1987)
B. Protection provides upto 6 years
C. Immunogenic, safe and effective
D. Cheaper
E. Over 90% of recipients of the vaccine mount perceptive antibody to HBV

96. This combined procedure passive active immunization is ideal both for prophylaxis of persons accidentally exposed to blood known to contain HBV and, for prevention of the carrier state in the newborn babies of carrier mothers.
A. True
B. False

97. Which is not true about hepatitis 'C' virus infection?
A. First identified in 1989
B. A single stranded DNA virus
C. Mainly transmitted through transfusion of contaminated blood or blood products
D. I.P. – 6 to 7 weeks
E. More than 50% develop chronic hepatitis

98. In India, screening for HCV has been made mandatory for all blood banks from July 1, 1997.
A. True
B. False

99. The only drug found useful in treatment of HCV infection is:
A. Levamisole
B. Ripasone
C. Interferon
D. Dactinomycin

100. The non A-non B hepatitis was 1st reported from which country?
A. Italy
B. India
C. Venezuela
D. South Africa

101. Regarding HEV, which of the following is/are false?
A. The infection was discovered in 1990
B. Essentially a water-borne disease
C. The 1st major epidemic was reported in New Delhi during winter in 1995-96
D. Diagnosis is made by the level of anti-HEV antibodies in the serum
E. Vaccine or specific immunoglobulin therapy is available

102. Delta hepatitis was 1st detected in 1977 in which country?
A. India
B. Italy
C. Hongkong
D. Denmark
E. Ethiopia

103. Following viruses cannot cause disease of its own independently:
A. HAV
B. HBV
C. HCV
D. HDV
E. HEV

104. Which communicable disease is mentioned as "Vishuchika" in Ayurveda and defined in "Susruta Samhita"?
A. Smallpox
B. Plague
C. Cholera
D. Tetanus
E. Rabies

105. Currently larger foci (80%) of cholera are seen in the following states, *except:*
A. Maharashtra
B. Tamil Nadu
C. Karnataka and Kerala
D. Delhi
E. Bihar

106. The code name given to a new strain of cholera in India is:
A. 0123
B. 0139
C. 0132
D. 0136
E. 0138

107. Now-a-days in India, most cases of cholera is due to:
A. Eltor biotype serotype ogawa
B. Eltor biotype serotype hikozima
C. Classical cholera
D. Eltor biotype serotype Inaba
E. Any of the above

108. The chances of development of clinical attack of cholera are more if the person consumes infected material on:

A. Empty stomach
B. Full stomach
C. Both of the above
D. Neither A nor B

109. Eltor vibrio may be distinguished from classical vibrios by the following:

A. Eltor vibrios agglutinate chicken and sheep red cells
B. Resistant to classical phage IV
C. The VP reaction and haemolytic test do not give consistent to classical phage IV
D. They are resistant to polymyxin B-50-unit disc
E. All of these

110. Vibrio cholerae are easily killed by following, *except:*

A. Heating at 56°C
B. Refrigerator ice box
C. Cresol
D. Boiling
E. Bleaching powder

111. The total number of hookworm cases in India is estimated to be:

A. 40 million
B. 200 million
C. 100 million
D. 400 million

112. Which is false in respect of cholera?

A. The human is the only known reservoir of cholera
B. A case of cholera is infectious for a period of 7 to 10 days
C. The chronic carrier state does not exist
D. Convalescent carriers are infectious for 2 to 3 weeks

113. The infectivity of an incubatory carrier of cholera lasts for:

A. 1 to 2 days
B. 1 to 5 days
C. Upto 1 week
D. 1 to 10 days

114. The I.P. of cholera is:

A. Few hours to 5 days
B. 1 days
C. 2 days
D. One week

115. The infectivity of a contact carrier in cholera lasts for:

A. 3 days
B. 5 days
C. 7 days
D. < 10 days

116. The infectivity of a convalescent case of cholera lasts for:

A. One week
B. Two weeks
C. 2 to 3 weeks
D. 4 weeks

117. The Eltor vibrio was 1st isolated from which nation?

A. India
B. Egypt
C. Indonesia
D. Taiwan
E. Bangladesh

118. Strike off whichever is not the cause for persistence of cholera vibrio during inter-epidemic period:

A. Long-term carriers
B. Low grade continuous transmission through asymptomatic cases
C. Persistence in altered form
D. Persistence in extra prehuman life

119. The main symptom of cholera is:

A. Abdominal pain
B. Vomiting
C. Diarrhea
D. All of the above
E. Both B and C

120. Adenylcyclase activity in intestine in cholera patient is activated by:

A. L. toxin
B. H. toxin

C. C-AMP
D. Increased peristalsis

121. The stool in cholera patients is:
A. Isotonic
B. Hypotonic
C. Hypertonic
D. All of the above

122. The appearance of stool in cholera patient is:
A. Aluminium paint
B. Toothpaste
C. Rice water
D. Currant jelly

123. The "stage of collapse" state of cholera shows the following, *except:*
A. Sunken eyes/hollow cheeks
B. Subnormal temperature
C. Absent pulse
D. Protuberant abdomen
E. Washerman's hand and feet

124. Vibrio cholerae enterotoxin produces isotonic diarrhoea by:
A. Increased peristalsis
B. Increasing secretion
C. Failure of Na^+ pump
D. Mucosal damage

125. Epidemiologically, Eltor cholera differs from classical cholera in the following respect, *but* one:
A. Low case fatality
B. Survive longer in extra intestinal environments
C. High infection to case ratio
D. Mild clinical manifestations
E. More secondary cases in affected families

126. Cholera is a notifiable disease upto what level?
A. Locally
B. State
C. Nationally
D. Internationally
E. All of the above

127. Under the IHR, cholera is notifiable to WHO within .... of its occurrence by the National Government.
A. 24 hours
B. 2 days
C. 3 days
D. 4 days
E. 7 days

128. The best method of collecting stools for detection of cholera is by:
A. Rectal swab
B. Rubber catheter
C. Disinfected stool
D. All of the above

129. An area is declared free of cholera when twice the I.P. (10 days) has elapsed since the death, recovery or isolation of the last case.
A. True
B. False

130. The culture media used for vibrio cholerae is:
A. VR medium
B. Alkaline peptone water
C. Cary Blair media
D. Bile salt agar medium
E. Any of the above

131. In cholera, following successful institution of rehydration therapy the mortality has brought down to less than:
A. 1%
B. 2%
C. 3%
D. 4%
E. 5%

132. The oral rehydration therepy (ORT) was introduced by W.H.O. in:
A. 1970
B. 1971
C. 1972
D. 1973
E. 1975

133. The amount of ORS required in 1st four hours by any individual with mild dehydration in ml/kg, body weight would be:
A. 30
B. 40
C. 50
D. 60
E. 70 ml/kg

134. In case of severe dehydration due to cholera or diarrhoea the recommended dose of intravenous Ringer Lactate or any other fluid in ml/kg body weight:
A. 50
B. 75
C. 100
D. 110 ml/kg

135. Which is not true regarding mild dehydration?
A. Tongue moist
B. Blood pressure low
C. Restlessness
D. Anterior fontanelle normal
E. Urine flow normal

136. It is true that in severe dehydration the patient:
A. BP is <80 mmHg or unrecordable
B. Tongue is very dry
C. Drowsy/may be comatose
D. Urine flow little or none
E. All of the above

137. Which is not true about composition of ORS-bicarbonate?
A. NaCl 3.5 gm
B. $NaHCO_3$ 1.5 gm
C. KCl 1.5 gm
D. Glucose (dextrose) 20 gm
E. Potable H_2O 1 liter

138. Composition of ORS-citrate includes the following *but* one:
A. NaCl 2.5 gm
B. Trisodium citrate dehydrate-2.9 gm
C. KCl-1.5 gm
D. Glucose 20 gm
E. H_2O 1 litre

139. In a cholera patient following antibiotic treatment, if diarrhoea persists after .... hours of treatment, resistance to antibiotic should be suspected.
A. 24
B. 48
C. 72
D. 96

140. The antibiotic of choice in pregnant women against cholera is:
A. Tetracycline
B. Doxycycline
C. Cotrimoxazole
D. Furazolidine

141. The antibiotic of choice for adults cholera patients is:
A. Tetracycline
B. Furazolidine
C. Cotrimoxazole
D. Doxycycline

142. The WHO International Centre for Vibrios (phage typing) is located at:
A. National Institute of Cholera and Enteric Diseases, Kolkata
B. National Institute of Communicable Diseases, Kolkata
C. All India Institute of Hygiene and Public Health, Kolkata
D. National Institute of Immunology, Mumbai

143. The most effective disinfectant for general use is a coal tar disinfectant with a Ridealwalker coefficient of 10 or more like cresol.
A. True
B. False

144. The DOIC for chemoprophylaxis against cholera is:
A. Ampicillin
B. Tetracycline

C. Cotrimoxazole
D. Doxycycline

145. The only specific prophylactic available against cholera is:
A. Sanitation measures
B. Chemoprophylaxis
C. Vaccination
D. All of these
E. Both A and B above

146. Reactions of cholera vaccine may be ameliorated by giving:
A. Ampicillin
B. Salicylates
C. Corticosteroids
D. None of these

147. The World Health Assembly abolished the requirement of a cholera vaccination certificate for international travel in:
A. May 1973
B. June 1977
C. April 1987
D. May 1995

148. In spite of international abolition of cholera certification, few nations still continue to demand cholera certificate includes:
A. Great Britain
B. Sudan
C. Libya
D. Both B and C
E. All of the above

149. The most effective prophylactic measure against cholera is perhaps health education which should be directed mainly towards:
I. The effectiveness and simplicity of oral rehydration therapy
II. The benefits of early reporting for prompt treatment
III. Food hygiene practices
IV. Handwashing after defecation and before eating
V. The benefit of cooked, hot foods and safe water

Select the true answer as per following code given below:
A. I, II and III
B. I, II, III and IV
C. I, II, III, IV and V All
D. I, III and V

150. Under Diarrhoeal Disease Control Programme:
A. The national management of diarrhoea in children undertaken
B. Breast feeding has been promoted
C. ORS is promoted as 1st line of treatment
D. All of these
E. Both A and B

151. Diarrhoea is defined as the passage of loose liquid or watery stools more than .... times a day.
A. 3
B. 5
C. 7
D. 10
E. 15

152. A diarrhoea is said to be chronic when it is lasted more than:
A. 1 week
B. 2 weeks
C. 3 weeks
D. 4 weeks
E. 6 weeks

153. Which of the following statements is/are false?
A. The WHO/UNICEF define "acute diarrhoea" as an attack of sudden onset, which usually lasts 3 to 7 days, but may last upto 10 to 14 days
B. Acute diarrhoea is caused by an infection of the bowel
C. The term "gastroenteritis" is most frequently used to describe acute diarrhoea
D. V. cholerae produce marked histological abnormality of small intestine
E. Blood mixed diarrhoea is called as dysentery

154. MODE (1991) survey conducted to ascertain incidence of diarrhoea in:
A. Bihar
B. J and K
C. Tamil Nadu
D. Both A and C
E. All of the above

155. According to SRS estimates, during 1992, the child mortality was about 26.5 per 1000 children under 5 years of age, out of which how much percentage of deaths were due to diarrhoeal diseases?
A. 5%
B. 10%
C. 20%
D. 25%
E. 30%

156. Following are recognised viral causes of diarrhoea, *but* one:
A. Astroviruses
B. Campylobacter jejuni
C. Norwalk group
D. Rotavirus

157. The most common pathogen of diarrhoea in children world over is:
A. Giardiasis
B. Enteroviruses
C. Campylobacter
D. Rotavirus
E. All of the above

158. Following protozoa may cause diarrhoea, *save* for one:
A. Entamoeba histolytica
B. Giardia intestinalis
C. Trichuriasis
D. Cryptosporidium species
E. None of these

159. Which bacteria is not associated with diarrhoea?
A. Staphylococcus
B. Shigella
C. Salmonella
D. Bacillus cereus

160. Most common bacteria implicated in acute diarrhoea in developing countries is:
A. Shigella
B. ETEC
C. Campylobacter jejuni
D. EPEC
E. Salmonella

161. Regarding ETEC (Enterotoxigenic Escherichia coli), which is correct?
A. It does not invade the bowel mucosa and diarrhoea is due to toxins
B. There are 2 ETEC toxins, heat labile (LT) and heat stable (ST)
C. The LT toxin is closely related to cholera toxin
D. ETEC is spread mostly by means of contaminated food and water
E. All of the above

162. Cryptosporidium is a coccidian parasite that causes diarrhoea in:
A. Infants
B. Immunodeficient patients
C. Domestic animals
D. All of these
E. Both A and C above

163. Infection caused by shigella dysenteriae type 1 are the most severe and often occur in epidemic form.
A. True
B. Partially true
C. False

164. Recognised causes of Parenteral diarrhoea (non-digestive origin) includes:
I. ENT infections.
II. Respiratory or urinary infections.
III. Malaria
IV. Bacterial meningitis
V. Simple teething
Select the true answer as per following code given below:
A. I, II and III
B. I, II, III and IV

C. I, II, III, IV and V All
D. I, III and V

165. According to the WHO definition of AIDS in children, persistent diarrhoea is defined as an episode of diarrhoea lasting more than:
A. 15 days
B. 30 days
C. 10 days
D. 20 days
E. 7 days

166. Recognised short-term intervention as recommended by WHO against diarrhoeal diseases control programme includes all, *but* one:
A. ORT
B. Appropriate feeding
C. Chemotherapy
D. Health education

167. The Diarrhoeal Disease Control Programme was started in India in:
A. 1978
B. 1980
C. 1985
D. 1986
E. 1990

168. Wordwide typhoid fever affects about 6 million people with more than 600,000 deaths a year.
A. True
B. Partially correct
C. False

169. Regarding typhoid fever, which of the following statement is false?
A. Typhoid (enteric fever) is caused mainly by salmonella typhi
B. Man is the only known reservoir of infection, cases or carriers
C. Typhoid Mary is a good example of a chronic carrier
D. Highest incidence of this disease occurs in 5 to 19 years of age group
E. The antibody to 'H' antigen is usually higher in diseased patient

170. The I.P. for enteric fever (typhoid) is:
A. < 7 days
B. 7 to 10 days
C. 10 to 14 days
D. > 15 days

171. Regarding Typhoid, all are true *save* for one:
A. The peak incidence reported in July, August and September
B. The salmonella typhi do multiply in water
C. Freezing does not destroy the bacilli
D. Typhoid bacilli grow rapidly in milk without altering in any way its taste or appearance

172. Presence of high titre of which antibody is diagnostic screening test for detection of typhoid carriers?
A. Hi-abs
B. O-abs
C. Vi-abs
D. All of these
E. Both A and B

173. Which communicable disease is regarded as the index of general sanitation in any country?
A. Typhoid fever
B. Amoebiasis
C. Cholera
D. Hookworm disease

174. The usual methods of control of reservoir are their:
A. Identification
B. Isolation
C. Treatment
D. Disinfection
E. All of these

175. Regarding treatment in Typhoid, which is true?
A. Chloramphenicol is still the DOIC
B. Co-trimoxazole, ampicillin, trimethoprim, is a good alternative

C. Patient who are seriously ill and profoundly toxic should be given an injection of hydrocortisone (100 mg) daily for 3 to 4 days
D. All of these
E. Both A and B above

176. One of the most radical ways of controlling Typhoid:
A. All patients of typhoid after full course of chlormycetin treatment should be treated with ampicillin 2 gm in divided doses for 7 days
B. Cholecystectomy associated with concomitant ampicillin therapy
C. Only cholecystectomy
D. All of these
E. Both A and C above

177. From the community point of view which type of typhoid carrier is most dangerous?
A. Intestinal
B. Biliary
C. Urinary
D. Temporary

178. Typhoid fever can be diagnosed by widal test earliest in:
A. 1st week
B. 2nd week
C. 3rd week
D. 4th week

179. The minimum diagnostic titre of 'O' antigen in widal test is:
A. 1 : 125
B. 1 : 175
C. 1 : 200
D. 1 : 225
E. 1 : 240

180. Immunization against Typhoid is recommended for all, *except* for:
A. People living in endemic area or in the same house with chronic carrier
B. Those on immunosuppressive therapy
C. Those attending melas or yatras
D. Groups exposed to risks of infection such as school children and hospital staff
E. Travellers proceeding to endemic areas

181. The vaccine of choice in India against Typhoid is:
A. Monovalent
B. Bivalent
C. TAB vaccine
D. All of the above

182. Which is the orally effective vaccine against Typhoid?
A. Monovalent
B. Bivalent
C. Live Ty 21a vaccine
D. TAB vaccine

183. Of the following foods which is commonly associated with salmonella type of food poisoning?
A. Rabdi
B. Boondi
C. Salad
D. Eggs
E. All of the above

184. Regarding salmonella food poisoning, which is false?
A. Extremely common form of food poisoning
B. I.P. is 12 to 24 hours
C. Man gets the infection from farm animals and poultry
D. Mortality is 11%

185. Concerning staphylococcal food poisoning which is untrue?
A. I.P. is 1 to 6 hours
B. Always associated with pyrexia of 38.5°C to 39°C
C. Preformed toxin
D. Toxin is heat resistant and act directly on intestine and CNS
E. Sudden onset of vomiting abdominal cramps and diarrhoea

186. All are true about botulism, *except* for one:
A. Most serious
B. Toxin is preformed
C. CNS symptoms are very mild
D. The food most frequently involved is homemade/canned vegetables smoked or picked fish, homemade cheese
E. GIT symptoms are very mild

187. Which is not true about clostridial perfringens food poisoning?
A. It is the most common organism associated with gas gangrene
B. I.P. is 8 to 24 hours
C. Diarrhoea, abdominal cramp, little or no fever
D. Nausea and vomiting are more prominent features

188. Along with other manifestations related to gastrointestinal tract in a case of food poisoning if there is fever too, then the infection is more likely to be:
A. Staphylococcal
B. Salmonella
C. B. cereus
D. Botulism

189. Regarding bacillus cereus food poisoning, which is false?
A. B. cereus is an aerobic, spore bearing motile gram negative rod
B. It has recently been recognised as a cause of food poisoning with increasing frequency
C. The toxin is preformed and stable
D. Diarrhoeal form with a longer I.P. (12 to 24 hours) resembling clostridial food poisoning
E. Emetic form has short I.P. (1 to 6 hours) resembling staphylococcal food poisoning

190. In cholera, following is not found, *but* one:
A. Nausea and vomiting
B. Leucocytosis
C. Headache
D. Tenesmus
E. Abdominal tenderness

191. Amoebiosis has been defined by W.H.O. as:
A. The condition associated with bulky foul smelling stool with griping
B. The condition associated with recent diarrhoea or loose motion 7 or more in a day with griping
C. The condition of harboring entamoeba histolytica with or without C/M
D. The condition of harboring entamoeba histolytic a with definite C/M and passage of 7 or more loose motions per day

192. Intestinal amoebiasis includes all, *but* one:
A. Amoebic dysentery
B. Amoeboma
C. Nondysenteric colitis
D. Perforation (intestinal)
E. Amoebic appendicitis

193. Regarding amoebiasis, which is false?
A. Affects 15% of world population
B. The normal habitat is the colon
C. Man is the only reservoir of infection
D. Isozyme electrophoretic mobility analysis have so far identified seven potentially pathogenic and 11 non pathogenic zymodems
E. Period of communicability lasts as long as vegetative forms are excreted

194. Following methods are employed in the prevention of amoebiasis, *except:*
A. Water filtration and boiling
B. Sanitary disposal of human excreta
C. Cysts are killed by chlorine in amounts added for water disinfection
D. Strict personal hygiene
E. Periodic examinations of food handler

195. NOT true about amoebiasis is:
A. Sand filters are quite effective in removing amoebic cysts

B. Uncooked vegetables and fruits can be disinfected with aqueous solution of acetic acid (5 to 10%) or full strength vinegar
C. Flies, cockroaches and rodents are recognised vectors
D. I.P. 1 to 3 days
E. Amoebiasis may occur at any age with no sex or racial difference

196. The most sensitive serological test against amoebiasis is:
A. Indirect haemagglutination test
B. ELISA technique
C. CIE
D. All of the above

197. Which of the following statement is/are true?
A. In amoebiasis, demonstration of trophozoites containing RBC is diagnostic
B. Serology is often negative in intestinal amoebiasis
C. Positive serological test may provide due to extraintestinal amoebiasis
D. All of these
E. Both A and B above

198. Regarding Ascariasis, all are true, *save* for one:
A. An infection of the GIT is caused by an adult worm
B. I.P. is 2 months
C. It is the most common helminthic infestations
D. About 1/4th of the world population is infected
E. None of these

199. Which is not true about Ascariasis?
A. Ascaris lumbricoides resides in the lumen of small intestine
B. The life span of adult worm is between 6 to 12 months
C. Man is the only reservoir of infection
D. Infective material is faeces containing the unfertilized eggs

200. The most favourable soil for the development of ascaris eggs is:
A. Moist porous soil
B. Alluvial soil
C. Clay soil
D. All of the above

201. All, *but* one, are associated with mode of transmission of Ascariasis:
A. Ingestion of unfertilized eggs along with food drinks and salads
B. By ingestion of infective eggs with food and drink
C. Pica
D. Polluted water
E. None of these

202. In present day context, which would be the best method to control Ascariasis in future?
A. Mass treatment with antihelminthic drugs
B. Sanitation improvement
C. Sanitation improvement and mass treatment
D. None of these

203. Which drug used against Ascariasis is effective in a single dose of 10 mg/kg of body weight with a maximum of 1 gm?
A. Piperazine citrate
B. Pyrantel pamoate
C. Levamisole
D. Mebendazole

204. During 1996 the global prevalence of hookworm infection was about:
A. 100 million
B. 151 million
C. 201 million
D. 251 million cases

205. Which state in India has the highest infestation of Ankylostomiasis?
A. Assam
B. Bihar
C. Orissa
D. Andhra Pradesh
E. West Bengal

206. Which index is used in epidemiological studies of hookworm disease?
A. Weinberg's index
B. Heidelberg's index
C. Chandler's index
D. Stephenson's index.
E. All of these

207. To become infective after excretion via faeces the Ascaris lumbricoides eggs need a time period of:
A. One week
B. One to two weeks
C. Two weeks
D. Two to three weeks

208. The single measure that depends on active community participation to prevent and control ascariasis and amoebiasis is:
A. Surveillance
B. Personal hygiene
C. Food hygiene
D. Potable water
E. Environmental hygiene

209. In Chandler's index, if the average number of hookworm eggs per gram of faeces for the entire community is about 300 then:
A. It is important public health problem
B. It is not of much significance
C. May be regarded as potential danger
D. Minor public health problem

210. Recently which species of hookworm is reported from Calcutta?
A. Necator Americanus
B. Ankylostoma ceylanicum
C. Ankylostoma duodenale
D. Necator pipensis

211. In southern India, hookworm disease is mainly due to:
A. A. duodenale
B. A. ceylanicum
C. Necator americanus
D. All of the above

212. In northern India, hookworm disease is mainly due to:
A. Ankylostoma ceylanicum
B. Ankylostoma duodenale
C. N. americanus
D. Both A and C
E. A, B and C All

213. Hookworms usually resides in:
A. Small intestine (jejunum)
B. Stomach
C. Appendix and caecum
D. Large intestine
E. Colon

214. The most common mode of transmission of hookworms is:
A. Faeco-oral
B. Vectorborne
C. Percutaneous
D. All of the above
E. Both A and B above

215. Use of Chandler's index is:
A. To initiate preventive measures
B. Severity of hookworm infection
C. Comparison of worm load in different population
D. Degree of egg reduction after treatment
E. All of the above

216. The infective stage of hookworm is:
A. Filariform larva (3rd stage)
B. Rhabditiform larva
C. Cercariform larva
D. Metacercaria
E. Adultworm as such

217. In endemic areas, the highest incidence of hookworm is found in which age group?
A. 1 to 5 years
B. 5 to 10 years
C. 10 to 15 years
D. 15 to 25 years
E. All ages

218. The most common presentation of hookworm disease is:
A. Anaemia

B. Malnutrition
C. Cachexia
D. Oedema
E. All of the above

219. Following *but* one, drugs are used in treatment of hookworms:
A. Albendazole
B. Mebendazole
C. Piperazine citrate
D. Levamisole
E. Pyrantel pamoate

220. Favourable environmental conditions are crucial for the survival of the hookworm larvae in the soil includes:
I. A damp, sandy or friable soil with decaying vegetation
II. A rainfall of 40 inches and above
III. O_2
IV. A temperature of 24 to 32° centigrade
V. Human habits
Choose the true answer as per code given below:
A. I, II and III
B. I, III and V
C. I, II, III and IV
D. I, II, III, IV and V All

221. Statement (S): Following infection, the prepatent period for necator americanus is 7 weeks while that for ankylostoma duodenale ranging from 5 weeks to 9 months.
Reasons (R): Because the invading larva of A. duodenale is capable of remaining arrested or dormant in the tissues of the host for as long as 9 months and then again resume development and migration.
A. Both (S) and (R) are true, but are related to cause and effect
B. Both (S) and (R) are true, but are not related to cause and effect
C. (S) is true, (R) is false
D. (R) is true, (S) is false
E. Both (S) and (R) are false

222. The only long-term solution to hookworm is:
A. Health education
B. Sanitary disposal of faeces
C. Chemotherapy
D. Correction of iron deficiency anemia
E. All of the above

223. In man, the adult guineaworm normally inhabits:
A. Subcutaneous tissue of head and neck
B. Small intestine
C. Lungs
D. Subcutaneous tissue of leg and foot
E. None of these

224. Worldwide, about .... people are estimated to be victims of guineaworm infection.
A. 5 million
B. 10 million
C. 20 million
D. 25 million
E. 1 million

225. Dracunculiasis occurs in the following nations, *save* for one:
A. India
B. USSR
C. Africa
D. Middle East
E. None of the above

226. In which nations, most cases of guineaworm are existing?
A. India
B. Middle East
C. West Indies
D. Sudan
E. Pakistan

227. Which Indian state is once endemic for guineaworm are now free from the disease?
A. Tamil Nadu
B. Andhra Pradesh

C. Gujarat
D. Maharashtra

228. In India, most of the Dracunculiasis cases are reported from:
A. Andhra Pradesh
B. Rajasthan
C. Gujarat
D. Maharashtra
E. M.P.

229. Regarding Dracunculiasis, which is false?
A. Man acquires infection by drinking water containing infected cyclops
B. An infected person harboring the gravid female is the reservoir of infection
C. The female worm grows to a length of 55 to 120 cm while male worm is just 2 to 3 cm
D. From step wells, the peak transmission occurs during rainy season

230. The transmission of guineaworm is effected after passage of egg/larvae through:
A. Faeces
B. Extra intestinal route
C. Both
D. Neither

231. For effective mass treatment for guineaworm infection among the different drugs available the one which is most suitable is:
A. Albendazole
B. Mebendezole
C. Niridazole
D. None of the above
E. All of the above

232. The best measure for control of guineaworm problem is:
A. Safe drinking water
B. Closure of step wells
C. Sanitary disposal of excreta
D. Early detection and treatment of case

233. The eradication strategy against guineaworm comprises the following:
I. Provision of safe drinking water
II. Control of cyclops
III. Health Education
IV. Surveillance
V. Treatment of cases
Select the most effective measures as per following code:
A. I only
B. I and II only
C. I, II and III
D. I, II, III and IV
E. I, II, III, IV and V All

234. Vaccine vial monitor is used in polio vaccine vials since:
A. 1998
B. 1999
C. 2000
D. 2003

235. If polio vaccine vial is exposed to higher temperature the colour of the white square becomes .... then the vaccine should be considered as ineffective.
A. Red
B. Blue
C. Yellow
D. Green

236. When was Hepatitis "G" (HGV) discovered?
A. 1996
B. 1997
C. 1998
D. 1999

237. The diarrhoeal diseases control programme of WHO was started since:
A. 1978
B. 1980
C. 1984
D. 1990

238. What % of Indian population has been suffering of amoebiasis? What is its prevalence rate?
A. 15%, 15%
B. 20%, 20%
C. 30%, 30%
D. 40%, 40%

239. The carriers of entamoeba histolytica can discharge upto how much cysts daily in stool?
A. 1000
B. 1.5×10^3
C. 1.5×10^5
D. 1.5×10^7 cysts

240. In India, the last reported case of guinea-worm was in the year:
A. 1996
B. 1997
C. 1999
D. 2000

241. India is declared by WHO in respect of dracunculiasis free in which year?
A. 1999 B. 2000
C. 2001 D. 2005

242. Entire Asian region has been declared guineaworm free or dracunculiasis free by:
A. 1999
B. 2000
C. 2001
D. 2002

243. Now-a-days which is regarded as a DOIC against typhoid?
A. Ampicillin
B. Contrimoxazole
C. Ciprofloxacin
D. Chloramphenicol

244. "Pea-soup" diarrhoea is associated with:
A. Typhoid
B. Cholera
C. Amoebiasis
D. Rotavirus

245. Following are recognised parasitic causes of diarrhoea, *except:*
A. Trichuriasis
B. Giardiasis
C. Campylobacter
D. Cryptosporidium

246. Which of the following viruses are not associated with diarrhoea?
A. Rotaviruses
B. Retroviruses
C. Astroviruses
D. Coronaviruses

247. Hepatitis 'G' virus (HGV) is a:
A. Picornavirus
B. Hepacivirus
C. Flavivirus
D. Calcivirus

248. HGV was discovered in which year?
A. 1995
B. 1996
C. 1997
D. 1998

249. Regarding HGV—which is false?
A. HGV commonly co-infects patients with HIV and curiously this dual infection is somewhat protective against HIV disease
B. It is transmitted by contaminated blood or blood products and possibly via sexual contact
C. The prevalence of HGV-RNA is blood donors ranges from 10 to 40%
D. HGV is not hepatotropic and does not cause elevations in serum transferases

250. VVM have been extensively used in the Pulse Polio Programme to assess the effectiveness of cold chain. According to the guidelines, the following changes in the VVM is an indication for discarding the vaccines:
A. Inner square is same colour as that of outer circle
B. Inner square is higher than outer circle

C. Outer square is higher than inner circle
D. Inner square is darker than outer circle

251. **Criteria for defining polio epidemic are all, *except:***
A. 2 or more cases
B. Cases occurring during 6 months period
C. Caused by same virus type
D. Cases should occur in same locality

252. **Typhoid vaccine efficacy is:**
A. 85%
B. 50%
C. 95%
D. 100%

253. **Case fatality rate of typhoid is:**
A. 10%
B. 20%
C. 30%
D. 50%

254. **The most effective way of treating typhoid carrier is:**
A. Cholecystectomy
B. Chemotherapy
C. Vaccination
D. Isolation

255. **Duration of immunity after typhoid vaccination is:**
A. 1 year
B. 2 years
C. 3 years
D. 5 years

3. ARTHROPOD BORNE INFECTIONS

1. **A prevalence of aedes aegypti and aedes albopictus together with the circulation of dengue virus of more than one type in any particular area tends to be associated with DHF/DSS.**
A. True
B. False

2. **Dengue affects more than 100 nations in the following continents *except:***
A. Asia
B. Australia
C. Africa
D. America
E. Europe

3. **The most common of all the arthropod borne viral disease is:**
A. Yellow fever
B. Dengue
C. KFD
D. Chikungunia fever

4. **The "break bone fever" is associated with the following:**
A. Yellow fever
B. KFD
C. Chikungunia
D. Dengue
E. All of the above

5. **In India the 1st recorded outbreak of dengue fever was in the year:**
A. 1912
B. 1923
C. 1812
D. 1898
E. 1995

6. **The "classical dengue fever" is due to following serotypes:**
A. 1
B. 2
C. 3
D. 4
E. All of the above

7. **In dengue fever, it is true that:**
A. The reservoir of infection is both man and mosquito
B. Epidemic outbreak of dengue fever have become frequent in recent years

C. The aedes mosquito becomes infective by feeding on a patient from the day before onset to the 5th day (viraemia stage) of illness
D. Both A and B above
E. All of these

8. The vector responsible for dengue fever is:
A. Aedes
B. Sandfly
C. Culex
D. Anopheles
E. Mansonia

9. Once the mosquito becomes infected it remains so for:
A. One week
B. Two weeks
C. Life
D. 3 weeks
E. None of these

10. Following *but* one, are true about classical dengue fever:
A. All ages and both sexes are susceptible
B. Children have severe disease than adults
C. The disease is characterised by the I.P. of 5 to 6 days
D. The onset is sudden with chills and high fever, intense headache, muscle and joint pains which prevents all movement
E. Fever lasts for about to 7 days

11. Regarding dengue haemorrhagic fever, all are true, *except* for one:
A. Severe illness is thought to be due to double infection
B. Arorexia, vomiting, epigastric discomfort, tenderness at the right costal margin and generalised abdominal pain are common
C. During the 1st few days the illness usually resembles classical DF, but maculopapular rash usually rubelliform type, is more common
D. Febrile convulsions may occur particularly in infants

12. The major pathophysiologic changes that determine the severity of disease in DHF and differentiate it from dengue fever (DF) is:
A. Plasma leakage
B. Abnormal homeostasis
C. Both A and B
D. Neither A nor B

13. Recognised haemorrhagic C/M in DHF includes:
A. Petechial, purpura, ecchymosis
B. Epistasis, gum bleeding
C. Haemetemesis/melena
D. Positive tourniquet test
E. All of the above

14. The severity of DHF has been classified into 4 grades according to following pathophysiological hallmarks like:
A. Shock
B. Bleeding
C. Fever
D. Both A and B
E. All of these

15. In which grade of DHF profound shock with undetectable blood pressure and pulse is kept?
A. Grade IV
B. Grade II
C. Grade I
D. Grade III

16. To establish a clinical diagnosis of DHF, following criteria has to be met, *save* for one:
A. Fever
B. Hepatomegaly
C. Hemorrhagic manifestations
D. Thrombocytopenia
E. Haemoconcentration

17. Regarding malaria, all are true, *save* for one:
A. A typical attack consists of cold state, hot state and sweating state

B. It is one of the oldest recorded disease in the world
C. In the 18th century, Italian considered it to be caused by "bad-air", hence the name
D. Laveran (1880) a French Army surgeon discovered the malarial parasite in Algiers, north Africa
E. None of these

18. Consider the following statements:

I. The main credit goes to Ronald Ross who discovered the transmission of malaria by Anopheline mosquitoes (1897) at Secunderabad, Andhra Pradesh, India
II. Ross found malarial parasites growing as cysts (Oocysts) on the stomach wall of an Anopheline mosquito which previously fed on an malaria patient
III. DDT was synthesized in 1874
IV. Paul Muller (1894) in Switzerland discovered the insecticidal properties of DDT for which he was awarded a Nobel prize

Select the true answer as per code given below:
A. I, II, III and IV All
B. I, II and III
C. I and IV only
D. I, II and IV
E. II, III and IV

19. Which country in the world first of all has launched a Malaria Eradication Programme and when?
A. U.S.A. in 1930
B. Venezuela in 1945
C. Canada in 1920
D. U.K. in 1928

20. From the year 1953 to 1961 India was heading towards malaria eradication. However thence the setback started and India had the highest number of cases in which of the following year after which the strategy changed?
A. 1958
B. 1966
C. 1971
D. 1976
E. 1979

21. In which year, W.H.O. convened a Ministerial Conference on Malaria in "Amsterdam at which the Government of both endemic and nonendemic nations signed a world declaration on the control of malaria and endorsed a global malaria control strategy, emphasizing the need to develop sustainable control programmes adapted to local needs?
A. 1970
B. 1978
C. 1992
D. 1989
E. 1985

22. Consider the following statement about malaria:

I. Malaria is occurring between 60° North and 40° South
II. Malaria is endemic in 91 countries
III. Epidemics are recurring in areas where transmission had been interrupted
IV. At present malaria is a major public health problem in the tropical developing nations

Choose the correct answer as per code given below:
A. I and IV
B. I, II and III
C. I and III
D. II and III only
E. I, II, III and IV All

23. Among all infectious diseases, which continues to be one of the biggest contri-

butors to disease burdens' in terms of deaths and suffering?

A. T.B.
B. Malaria
C. Measles
D. Dengue
E. All of these

24. Those at greatest risk of dying from the malaria includes:

I. Children under 5 years in malaria endemic areas
II. Pregnant women
III. People moving from non-malarious zones for reasons of work, migration refuge, war or tourism
IV. Travellers who visit endemic countries and return home with the disease

Select the true answer as per code given below:

A. I, II, III and IV All
B. I, II and III
C. I and IV
D. II, III and IV
E. I and III only

25. In India "Tribal malaria" is mainly due to:

A. Plasmodium vivax
B. Plasmodium malariae
C. Plasmodium falciparum
D. Plasmodium ovale

26. The main vector of "rural malaria" is:

A. Anophelis stephensi
B. Anophelis culcifacies
C. Anophelis fluviatilis
D. Anophelis minimum
E. All of the above

27. In rural areas, which species of malarial parasite is predominant during lean period?

A. P. falciparum
B. P. ovale
C. P. vivax
D. P. malariae

28. The main vector for "Urban malarial parasite" is:

A. Anophelis culcifacies
B. An stephensi
C. An. minimus
D. Anophelis fluviatilis
E. All of these

29. Which species of malarial parasite has the widest geographic distribution throughout the world?

A. P. ovale
B. P. vivax
C. P. malariae
D. Plasmodium falciparum

30. Less than 1% of malarial infection in India is reported to be due to:

A. P. ovale
B. P. vivax
C. P. malaria
D. P. falciparum

31. The largest focus of P. malariae in India is reported to be in Tumkur and Hassan districts of Karnataka.

A. True
B. False

32. "Plasmodium ovale" is not seen in:

A. Tropical Africa
B. India
C. Vietnam
D. Both A and B
E. All of the above

33. "Cerebral malaria" is caused by:

A. P. ovale
B. P. vivax
C. P. falciparum
D. P. malariae
E. All of the above

34. About 70% of malarial parasite infection reported to be due to:

A. P. vivax
B. P. falciparum

C. P. ovale
D. P. malariae

35. A plasmodium causing nephrotic syndrome is:
A. P. ovale
B. P. malariae
C. P. falciparum
D. P. vivax
E. All of the above

36. A plasmodium causing "Black water fever" is:
A. P. vivax
B. P. ovale
C. P. falciparum
D. P. malariae

37. Younger RBC are parasitised by which plasmodium?
A. P. vivax
B. P. ovale
C. P. malariae
D. P. falciparum

38. The developmental cycle of plasmodium which takes place in mosquitoes is:
A. Asexual
B. Sexual
C. Both of the above
D. Neither A nor B

39. The exoerythrocytic phase of development is absent in:
A. P. vivax
B. P. ovale
C. P. falciparum
D. P. malariae

40. In each plasmodium infection intrahepatic schizont burst at different times, *except* for:
A. P. vivax
B. P. ovale
C. P. malariae
D. P. falciparum

41. Which plasmodial sporozoite gives rise to highest number of merozoites?
A. P. falciparum
B. P. ovale
C. P. vivax
D. P. malariae

42. "Sporozoites" demonstrated by whom?
A. Ronald Ross
B. Bastianelli and Grassi
C. Charles Laveran
D. Manson

43. The infective agent of Malarial Parasite for human is:
A. Female anopheles mosquito
B. Trophozoites
C. Sporozoites
D. Schizonts

44. The duration of the erythrocytic cycle is constant for each species of malarial parasite, *save* for one:
A. P. falciparum
B. P. vivax
C. P. ovale
D. P. malariae
E. None of the above

45. The infective stage of plasmodium (MP) for female anopheles mosquito is:
A. Sporozoites
B. Male gametocytes
C. Female gametocytes
D. Schizonts
E. Both B and C above

46. The 1st event to take place in the stomach of the mosquito is:
A. Exflagellation of male gametocyte
B. Release of schizonts
C. Exflagellation of female gametocyte
D. Liberation of merozoites

47. Which penetrates the stomach wall of the mosquito and develops into an oocyst on the outer surface of the stomach?
A. Zygote
B. Ookinete
C. Microgametes
D. Macrogametes
E. All of the above

48. The extrinsic I.P. of malaria in the body of female anopheles mosquito is:
- A. 5 to 10 days
- B. 5 to 15 days
- C. 10 to 20 days
- D. 10 to 25 days
- E. 10 to 30 days

49. Regarding reservoir of infection against malaria, which is false?
- A. Chimpanzes in tropical Africa that may carry the infection with P. malariae
- B. A human reservoir is one who harbours the sexual forms (gametocytes) of the malarial parasite
- C. A patient can be a carrier of several plasmodial species at the same time
- D. Children are more likely to be gametocyte carriers than adults
- E. None of these

50. Certain conditions must be met before a person can serve as a reservoir:
- **I. The person must harbour both the sexes of the gametocytes in his blood**
- **II. The gametocytes must be mature**
- **III. Gametocytes take 2 to 4 days to attain maturity**
- **IV. The gametocytes must be viable**
- **V. The gametocytes must be present in sufficient density to infect mosquitoes**

Select the true answer as per code given below:
- A. I, II and III
- B. I, III and V
- C. I, II, III and IV
- D. I, II, III, IV and V All

51. Consider the following statements:
- **I. Malaria is communicable as long as mature, viable gametocytes exist in the circulating blood in sufficient density to infect vector mosquitoes**
- **II. In vivax infections, gametocytes appear in blood 4 to 5 days after the appearance of the asexual parasite**
- **III. In falciparum infections, they do not appear until 10 to 12 days after the 1st appearance of asexual parasites**
- **IV. Gametocytes are the most numerous during the early stages of the infection when their density may exceed 1,000 per cmm of blood**

Select the true answer as per code given below:
- A. I, II, III and IV All
- B. I, II and III
- C. I, II and IV
- D. I and IV
- E. I and III

52. Relapses are earliest to go after 1 to 2 years in which species of malarial parasite infection?
- A. P. malariae
- B. P. falciparum
- C. P. ovale
- D. P. vivax

53. "Sporozoite induced" relapses in malaria are seen in the following:
- A. P. vivax
- B. P. ovale
- C. P. malariae
- D. Both A and B
- E. All of the above

54. Following statements are true regarding the host factors in malaria, *save* for one:
- A. New born infants are quite susceptible to infection with P. falciparum
- B. High concentration of HbF suppresses infection with P. falciparum
- C. Individuals with AS hemoglobin (sickle-cell trait) have a milder illness with falciparum infection than do those with normal (AA) haemoglobin
- D. Persons whose RBCs are "Duffy negative" are resistant to P. vivax infection
- E. Malaria during pregnancy may cause intrauterine death of the foetus

55. Regarding immunity in malaria, which of the following is/are false?
A. Infants born of immune mothers are generally protected during the 1st 3 to 5 months by maternal IgG antibody
B. Infants born of semi-immune mothers are only partially protected
C. Immunity against one strain does not protect against another
D. Semi-immune individuals may harbour malaria parasites without presenting any symptoms of disease
E. Only humoral factors play a role in malaria protection

56. Regarding environmental factors in malaria, which is false?
A. In most parts of India, the maximum cases are seen from July to November
B. A relative humidity of 60% is necessary for mosquitoes to live normal span of life
C. Malaria is also seen at altitudes above 2000 to 2500 meters
D. The parasite ceases to undergo development in the mosquito if the mean temperature is below 16°C
E. None of these

57. The optimum temperature for the development of the malarial parasite in the insect vector is between:
A. 5 to 10°C
B. 10°C to 15°C
C. 16°C to 20°C
D. 20°C to 30°C
E. 30° to 40°C

58. In India, how many species of Anopheline mosquitoes are seen?
A. 11 B. 45
C. 25 D. 35
E. Only four

59. Which is the most efficient vector of malaria?
A. Anopheles fluviatilis
B. An. stephensi
C. An. culcifacies
D. An. minimum

60. Consider the following statements:
I. The key factor in the transmission of malaria is the life span of the vector
II. The vector mosquito must live for at least 10 to 12 days after an infective blood meal to become infective
III. The strategy in malaria eradication is to shorten the life span of mosquitoes to less than 10 days by insecticides

Choose the correct answer as per following code:
A. I and II
B. I and III
C. I, II and III All
D. II and III only

61. "Man made malaria" means:
A. Person to person transmission
B. Artificial conditions
C. Blood borne transmission mosquitogenic
D. All of these
E. Both A and C above

62. An effective reservoir of malaria does not possess the following characteristics:
A. Presence of male and female gametocytes in blood
B. Mature and viable gametocytes in blood
C. Number of male gametocytes less than female gametocytes
D. Minimum gametocyte density of 12/cmm.
E. Minimum 12 hours old gametocytes in blood

63. The I.P. of naturally mosquito transmitted malaria is:
A. P. falciparum 12 days
B. P. vivax 14 days
C. Quartan malaria 28 days
D. P. ovale 17 days
E. All of these

64. The typical attack of malaria comprises following:

I. Cold stage
II. Hot stage
III. Sweating stage
IV. Afebrile period

Select the true sequence as per code given below:

A. I, IV, III and II
B. I, II, III and IV
C. II, I, III and IV
D. IV, III, II and I
E. I, III, II and IV

65. Recognised complications of P. falciparum malaria is:

I. Cerebral malaria
II. Acute renal failure
III. Liver damage
IV. GIT symptoms, dehydration, collapse
V. Anaemia and black water fever

Select the true answer as per code given below:

A. I, II, III, IV and V All
B. I, II, III and IV
C. I, II and III
D. I, III and V

66. P. vivax is the most common species of malaria in South-East Asia but rare in Africa.

A. True
B. False

67. Recognised complications of P. vivax, P. ovale, and P. malariae infections are the following, *save* for one:

A. Anaemia
B. Black water fever
C. Hepatosplenomegaly
D. Herpes
E. Renal failure

68. Which test is of the greatest value in epidemiological studies and in determining whether a person has had malaria in the past?

A. Thin blood film
B. Thick blood film
C. Malarial fluorescent antibody test
D. Dipstick or antigen capture assay test

69. Spleen rate is defined as the % of children between .... of age showing enlarge ment of spleen.

A. < 1 year
B. 1 to 2 years
C. 1 to 1½ years
D. 2 to 10 years
E. 5 to 10 years

70. Which is widely used for measuring the endemicity of malaria in a community?

A. Average enlarged spleen
B. Spleen rate
C. Infants parasite rate
D. Proportional case rate
E. Parasite density index

71. The most sensitive index of recent transmission of malaria in a locality is:

A. Infant parasite rate
B. Proportional case rate
C. Spleen rate
D. Parasite density index
E. Average enlarged spleen

72. A sophisticated measure of malaria incidence in a community is:

A. AFI
B. ABER
C. API
D. SPR
E. SFR

73. An index of operational efficiency is:

A. AFI
B. ABER
C. API
D. SPR
E. SFR

74. The WHO expert committee on Malaria (1964) recommended that the monthly

number of slides examined should amount to atleast .... of the population.

A. 1%
B. 2%
C. 3%
D. 4%
E. 5%

75. The degree of "anthrophism" in malarial vector indices is shown by:

A. Sporozoite rate
B. Mosquito density
C. Human blood index
D. Man biting rate
E. Inoculation rate

76. "Stable malaria" means what?

A. Mosquitogenic conditions is stable
B. Malaria in stable population
C. Mosquitogenic condition round the year for transmission
D. All of these
E. Both A and B above

77. In which year, Government of India launched the NMCP?

A. April 1953
B. April 1963
C. May 1958
D. June 1966

78. In which year NMEP was launched?

A. 1953
B. 1958
C. 1960
D. 1968
E. 1978

79. The global programme of malaria eradication commenced in which year under the aegis of WHO?

A. 1953
B. 1955
C. 1957
D. 1958
E. 1960

80. What were the strategies taken in NMEP?

A. Attack phase
B. Preparatory phase
C. Consolidation phase
D. Maintenance phase
E. All of these

81. In NMEP infant parasite rate =

A. Infants +ve for M.P. + Total number of peripheral blood slide of infants × 100
B. Infants +ve for M.P. + Total number of infants in population × 100
C. Infants +ve for M.P. + Total number of febrile infants × 100
D. None of these

82. In NMEP, Annual Blood Examination Rate (ABER):

A. Number of slides examined ÷ fever cases × 100
B. Number of slides examined ÷ population × 100
C. Number of fever cases ÷ population × 100
D. None of these

83. In NMEP, API =

A. Confirmed cases of malaria ÷ fever cases × 100
B. Confirmed cases of malaria ÷ slides examined × 100
C. Confirmed cases of malaria ÷ population × 1000
D. None of these

84. Under Modified Plan of operation, the strategy for spraying with DDT/BHC is:

A. 2 or 3 rounds in a year for areas with API more than 2 and focal spraying for areas with API less than 2
B. 2 or 3 rounds in a year for areas with API more than 5 and focal spraying for areas with API less than 5
C. 2 or 3 rounds in a year for areas with API 1 or more and focal spraying in areas with API less than 1
D. None of these

85. The minimum prescribed annual target of ABER under Modified Plan of NMEP is:
A. 5%
B. 10%
C. 15%
D. 20%
E. 30%

86. Recognised causes of setback in NMEP was:
A. Technical failure
B. Administrative failure
C. Operational failure
D. All of these
E. Both B and C above

87. Fever treatment depots (FTD) collected the blood slides in addition to the distribution of antimalarial tablets. How many FTD are functioning all over the country in rural areas?
A. 1 lakh
B. 2 lakh
C. 3.57 lakh
D. 5 lakh
E. 7.5 lakh

88. The urban malaria scheme was launched in which year to reduce or interrupt malaria transmission in town and cities?
A. 1953
B. 1958
C. 1961
D. 1971
E. 1981

89. P. falciparum containment programme has been introduced from October 1977 through the assistance of:
A. Swedish International Development Agency (SIDA)
B. W.H.O.
C. Red Cross Society
D. Government of India

90. Currently P. falciparum contaiment programme is operating in the following Indian states, *save* for one:
A. Orissa
B. Punjab
C. Bihar, West Bengal and MP
D. Andhra Pradesh
E. Gujarat, Maharashtra and Rajasthan

91. For how many peoples residing in a malarious locality each MPW has been appointed?
A. 5000
B. 3500
C. 10000
D. 1000
E. 7500

92. The surveillance worker/MPW collects a blood film and administers a single dose of chloroquine according to prescribed NMEP schedule. This is known as:
A. Presumptive treatment
B. Radical treatment
C. Chemoprophylaxis
D. All of the above

93. The search for malaria cases by the local health agencies such as the PHC, sub-centres, hospital dispensaries and local medical practitioners is known as:
A. Active surveillance
B. Passive surveillance
C. Both of the above
D. Neither A nor B

94. The following parameters are widely used in the epidemiological surveillance of malaria:
I. API
II. ABER
III. AFI
IV. SPR
V. SFR

Select the true answer as per code given below:
A. I, II and III
B. I, II, III and IV
C. I, II, III, IV and V All
D. I, III and V
E. I only

95. Which of the following statements is/are false about presumptive treatment?
A. It means that all fever cases are assumed to be due to malaria
B. The aim of such treatment is to relieve symptom due to malaria and to reduce mortality and morbidity
C. A single dose can save lives in all types of malaria
D. Such treatment given to all age groups including pregnant women in any month of pregnancy or during postpartum period
E. None of the above

96. A single dose of 600 mg chloroquine and 15 mg primaquine on the 1st day followed by 15 mg primaquine daily for the next four days (adult dose) brings about radical cure in the following, *but* one:
A. P. vivax
B. P. malariae
C. Mixed infections
D. P. falciparum
E. None of the above

97. In areas with chloroquine resistance the presumptive treatment for falciparum infection recommended is:
A. Sufaldoxine-pyrimethamine + primaquine
B. Chloroquine + Primaquine
C. Chloroquine + sulfadoxine pyrimethamine
D. None of the above

98. For radical treatment of P. vivax infection in an infant aged 9 months the daily dose of primaquine would be:
A. 2.5 mg
B. 7.5 mg
C. 15 mg
D. None of these

99. The dose of chloroquine base in presumptive treatment for malaria in a month old child would be:
A. 75 mg
B. 150 mg
C. 7.5 mg
D. 300 mg
E. 600 mg

100. Mass drug administration under NMEP is advocated for areas with API:
A. 2 or more
B. 5 or more
C. 10 or more
D. None of these

101. Suppose you are working as a Districal Malaria officer (DMO) and few outbreaks of malaria ensues in that locality, before, prescribing chloroquin what instructions would you like to provide to the patient?
A. Nausea and vomiting may not occur
B. Blurring of vision and headaches may not seen
C. Chloroquine should not be taken on empty stomach
D. All of these
E. Both A and B above

102. New drugs in malaria includes all, *but* one:
A. Artemisinin
B. Mefloquine
C. Halofantrine
D. Sulphalene

103. The DOIC for chemoprophylaxis against Malaria is:
A. Pyimethamine
B. Primaquine
C. Chloroquine
D. Halofantrine

104. In chemoprophylaxis, WHO recommended the prescribed dose of chloroquin for adult is:
A. Chloroquine 300 mg base once weekly
B. Chloroquine 600 mg base once daily
C. Cloroquine 300 mg base once daily
D. None of these

105. A chemoprophylaxis should begin a week before arrival in the malarious area and

continued for how many weeks after leaving a malarious area?

A. 1 to 2 weeks
B. 2 to 3 weeks
C. 3 to 4 weeks
D. 4 to 6 weeks
E. Just 1 week

106. Regarding antimalarial vaccines, which among the following seems to be more promising?

A. Sporozoite
B. Merozoite
C. Schizonticide
D. Microgamete vaccine

107. Consider the following statement:

I. Dr. M. Patarroyo (Colombia) developed a synthetic "cocktail" vaccine for plasmodium falciparum called SP 166

II. SP 166 has been tested in South, America, Africa and South-East Asia

III. A recent field study among children under age 5 in the United Republic of Tanzania showed that the vaccine was safe, induced antibodies and reduced the risk of clinical malaria by about 30%

IV. Pfs 25 is a transmission blocking vaccines against malaria

Choose the true answer as per code given below:

A. I and II
B. II and III
C. III and IV
D. I, II and III
E. I, II, III and IV All

108. "Filariasis" is caused by the following:

A. Protozoon
B. Nematodes
C. Cestodes
D. Flukes

109. According to WHO expert committee .... people are actually infected with filariasis.

A. 62 million
B. 120 million
C. 174 million
D. 236 million

110. Numerically, the lymphatic filariasis cases are greatest in the following various/regions of the world, *except* for one:

A. Latin America
B. China
C. India
D. Indonesia

111. Which was the 1st disease proved to be transmitted by insects?

A. Malaria
B. Kala-azar
C. Filariasis
D. Dengue

112. In world area, if 1-1 billion people are at risk of infection due to filariasis, then what should be the number of such in India?

A. 64 million
B. 136 million
C. 236 million
D. 304 million
E. 467 million

113. All are the heavily infected areas due to filariasis, *except:*

A. U.P. and Bihar
B. J and K
C. Andhra Pradesh and Orissa
D. Tamil Nadu and Kerala
E. Gujarat

114. In India 98% of filariasis is due to:

A. Wuchereria bancrofti
B. Brugia malayi
C. Brugia timori
D. All of the above
E. Both B and C above

115. W. bancrofti diurnal sub-periodic form has been reported from:
A. M.P.
B. Orissa
C. Nicobar group of Islands
D. Delhi

116. Following filarial worms cause lymphatic filariasis, *but* one:
A. W. bancrofti
B. Brugia malayi
C. Brugia tirmori
D. Loa-loa
E. None of these

117. The maximum density of Mf in blood is reported between:
A. 6 AM to 10 AM
B. 10 AM to 2 PM
C. 10 PM to 2 AM
D. 2 PM to 6 PM

118. Subperiodic Brugia malayi is found in:
A. India
B. Malaysia
C. Indonesia
D. Both B and C
E. All of the above

119. In lymphatic filariasis, prepatent period means time between:
A. Invasion of infective larvae and C/M
B. Inoculation of infective larvae and the appearance of Mf. in blood
C. Occurrence of 1st case and secondary case
D. None of these

120. It is true about filariasis that:
A. The adult worm are usually found in lymphatic system of man
B. The females are viviparous and gave birth to as many as 50,000 Mf per day
C. The life span of Mf is not exactly known
D. The adult worms may survive for 15 years or more
E. All of these

121. Animal reservoirs of Brugia present in all, *but* one:
A. Rats
B. Monkeys
C. Cats
D. Dogs
E. None

122. Which of the following statement is/are NOT true about filariasis?
A. In humans the source of infection is a person with circulating Mf in peripheral blood
B. In filarial disease (late obstructive stage) Mf are found in the blood
C. A man with one Mf per 40 cmm of blood was infective to 2.6% of the mosquitoes fed on him
D. The maximum prevalence of culex quinquefasciatus was observed when the temperature was between 22 to 38°C and optimum longevity when the relative humidity was 70%
E. None of these

123. Tropical pulmonary eosinophilia is the best known example of:
A. Lymphatic mariasis
B. Occult mariasis
C. Cryptic filariasis
D. Both B and C above
E. All of these

124. Which is false about lymphatic filariasis?
A. The chronic stage usually develops 1 to 15 years from the onset of the 1st acute attack
B. The term occult or cryptic filariasis refers to filarial infections in which the classical C/M are not present and Mf are not found in the blood
C. In Brugian filariasis genitalia are mainly involved
D. In Ethiopia endemic leg elephantiasis is caused by silica in the iliac lymph glands
E. None of these

125. Following may cause elephantiasis:
I. T.B.
II. Tumours
III. Surgery
IV. Irradiation
V. Lymphatic filarial infection

Choose the true answer as per code given below:

A. I, II and III
B. I, III and V
C. I, II, III and IV
D. I, II, III, IVand V All
E. V only

126. "Microfilaria rate" is the percentage of persons:

A. Showing Microfilaria in peripheral blood (20 cmm)
B. Showing Microfilaria or disease
C. Showing Microfilaria and disease
D. All of these

127. "Filaria endemicity rate" is the percentage of persons:

A. Showing Mf in their blood
B. Mf in blood or disease manifestation or both
C. Mf and disease
D. None of these

128. The most sensitive method currently available for detecting low-density microfilaraemia is:

A. Thin
B. Thick film
C. Membrane filter concentration methods
D. Serological tests
E. Xenodiagnosis

129. Mf can be induced to appear in blood during daytime by giving Diethylcarbamazine (DEC) 100 mg orally.

A. True
B. False

130. The total dose of DEC for treating bancroftian filariasis is:

A. 36 mg/kg body wt
B. 72 mg/kg body wt
C. 100 mg/kg body wt
D. 6 mg/kg body weight per day orally for 12 days

131. In India, maximum prevalence of Brugia malayi filariasis is found in the state of:

A. Assam
B. A.P.
C. Tamil Nadu
D. Kerala
E. Karnataka

132. The genital lesions are common with the disease due to:

A. Loa-loa
B. Brugia malayi
C. W. bancrofti
D. B. timori

133. Brugia malayi has been restricted to certain parts of the country because of following facts:

A. Typical climate
B. Mosquitogenic conditions
C. Social customs
D. Occupational/economic reasons
E. All of the above

134. Filariasis does not assume epidemic proportion because of the following, *but* one:

A. Universal acceptability of medicated salt
B. There is no multiplication of parasites in insect vector
C. Infective Mf donot multiply in human host
D. Lifecycle of parasite is long
E. None of the above

135. DEC is still the only drug available for chemotherapeutic control of filariasis. It is given in the following ways:

A. Mass therapy
B. Selective treatment
C. DEC medicated salt
D. All of the above
E. Both A and B

136. Which is a semisynthetic macrolide antibiotic with a broad spectrum of activity against a variety of nematodes and ectoparasites?
A. Erythromycin
B. Ivermectin
C. Cilastin
D. Both A and C
E. All of the above

137. The flight range of culex quinquefasciatus is about:
A. 1 km
B. 2 km
C. 3 km
D. 4 km
E. 5 km

138. In India, the 1st commercially prepared DEC salt went on sale, at about twice the price of ordinary salt in which year?
A. 1991
B. 1992
C. 1993
D. 1994
E. 1998

139. The most effective method for vector control is:
A. Minor environmental measures
B. Antiadults measures
C. Antilarval measures with larvicides
D. Removal of Pistia plant

140. Following is useful in detecting low density microfilaraemia:
A. Immunofluoresenrt test
B. Xenodiagnosis
C. DEC provocation test
D. Membrane filter concentration method

141. The Village Health Guide is the key person who should be trained and involved in anti-filaria activities, with community support at the village level.
A. True
B. Partially true
C. False

142. Statement (S): The current approach against filariasis in India is to restrict the antilarval measures to urban areas. Reasons (R): Because it is operationally difficult and very costly to cover the vast rural areas of the country.

Select the correct response as per code given below:
A. Both (S) and (R) are true but are not related to each other
B. Both (S) and (R) are true and are related to each other
C. (S) true, (R) false
D. (R) true, (S) false
E. Both (S) and (R) are false

143. Which of the following statement is/are correct?
A. The vector mosquitoes of filariasis have become resistant to DDT, HCH, and dieldrin
B. The most effective preventive measures is avoidance of mosquito bites by using mosquito nets
C. Mosquito larvicidal oil is active against all pre-adult stages
D. All of these
E. Both A and B above

144. A combination of DEC and ivermectin as a single dose if given 2 years after treatment, reduces microfilaraemia by what percentage?
A. 25%
B. 60%
C. 95%
D. Almost 100%

145. In India, the incidence rate for malaria is highest in:
A. Arunachal Pradesh
B. Orissa
C. Mizoram
D. Rajasthan

146. "Rollback Malaria" initiative was launched by—WHO, UNICEF, UNDP and World Bank in 1998.
A. Partially true
B. True
C. False

147. The major malaria endemic areas in India includes all, *except:*
A. Andhra Pradesh
B. Gujarat
C. Bihar
D. Jharkhand

148. In India majority of P. falciparum cases are seen as:
A. Tribal malaria
B. Border malaria
C. Rural malaria
D. Urban malaria

149. The majority of mortality and DALY's lost due to malaria worldwide (2002) is seen in which region?
A. SEAR
B. Africa
C. East Mediterranean
D. Western Pacific

150. Predominant causative agent for malaria in SEAR is:
A. Plasmodium falciparum
B. P. malariae
C. P. ovale
D. P. vivax

151. Most of the countries of SEAR have experienced large outbreaks of the disease (Malaria) by:
A. 1995
B. 1997
C. 1999
D. 2001

152. Currently dengue fever/DHF endemic in:
A. Bangladesh and Myanmar
B. India, Maldives, Srilanka
C. Indonesia and Thailand
D. All of these

153. The case fatality rate for dengue in major endemic nations is:
A. 1%
B. 2%
C. 3.5%
D. 4.5%

154. Dengue/DHF is widely prevalent in India and how many serotypes of dengue has been found in India?
A. One
B. Two
C. Three
D. Four

155. Following Indian states are dengue/DHF prone as per 2003 data, *except:*
A. Bihar and Orissa
B. AP and Tamilnadu
C. Karnataka and Kerala
D. Delhi, Haryana and Punjab

156. In India human infection has been reported with dengue virus type:
A. Type 1 and 2
B. Type 1 and 3
C. Type 2 and 4
D. All 4 types

157. Which is not monitored in malaria surveillance now?
A. ABER
B. Infant parasite rate
C. Annual parasite incidence
D. Slide positivity rate

158. Rollback malaria programme is:
A. Encourage the development of mere effective and new antimalarial drugs and vaccines
B. Encourage the proper and expanded use of insecticide treated mosquito nets
C. Training of village health workers and mother on early and appropriate treatment of malaria
D. All of the above

159. The current global strategy for malaria control is called:

A. Modified plan of opeartion
B. Rollback malaria
C. Malaria control programme
D. Malaria eradication programme

160. For a person visiting chloroquine resistant malaria, endemic area the best prophylaxis is:

A. Chloroquine and daily proguanil
B. Chloroquine only
C. Sulfadoxine and pyrimethamine
D. All of the above

161. I.P. for filariasis is:

A. 18 to 24 months
B. 1 to 8 months
C. 8 to 16 months
D. > 24 months

4. ZOONOSES

1. Statement (S): Zoonoses and human health are matters of particular concern in India.
Reason (R): Because nearly 80% of India's population is rural and live in close contact with domestic animal, and often not far from wild ones.

A. Both (S) and (R) are true and are related to cause and effect
B. Both (S) and (R) are true but are unrelated to cause and effect
C. (S) is true, (R) is false
D. (R) is true, (S) is false
E. Both (S) and (R) are false

2. A infections maintained in both man and lower vertebrate animals threat may be transmitted in either direction is:

A. Anthropozoonoses
B. Amphixenoses
C. Zooanthroponses
D. All of the above

3. Recognised examples of direct zoonoses include the following:

A. Rabies
B. Brucellosis
C. Trichinosis
D. All of the above

4. The type of zoonoses that require more than one vertebrate host species but no invertebrate host, in order to complete the development cycle of the agent is called as:

A. Sapro-zoonoses
B. Metazoonoses
C. Cyclozoonoses
D. Direct zoonoses

5. Pentastomid infections is:

A. Cyclozoonosis
B. Metazoonoses
C. Sapro-zoonoses
D. Direct zoonoses

6. Infection transmitted biologically by invertebrate vectors includes all, *except:*

A. Arboviral infections
B. Taeniasis
C. Plague
D. Schistosomiasis

7. Rabies is caused by:

A. Lyssavirus type 1
B. Lyssavirus type 2
C. Lyssavirus type 3
D. Lyssavirus type 4

8. The only communicable disease of man that is always fatal includes:

A. Smallpox
B. Tetanus
C. Cholera
D. Rabies
E. All of the above

9. Which appears to be the most effective natural barrier to rabies?

A. Air
B. Water
C. UVR
D. Soil
E. SUN

10. Which place of Indian union is free of rabies?

A. Andaman and Nicobar Island
B. Bihar
C. Lakshadeep
D. Both A and C

11. "Canine rabies" accounts for what % of all human rabies cases?

A. 33%
B. 53%
C. 66%
D. 87%
E. 99%

12. Globally each year, ... people require post-exposure treatment for rabies.

A. 3 million
B. 7 million
C. 10 million
D. 15 million
E. 20 million

13. The India, how many people receive rabies post-exposure prophylaxis each year?

A. 1.2 million
B. 3 million
C. 6 million
D. 8 million
E. 10 million

14. The rabies virus freshly isolated from naturally occurring cases it is known as:

A. Street virus
B. Fixed virus
C. Both
D. Neither

15. Characteristic "Negri bodies" are usually not produced by:

A. Street virus
B. Fixed virus
C. Both of the above
D. Neither A nor B

16. Regarding "Fixed virus", all are true, *but* one:

A. Used to prepare antirabies vaccine
B. I.P. 4 to 6 days
C. Not multiplies in extra neural tissues
D. Negribodies are formed if injected intracerebrally in suitable animal

17. Recently, rabid bats have been found in following nations, *except:*

A. Holland
B. Germany
C. India
D. Denmark
E. None of the above

18. Recognised mode of transmission of rabies includes:

A. Animal bites
B. Licks
C. Aerosols
D. Person to person
E. All of these

19. The statement, "It is a rule that saliva of every rabid animal have rabies viruses" is.

A. Correct
B. Partially true
C. Incorrect

20. Following is/are not true about fixed rabies virus.

A. Poor invasiveness
B. Nagri bodies not produced
C. Definite fixed I.P.
D. No multiplication salivary glands
E. None of the above

21. Epidemiologically rabies does not exist as:

A. Avian

B. Bat
C. Wildlife
D. Urban
E. All of the above

22. The I.P. of rabies in man does not depend upon:
A. Site of bite
B. Shape of bite
C. Severity and species of biting animal
D. Protection by clothing and local treatment received
E. Time of bite with relation to bout of biting

23. Regarding pathogenesis of rabies, which is false?
A. Rabies virus replicates locally at the site of bite in a muscle or connective tissue cells
B. It spreads from the site of infection centripetally via the peripheral towards the CNS
C. Following infection of CNS the virus spreads centrifugally in peripheral nerves to many tissues including skeletal and myocardial muscles, adrenal glands and skin
D. The salivary glands invasion is crucial for the transmission of the virus to another animal to human
E. None of the above

24. The only prodromal symptom in rabies which is considered reasonably specific is:
A. Hydrophobia
B. Pain and tingling at the site of bite
C. Headache only
D. Fever, malaise only
E. Sore throat

25. The pathognomonic rabies in man is:
A. Aerophobia
B. Hydrophobia
C. Convulsions
D. Salivation
E. Irritability

26. In rabies patients neutralising antibodies are not usually detectable in serum or CSF before:
A. 3 days
B. 5 days
C. 8 days
D. 12 days
E. 20 days

27. To date, how many people are on record who have been stricken with rabies and have survived?
A. Only one
B. Three
C. Five
D. Seven
E. Twelve

28. Statement (S): Patients with rabies are potentially infectious.
Reason (R): Because the virus may be present in the saliva, vomits, tears, urine or other body fluids.

Select the true response as per following code given below:
A. Both (S) and (R) are true, and are related to cause and effect
B. Both (S) and (R) true, but are unrelated to cause and effect
C. (S) true, (R) false
D. (R) true, (S) false
E. Both are false

29. Which rabies vaccine in not available in India?
A. Nervous tissue vaccine
B. Duck embryo vaccine
C. Cell culture vaccine
D. Both A and C above
E. None of these

30. Which is false about suckling mouse brain vaccine?
A. The brains of suckling mice less than 9 days old are used
B. This vaccine is regarded as devoid of neuroparalytic effect

C. This vaccine is given in 10 daily doses, plus booster dose, 10 and 20 days after the end of the primary series
D. This vaccine is extensively used in China

31. "Semple vaccine" is prepared from the brains of:
A. Adult sheep
B. Suckling mouse
C. Duck embryo
D. Cell culture

32. Recognised advantages of cell culture vaccine include all, *except:*
A. More potent
B. Much safer than nervous tissue vaccine
C. Cheaper
D. Relatively fewer side effects
E. Immunization requires fewer injections of smaller volume

33. Regarding duck embryo vaccine, which is untrue?
A. It is free of allergic reactions
B. It is not available in India
C. It has developed to eliminate neuroparalytic factors
D. Persons known to be sensitive to egg protein should not be given vaccines of avian origin
E. DEV was used in U.S.A. and U.K. in the recent past

34. Not true about human diploid cell vaccine (HDCV) is:
A. It is generally safe and highly potent vaccine
B. It is prepared in human diploid fibroblast cells
C. It is now used in India for both pre and post exposure immunization
D. It is prepared from street virus

35. The 2nd generation tissue culture vaccine includes:
A. Foetal bovine kidney
B. Chick embryo fibroblasts
C. Dog kidney cells
D. Hamster kidney cells
E. All of the above

36. Non tumorigenic continuous cell lines vaccines is:
A. Hamster kidney cell
B. Vero cell
C. Chick embryo
D. Foetal bovine kidney

37. Treatment of fresh wounds caused by rabid dog involves the following measures, *but* one:
A. Povidone I_2
B. Washing the wound with soap and water
C. Chemical cautery
D. Thorough debridement
E. Local application of antirabies serum

38. All the following are regarded as class I wounds for rabies management, *save* for one:
A. Bite on calf
B. Lick on healthy skin
C. Scratches without oozing of blood
D. Use of unboiled milk of suspected animal

39. Bites on following sites are regarded as class III bites, *but* one:
A. Head
B. Toes
C. Face
D. Fingers
E. None of the above

40. Following is regarded as a class III bite:
A. Lacerated wounds on any part of body
B. Multiple wounds
C. Bites from wild animals
D. All of the above
E. Both B and C

41. Multiple wounds more than in number are classified under class III (severe risk):
A. Two
B. Three
C. Five

D. Seven
E. Eleven

42. If under class I treatment, rabies vaccine is given for 7 days, then it has to be given for how many days in class II or class III bites?
A. 7 days
B. 10 days
C. 14 days
D. 16 days

43. The only vaccine which is given after exposure to infection is:
A. Tetanus
B. Measles
C. Pertussis
D. Rabies
E. All of the above

44. The 1st successful human anti-rabies vaccination was performed by whom and when?
A. Louis Pasteur (1883)
B. Edward Jenner (1773)
C. Chapman (1860)
D. von Behring (1886)
E. von Pirquet (1902)

45. Recognised indications of anti-rabies treatment includes:
I. If animals show sign of rabies or dies within 10 days of observation
II. If the biting animal cannot be traced or identified
III. Unprovoked bites
IV. All bites by wild animals
V. Lab tests (Fluorescent test for rabies antibody or test for Negri bodies) are positive for rabies

Choose the true answer as per code given below:
A. I, III and IV
B. I, II, III, IV and V All
C. I, III and V
D. I, II, III and IV

46. "Semple vaccine" is given:
A. Anterior abdominal wall
B. Deep subcutaneously
C. Intradermally
D. Both A and B
E. Both A and C

47. Following anti-rabies immunization, serum antibodies appear after how many days of vaccination?
A. 3 days
B. 5 days
C. 7 days
D. 11 days
E. 15 days

48. Following anti-rabies vaccination, it takes how many days to achieve a maximum level of immunity?
A. 7 days
B. 14 days
C. 21 days
D. 30 days
E. None of the above

49. Number of booster doses of semple vaccine in class II bites is:
A. Nil
B. Only one
C. Two
D. Ten
E. Five

50. A 5-year-old child was bitten by a stray dog. The following is the appropriate management of this case:
A. Anti-rabies serum, suturing of wound, vaccine
B. Vaccine + leave wound open
C. Vaccine, leave wound open, TT, anti-rabies serum
D. Antirabies serum, suturing of wound, TT

51. In nervous tissue vaccine, neuroparalytic factors seen is myelin.
A. True
B. False

52. Allergic reaction of nerve tissue vaccine (semple) includes all, *except:*
A. Urticaria
B. Angioneurotic oedema
C. Anaphylactic reaction
D. Syncope
E. None

53. Neuroparalysis ensues almost always in 88% of cases within how many days of vaccination with anti-rabies vaccine?
A. 7 days
B. 10 days
C. 20 days
D. 30 days
E. 90 days

54. The case management of neuroparalysis following anti-rabies vaccination includes:
I. Strict bed rest
II. Administration of corticosteroids
III. Anti-neuritic vitamins
IV. Bladder and bowel and general care

Choose the true answer as per code given below:
A. I, II and III
B. I, II, III and IV All
C. I and IV
D. II and IV only
E. I, II and IV

55. It is true that all patients undergoing anti-rabic treatment should be advised as follows:
I. They should abstain from alcohol during and a month after completion of anti-rabic treatment since it may precipitate paralytic accidents or facilitate lighting up the infection
II. Undue physical and mental strain and late night should be avoided
III. Corticosteroids and other immuno-suppressive agents should not be used
IV. Rabies may develop following inade-quate immunization

Choose the true answer as per code given below:
A. I, II, III and IV All
B. I, II and III
C. I and IV
D. III and IV
E. I, III and IV

56. Following are recognised advantages of cell culture vaccine, *except:*
A. Six doses (0, 3, 7, 14, 30 and booster at day 90) are given
B. The 1 ml injection are given IM in the deltoid not in buttock
C. Its high cost only
D. Efficacy and safety

57. Recognised advantages of intradermal multi site vaccination includes all the following, *but* one:
A. Multisite intradermal vacccination has been used in India, Kenya and Thailand
B. It is also known as 2-2-21-1, regimen as per WHO recommendations
C. It consists of one dose (0.1 ml) of vaccine given at each of two sites on days 0, 3 and 7 and at one site on days 30 and 90
D. The multisite regimen lower the cost of vaccination by around 70% compared with the conventional IM schedules
E. None of the above

58. Post-exposure treatment of person who have been vaccinated previously against rabies includes:
A. If the patients antibody titre is unknown, or if the bite is severe, three 1 ml. IM doses of HDC vaccine are given on days 0, 3 and 7
B. If the titre is > 0.5 IU/ml and the bite is not severe, only 2 doses are needed on days 0 and 3
C. Both of the above
D. Neither

59. Topical application of anti-rabic serum where indicated is of use if given within:
A. 12 hours
B. 24 hours
C. 36 hours
D. 48 hours
E. 72 hours of bite

60. The I.P. of rabies in dogs, is:
A. 3 weeks
B. 6 weeks
C. 3 to 8 weeks
D. 3 to 6 weeks

61. The rabid dog after biting usually dies within:
A. 3 days
B. 7 days
C. 14 days
D. 3 to 10 days

62. Antemortem lab. examination for diagnosis of rabies can be done with:
A. Fluorescent antibody test
B. Corneal test
C. Biological test
D. Negri bodies inspection
E. All of the above

63. For class II bite by a rabid dog the dose of BPL vaccine for an adult for 10 days includes:
A. 3 ml
B. 5 ml
C. 7 ml
D. 10 ml
E. 12 ml

64. If a person is bitten by a rabid dog (known) the recommended action is:
A. Observe the dog for 10 days
B. No need to do anything
C. Kill the dog as humanly as possible at the earliest and send the brain to laboratory for examination
D. Hold the animal till it dies and then send the brain for lab examination

65. A person has been bitten by a confirmed rabid dog three weeks earlier. There were two scratches on flexor aspect of left forearm without drawing blood. The case will be treated as class:
A. I
B. II
C. III
D. None of these

66. Furious rabies or "mad dog syndrome" is characterized by the following, but one:
A. No change in behaviour
B. Running amuck
C. Change in voice
D. Paralytic stage
E. Excessive salivation

67. Which is predominantly paralytic?
A. Furious rabies
B. Mad dog syndrome
C. Dumb rabies
D. All of the above

68. Fluorescent antibody test is a highly reliable and the best single test currently available for the rapid diagnosis of rabies viral antigen in infected specimens within few hours.
A. True
B. Partially true
C. False

69. For immunization of dogs with BPL inactivated nervous tissue vaccine the dose is:
A. 3 ml followed by one injection after 6 months and every year thence
B. 5 ml followed by one injection after 6 months and every year thence
C. 5 ml every six months
D. 10 ml every 6 months

70. Most cost effective method for control of urban rabies includes:
A. Health education
B. Licensing of all domestic dogs
C. Immunization of all dogs
D. Killing of stray dogs

71. Following measures are essential to control rabies in urban areas, *save* for one:
A. Restraint of dogs in public places
B. Health education about rabies
C. Early diganosis and treatment
D. Quarantine for 6 months of imported dogs
E. Immediate destruction of dogs and cats bitten by rabid animals

72. Oral rabies vaccine is developed for immunizing:
A. Vampire bats
B. Man
C. Dogs
D. Foxes
E. All except 'B'

73. Regarding yellow fever, which is false?
A. Caused by arbovirus
B. Transmitted by culcine mosquitoes
C. In severe cases, the case fatality rate may reach 80%
D. In general death occurs between the 5th and 10th day of illness
E. Survivers exhibits no lasting immunity

74. The 1st epidemic of yellow fever was recorded in Kenya in the year:
A. 1991
B. 1992
C. 1993
D. 1994
E. 1995

75. Regarding yellow fever, all are true, *but* one:
A. The causative organism is flavivirus fibricus
B. In forest areas, the reservoir of infection is monkeys and mosquitoes
C. In urban areas, the reservoirs of infection is man and Aedes mosquitoes
D. A single attach of yellow fever does not provide lasting immunity
E. Blood of patient is infective during the 1st 3 to 4 days of illness

76. Under IHR, the I.P. of yellow fever is recognised as:
A. 1 day
B. 3 days
C. 6 days
D. 9 days
E. 12 days

77. Which of the following statement is/are true about yellow fever?
A. One attach of yellow fever provide life long immunity
B. Infants born to immune mother have antibodies upto 6 months of life
C. There are two cycles, the jungle (Sylvan) cycle and urban cycle
D. All of these
E. Both A and C above

78. Following 17D vaccination, against yellow fever, immunity begins on:
A. 1st day
B. 3rd day
C. 5th day
D. 2nd day
E. 7th day

79. For international travel, WHO recommends 17D vaccination after:
A. 5 years
B. 10 years
C. 15 years
D. 25 years
E. 30 years

80. Concerning yellow fever vaccination, which is false?
A. 17 D is a live attenuated vaccine prepared from a non-virulent strain (17D) which is grown in chick embryo and subsequently freeze-dried
B. Anaphylaxis occurring mainly in those allergic to eggs
C. The vaccine is given intramuscularly in a single dose of 0.5 ml irrespective of age
D. Cholera and yellow fever vaccine should not be given simultaneously

81. The most effective control strategy for urban yellow fever is:

A. Vaccination
B. Vector control
C. Surveillance
D. All of the above

82. Regarding Aedes aegypti index, which is false?

A. WHO uses this index
B. It is a house index
C. It is defined as "the percentage of houses and their premises, in a limited well defined area, showing actual breeding of Aedes aegypti larvae"
D. This index should not be > 1% in town and seaports in endemic areas to ensure freedom from the disease
E. None of the above

83. In India, the travellers visiting this country has to produce a certificate of yellow fever, vaccination, if no such document is available, the traveller is placed on quarantine for:

A. 3 days from the date of leaving an infected area
B. 6 days from the date of leaving an infected area
C. 10 days from the date of leaving an infected area
D. 16 days from the date of leaving an infected area

84. The validity of yellow fever vaccination certificate begins 10 days after the date of vaccination and extends upto:

A. 3 years
B. 5 years
C. 10 years
D. Life long

85. Following is the recognised yellow fever reference centres in India:

I. National Institute of Virology, Pune
II. Central Research Institute, Kasauli
III. Institute of Communicable Diseases, Kolkata
IV. AIIMS, New Delhi

Choose the correct answer as per following code given below:

A. I and II only
B. I, II and III only
C. I, II, III and IV All
D. I and IV
E. II and IV

86. The virus of yellow fever could get imported into India by following ways:

A. Through infected persons
B. Through infected mosquitoes
C. Both A and B
D. Neither A nor B

87. India is regarded as yellow fever "receptive" zone, owing to following reasons, *save* for one:

A. The vector is found in abundance (Aedes aegypti)
B. The virus is not found in India
C. The common monkey of India is susceptible to yellow fever
D. The climatic conditions are favourable in most parts of India for its transmission
E. The population of India is unvaccinated and susceptible to yellow fever

88. Following are recognised group 'B' arboviruses, *but* one:

A. Dengue
B. KFD
C. Chikungunya
D. West Nile
E. J. Encephalitis

89. Viruses responsible for hemorrhagic fevers in India 'include:

A. Dengue
B. Chikungunya
C. KFD
D. All of the above
E. Both A and C above

90. In 1951, the number of arboviruses known in India is:
A. Only one B. Two
C. Three D. Four
E. Seven

91. The following arboviruses has been known in India since 1951:
A. Dengue
B. Sandfly fever
C. Chikungunya
D. Both A and B
E. All of the above

92. Group 'A' arbovirus includes the following:
A. Sindbis
B. West Nile
C. Chikungunya
D. All of the above
E. Both A and C

93. Following clinical syndrome has been related to arboviral infections:
I. Febrile group
II. Hemorrhagic fever
III. Encephalitis
Select the most common group as per code given below:
A. I only
B. I and II
C. I and III
D. I, II and III All
E. II and III

94. Following viruses are known to cause febrile group of illnesses in India, *but* one:
A. Sindbis
B. KFD
C. Chikunguniya
D. Dengue

95. Viruses associated with hemorrhagic fever in India is:
A. Dengue
B. Chikunguniya
C. KFD
D. All of the above
E. Both A and B

96. Most frequently, Japanese Encephalitis involves:
A. Infants
B. Children < 5 years of age
C. Children < 15 years of age
D. Young adults
E. Elderly group

97. In India, the recognition of Japanese encephalitis (JE) was 1st made in 1955 in which state?
A. Assam
B. Bihar
C. Karnataka
D. Tamil Nadu

98. "Japanese Encephalitis" is not reported from which Indian states?
A. J and K
B. A.P.
C. Bihar
D. Goa
E. Pondicherry

99. Basic cycle of transmission of JE is:
A. Pig-human-pig
B. Pig-mosquito-pig
C. Man-mosquito-pig
D. Bird-mosquito-pig

100. Which of the following domestic animals may show C/M of JE infection?
A. Horses
B. Buffaloes
C. Cattle
D. Dogs and pigs
E. All of these

101. The most important vector for JE in South India is:
A. Culex vishnui
B. C. tritaeniorhynchus
C. C. gelidus
D. Anopheles paptasi
E. All of the above

102. The rice-fields are probably the most important breeding places for culex tritaeniorhynchus.
A. True
B. Partially true
C. False

103. The course of the disease (JE) in man may be divided into 3 stages. In which stage, high fever is usually seen?
A. Prodromal stage
B. Acute encephalitic stage
C. Late stage
D. Sequelae
E. All of these

104. After how many days of infected meal a female mosquito can transmit the virus to other hosts?
A. 6 days
B. 9 days
C. 9 to 12 days
D. 12 to 18 days

105. Most important animal host involved in transmission of JE is:
A. Monkey
B. Horses
C. Cattle
D. Dog
E. Pigs

106. In JE, the average period between the onset of illness and death is:
A. 9 days
B. 12 days
C. 15 days
D. 18 days
E. 28 days

107. Following is not acute encephalitis JE:
A. Arthritis
B. Nuchal rigidity
C. Focal neurological signs
D. Convulsions
E. Altered sensorium progressing to coma

108. In JE, the case fatality rate may reaches upto how much?
A. 20% B. 40%
C. 58% D. 75%
E. 80%

109. The major deterrent to JE eradication is:
A. Numerous animal hosts
B. The breeding places of vector
C. No effective vaccine
D. Large number of inapparent infections

110. Regarding vaccination against JE, following are true, *except* for:
A. A killed "mouse-brain" is available
B. For primary immunization 2 doses of 1ml each (0.5 for children less than 3 years old) should be given IM at an interval of 7 to 14 days
C. A booster injection of 1ml should be given before one year in order to provide full protection
D. Protective immunity develops in about a month's time after the second dose
E. Revaccination may be given after 3 years

111. KFD was 1st recognised in 1957 in which Indian states?
A. Karnataka
B. Kerala
C. Pondicherry
D. Tamil Nadu

112. Deaths of which animals are considered as heralders of this disease in endemic areas?
A. Pigs
B. Rats
C. Monkeys
D. Dogs
E. Sheep

113. A prolonged viraemia in man for about 10 days or more has not been seen in following arbovial infections:
A. West Nile encephalitis
B. JE

C. Chikungunya
D. KFD

114. The main reservoirs of KFD virus is:
A. Rats
B. Squirrels
C. Cat
D. Both B and C
E. Both A and B

115. The amplifying hosts for KFD virus is:
A. Monkeys
B. Rats
C. Cat
D. Dogs
E. Pigs

116. The vector for KFD includes:
A. Aedes mosquitoes
B. Haemophysalis
C. Culex
D. Xenopsylla

117. The transmission cycle in KFD involves:
A. Monkey and pigs
B. Pigs and cattle
C. Monkeys and ticks
D. Dog and ticks

118. The KFD is transmitted by the bite of infected:
A. Mouse
B. Mosquitoes
C. Soft ticks
D. Nymphal ticks

119. The I.P. of KFD is:
A. 3 days
B. 5 days
C. 5 to 15 days
D. 3 to 5 days
E. 3 to 8 days

120. Following C/F does not seen in KFD:
A. Fever, headache and severe myalgia
B. GIT disturbances
C. In severe case hemorrhages from nose, gums, stomach and intestine may ensue
D. Mild meningoencephalitis may occur
E. Diagnosis is established by doing TLC/ DLC and ESR

121. "Hot spot" in KFD control refers to areas where:
A. There is high endemicity of KFD
B. Monkey deaths are reported
C. KFD death in man are reported
D. All of the above

122. Following, but one, measures used for KFD control:
A. Vector control in forests
B. Immunization with KFD vaccine
C. Use of insect repellants
D. Health education
E. None of these

123. Chikungunia virus is transmitted by all, *but* one:
A. Anopheles
B. Mansonia
C. Culex
D. Aedes mosquitoes

124. Which is false about chikungunia fever?
A. A dengue like fever caused by group 'A' virus
B. It is manifested by high fever and severe articular pains in the limbs and spinal column
C. In India, the virus activity is still prevailing
D. The virus is 1st isolated from patients and mosquitoes during an epidemic in Tanzania in 1952-53
E. Chikungunia is a local word meaning "doubling up" owing to excruciating joint pains

125. "West Nile Fever" is not endemic in:
A. India
B. South America
C. Africa
D. Middle East
E. South West Asia

126. The sandfly fever virus was isolated in Aurangabad (Maharashtra) from febrile illness cases in 1967.
A. True
B. False

127. Brucellosis in humans is also known as the following, *except:*
A. Undulant fever
B. Oroya fever
C. Malta fever
D. Mediterranean fever

128. Not a feature of Brucella species is:
A. Gram negative rod
B. Non-motile
C. Sporing
D. Intracellular

129. The most virulent and invasive species of Brucellosis is:
A. Brucella abortus
B. B. canis
C. B. suis
D. B. militensis

130. The most common mode of transmission of Brucellosis is through:
A. Contact
B. Food-borne
C. Air-borne infection
D. All of the above

131. Majority of Brucellosis cases are reported from middle east nations.
A. True
B. Partially true
C. False

132. Brucella melitensis usually infects the following:
A. Sheep
B. Goat
C. Cattle
D. Dog
E. All of the above

133. Brucella suis chiefly infects:
A. Sheep
B. Goat
C. Pigs
D. Dog

134. In animals, Brucellosis may cause the following:
A. Abortion
B. Premature expulsion of foetus
C. Foetal death
D. All of these
E. Both A and B above

135. Regarding Brucellosis, all are true statements *save* for one:
A. Human brucellosis is predominantly disease of adult males
B. Immunity does not develop following infection
C. Main reservoirs of human infection includes cattle, sheep, goat, swine, buffaloes, horses and dogs
D. The infected animals excrete brucella in the urine, milk, placenta, uterine and vaginal discharges particularly during a birth or abortion
E. The animals may remain infected for life

136. Following condition favour the spread of Brucellosis:
A. Overcrowding of herds
B. High rainfall
C. Lack of exposure to sun-light
D. Unhygienic practices in milk and meat production
E. All of the above

137. In Brucellosis, the following joints are chiefly involved, *except:*
A. Phalangeal joints
B. Hip joint
C. Knee joint
D. Shoulder joint
E. Ankle joint

138. Recognised C/M of Brucellosis includes all, *but* one:
A. Swinging pyrexia (40 to 41°C), rigors, and sweating

B. Low back pain
C. Headache, insomnia
D. Small firm splenomegaly and hepatomegaly
E. Leukocytosis with relative lymphocytosis

139. Diagnosis of Brucellosis is established by isolation of organisms from:
A. Blood culture
B. Bone marrow
C. Exudate and biopsy
D. All of these
E. Both A and C above

140. The only satisfactory solution aimed at eradication of Brucellosis includes:
A. Killing of infected animals
B. Case finding
C. T/t of animals
D. Vaccination
E. All of these

141. In humans, the Brucellosis is:
A. Penicillin
B. Tetracycline
C. Cyclophosphamide
D. Ofloxacin

142. Vaccine of B. abortus strain 19 is commonly used for young animals:
A. True
B. Partially true
C. False

143. Skeletal Brucellosis is best treated with:
A. Tetracycline
B. Minocycline
C. Streptomycin
D. Doxicycline

144. Human live vaccine of B. abortus strain 19-BA is available.
A. True
B. Partially true
C. False

145. The national and international centre for Brucellosis is located at FAO/WHO Brucella Reference Centre, Indian Veterinary Research Institute at IZATNAGAR in:
A. Assam
B. Bihar
C. U.P.
D. M.P.
E. Rajasthan

146. The 1st recorded outbreak of plague in India occurred in the year 1031-32 AD.
A. True
B. False

147. Plague reached India from central Asia following invasion by:
A. Sultan Mohammad
B. Mohammad Tuglaq
C. Taimur Lung
D. All of these
E. Both A and C above

148. Plague epidemics was mentioned in following books:
A. Rigveda
B. Bhagwatpuran
C. Bible
D. All of the above
E. Both B and C

149. In India, plague has reappeared in 1994 after a silent period of:
A. 10 years
B. 20 years
C. 28 years
D. 38 years
E. 68 years

150. Justinian plague occur in the year .... claiming 100 million deaths.
A. 342
B. 542
C. 1346
D. 1984
E. 1930s

151. Plague reached its peak in India in which year?
A. 1325

B. 1403
C. 1896
D. 1907
E. 1940

152. U.P., which was one of the plague-active states in India, become free of plague in which year?
A. 1949
B. 1959
C. 1960
D. 1962
E. 1968

153. In 1994, in Beed (Maharashtra), the type of plague seen is:
A. Bubonic
B. Pneumonic
C. Septicemic
D. All of the above

154. In 1994, in Surat (Gujarat), the type of plague seen is:
A. Bubonic
B. Pneumonic
C. Septicemic
D. All of the above

155. The causative organism of plague is best demonstrated by:
A. Leishman stain
B. Levaditi stain
C. Wayson's stain
D. All of the above

156. The virulence of the plague bacilli is related to its ability to produce:
A. Exotoxin
B. Endotoxin
C. Fraction 1
D. All of the above
E. Both A and B above

157. In India, the main reservoir of plague is:
A. Rattus rattus
B. Rattus norvegicus
C. Tatera indica
D. All of the above

158. Recognised source of infection of plague is:
A. Infected rodents
B. Infected fleas
C. A case of pneumonic plague
D. All of these
E. Both A and C above

159. The most common and the most efficient vector of plague is the ratflea:
A. Xenopsylla cheopsis
B. X. brasiliensis
C. X. astia
D. Pulex irritans
E. All of these

160. Following is the efficient transmitter vector for plague:
A. Starved flea
B. Partially blocked flea
C. Blocked flea
D. All of the above

161. Should a plague outbreak occur, which index is regarded as indicative of potential explosiveness of the situation?
A. Total flea index
B. Burrow index
C. Cheopsis index
D. Specific percentage of fleas

162. Persons handling infected rats are exposed to the risk of pneumonic plague and this danger should be borne in mind:
A. True
B. Partially true
C. False

163. When a guinea pig a white mouse is inoculated with a suspected specimen of plague, the guinea pig will die in 7 days and the white mouse in:
A. 1 day
B. 2 days

C. 5 days
D. 7 days

164. Human plague is most frequently acquired from:
A. The bite of an infected flea
B. By droplets from pneumonic plague
C. By direct contact with tissues of infected animal
D. All of the above

165. In human the most common variety of plague is:
A. Septicemic plague
B. Bubonic
C. Pneumonic
D. All of the above

166. Plague bacilli can be demonstrated by staining with:
A. Giemsa's stain
B. Wayson's
C. Both of the above
D. None of the above

167. The I.P. of which type of plague is 2 to 7 days?
A. Bubonic
B. Septicemic
C. Pneumonic
D. Both A and B above
E. All of the above

168. The DOIC against plague is:
A. Tetracycline
B. Streptomycin
C. Sulphonamides
D. PG
E. Both A and B above

169. The I.P. of pneumonic plague is:
A. 1 day
B. 2 days
C. 1 to 3 days
D. 2 to 5 days
E. 2 to 7 days

170. The incidence of pneumonic plague is usually below:
A. 1% B. 1.9%
C. 2.1% D. 3.3%
E. 4.4%

171. Unless promptly treated, pneumonic plague have a mortality of:
A. 50% B. 75%
C. 80% D. 90%
E. 100%

172. Within 48 hours of application of insecticides, the flea index should drop down to zero.
A. True
B. Partially true
C. False

173. Regarding plague vaccine/vaccination:
I. Haffkine (1897) developed a killed plague vaccine while working in India and inoculated himself with this experimental vaccine
II. The currently used vaccine is that of Haffkine, modified by sokhey
III. It is a formalin killed vaccine containing 2000 million killed organisms per ml
IV. The vaccine is given subcutaneously in two doses of 0.5 and 1.0 ml at an interval of 7 to 14 days
V. Immunity starts 5 to 7 days after inoculation, and lasts for about 6 months

Select the true answer as per code given below:
A. I, II and III
B. I, II, III, IV and V All
C. I, III and IV
D. II, III and V
E. I, II, III and IV

174. The DOIC for chemoprophylaxis against plague is:
A. Streptomycin
B. PG
C. Tetracycline
D. Sulfonamides

175. Medical practitioner should keep plague in mind in D/d of any cases of fever with lymphadenopathy, or when multiple cases of pneumonia ensues.
A. True
B. Partially true
C. False

176. The most common C/M of salmonella infection is:
A. Paratyphoid fever
B. Gastroenteritis
C. Typhoid fever
D. Septicemia with focal lesions

177. Following salmonella species predominantly affects man, *but* one:
A. S. typhi
B. S. paratyphi 'A'
C. S. paratyphi 'B'
D. S. paratyphi 'C'

178. Salmonella is sensitive to heat and will not survive temperature above 70°C.
A. True
B. Partially true
C. False

179. Salmonella have been isolated from following foods:
A. Chocolate
B. Biscuits
C. Coconut
D. Species
E. All of the above

180. Which salmonella species is responsible for upto 50% or more of all human salmonella infections all over the world?
A. S. typhi
B. S. typhimurium
C. S. paratyphi A and C
D. All of the above

181. "BEEF" is the main source of salmonella infection in:
A. UK
B. Brazil
C. Canada
D. USA

182. Regarding salmonellosis, which is correct?
A. The main reservoir of salmonella is GIT of man and animals
B. Foods of animal origin like meat, poultry and egg products are considered to be the primary sources of salmonellosis
C. Carriers occur among both man and animals
D. Salmonella can survive in soil for months
E. All of these

183. In which of the following rickettsial disease insect vector is not seen?
A. RMSF
B. Q fever
C. Epidemic typhus
D. Endemic typhus

184. Mammalian reservoir for Trench fever is:
A. Humans
B. Cattle
C. Sheep
D. Goats
E. All of the above

185. Rickettsia tsutsugamushi causes what?
A. Trench fever
B. Q. fever
C. Scrub typhus
D. RMSF

186. Insect vector for RMSF is:
A. Louse
B. Flea
C. Mite
D. Tick
E. Nil

187. With Giemsa's stain, rickettsia are seen as:
A. Yellow
B. Blue
C. Crimson
D. Velvety
E. Green

188. Which antibiotic enhance the rickettsial growth?
A. Tetracycline
B. PG
C. Cephalosporin
D. Doxicycline
E. Sulfonamides

189. No skin lesion is observed in following rickettsial infection:
A. Q. fever
B. Scrub typhus
C. Murine typhus
D. Indian tick typhus

190. The DOIC for all rickettsial infection is:
A. PG
B. Tetracycline
C. Cotrimoxazole
D. Streptomycin

191. The most widespread of all rickettsial disease affecting man is:
A. Q. fever
B. RMSF
C. Scrub typhus
D. Epidemic typhus

192. Regarding scrub typhus which is false?
A. It resembles RMSF clinically
B. A macular rash appears around 8th day of illness
C. Generalised lymphadenopathy and lymphocytosis are common
D. One typical feature is the punched out under covered with a blackened scale which indicates the location of the mite bite
E. The fever falls by lysis in the 3rd weeks in untreated cases

193. The Weil Felix reaction is strongly positive with the proteins strain OXK in which rickettsial infection?
A. Murine typhus
B. Scrub typhus
C. Q. fever
D. All of the above

194. Which is not true regarding murine (endemic) typhus?
A. It is caused by R. typhi
B. Rats are the reservoir of infection
C. The flea can transmit the rickettsiae transovarially
D. The Weil-Felix reaction with proteins OX-13 becomes positive in 2nd week

195. Following, *but* one, are true about India tick typhus:
A. The causative agent is R. conorii
B. The tick is the reservoir of infection
C. Man is only an accidental host and get infection by bite of mite
D. A maculopapular rash appears on 3rd day
E. The clinical syndrome may be confused with atypical measles

196. All are true about Q fever, *save* for one:
A. It is a highly infectious zoonosis having worldwide distribution
B. It is seen in population of Haryana, Punjab, Delhi, Rajasthan
C. The causative agent is coxiella burnetti
D. The I.P. is 2 to 5 days
E. The infection can cause endocarditis + Pneumonia + hepatitis

197. No cases of epidemic typhus have been reported from South-East Asia since 1978.
A. True
B. False

198. "Brill-Zinsser disease" is associated with which rickettsial infection?
A. Endemic typhus
B. Q. fever
C. Trench fever
D. RMSF
E. Epidemic typhus

199. Regarding Rickettsial pox, all are true, *but* one:
A. Man gets the infection through the bite of ticks found on Mus. musculus
B. Transovarial transmission occurs in the mite

C. The mouse acts as true reservoir as well as vector
D. It may be confused with atypical case of chickenpox (varicella)

200. Statement (S): T. saginata and T. solium is classified as cyclozoonoses.
Reason (R): Because they require more than one vertebrate host species to complete their developmental cycles.
A. Both (S) and (R) are true but are not related to each other
B. Both (S) and (R) are true and are related to each other
C. (S) true, (R) false
D. (R) true, (S) false
E. Both are false

201. Low endemic areas for T. saginata includes all *except*:
A. Australia
B. USA
C. Canada
D. USSR

202. "Neurocysticercosis" may produce following C/M, *but* one:
A. Epilepsy
B. Intracranial hypertensive syndromes
C. Hydrocephalus
D. Psychiatric disease or death
E. None of the above

203. Drugs used against Taeniasis includes:
A. Mepacrin
B. Praziquantal
C. Niclosamide
D. All of the above
E. Both B and C above

204. In India, highest prevalence of hydatid disease is reported from:
A. Andhra Pradesh
B. Bihar
C. Tamil Nadu
D. Both A and C above

205. "Polycystic hydatidosis" is caused by:
A. E. granulosus
B. E. vogeli
C. E. oligarthus
D. E. multilocularis

206. "Unilocular" type of echinococcosis is caused by:
A. E. granulosus
B. E. multilocularis
C. E. oligarthus
D. E. vogeli

207. The definitive host for echinococcosis is:
A. Man
B. Sheep
C. Dog
D. All of the above
E. Both A and B above

208. More than 70% of hydatid cysts is located in the:)
A. Lungs
B. Liver
C. Brain
D. Peritoneum
E. Long bones

209. Casoni's test is used to diagnose:
A. Hydatid cysts
B. Taeniasis
C. Leishmaniasis
D. All of the above

210. The most sensitive and specific tests against hydatid cysts is:)
A. X-ray
B. Ultrasound
C. CAT scan
D. Indirect immuonofluorescent test

211. The most promising drugs against hydatidosis is:
A. Niclosamide
B. Praziquantel
C. Mebendazole
D. All of the above

212. Leishmaniasis is transmitted to man by the bite of female sandfly.
A. True

B. Partially true
C. False

213. Nine out of 10 cases of visceral leishmaniasis occur in:
A. Bangladesh
B. Brazil
C. India
D. Sudan
E. All of the above

214. Currently leishmaniasis is endemic in 88 nations.
A. True
B. False

215. In India, the peak age for Kala-azar is:
A. < 1 years
B. 5 years
C. 5 to 9 years
D. < 15 years

216. Currently kala-azar is endemic in .... districts of Bihar, ... districts of West Bengal and .... districts of U.P.
A. 20, 5, 1
B. 33, 10, 2
C. 10, 8, 1
D. 15, 9, 1

217. "Kala-azar" is caused by:
A. Leishmania donovani
B. L. brasiliensis
C. L. tropica
D. All of the above

218. "Oriental sore" is caused by:
A. L. donovani
B. L. brasiliensis
C. L. tropica
D. All of the above

219. Cutaneous leishmaniasis is transmitted by:
A. P. argentipes
B. P. papatasi
C. P. sergenti
D. Both B and C
E. All of the above

220. Mode of transmission of kala-azar is:
A. Person to person by the bite of the female phlebotmine sandfly
B. By contamination of bite wound
C. Blood transfusion
D. By contact when the insect is crushed during the act of feeding
E. All of the above

221. The classical C/F of kala-azar includes all the following, *save* for one:
A. Fever
B. Splenohepatomegaly
C. Lymphadenopathy
D. Anaemia
E. Weight loss

222. PKDL is common in which country?
A. India
B. Britain
C. Canada
D. Denmark
E. Ethiopia

223. "Leishmanin" is a preparation of 10 per ml washed .... of leishmania suspended in 0.5% phenol saline or merthiolate.
A. Amastigotes
B. Promastigotes
C. Both of the above
D. Neither A nor B above

224. Leishmanin (Montenegro) test is usually positive 4 to 6 weeks after onset in cases of CL and MCL.
A. True
B. Partially true
C. False

225. Leishmanin test is usually negative in the active phase of kala-azar and becomes positive in 75% patients within one year of recovery.
A. Partially true
B. True
C. False

226. Which test is used for diagnosis as well as for epidemiological field surveys of kala-azar?
A. Aldelyde test
B. IFAT
C. ELISA
D. All of the above

227. "L-D bodies" are the .... of Leishmania Donovani.
A. Amastigote form
B. Promastigote form
C. Sandfly
D. All of these
E. Both A and B above

228. The best specimen for demonstrating LD bodies is:
A. Bone marrow
B. Spleen
C. Lymph nodes
D. Skin

229. Aldehyde test reverts back to negative .... after cure.
A. 3 months
B. 4 months
C. 6 months
D. 9 months
E. 1 year

230. Following hematological findings are seen in kala-azar, *except*:
A. Progressive leucopenia
B. Anaemia
C. Reversed A-G ratio
D. Greatly increased IgM
E. Raised ESR

231. Usual time for symptoms to appear in Rabid animal is:
A. 2 days B. 7 days
C. 10 days D. 30 days

232. The breeding ground for the vectors of Japanese B virus is:
A. Paddy field
B. Mixed garbage
C. Cooler water
D. Stale food

233. KFD is transmitted by:
A. Aedes
B. Haemaphysalis spinigera
C. Culex vishnui
D. Anopheles

234. Which is true regarding leprosy is India?
A. Estimated 10 million cases
B. Eradicated in Orissa
C. Vaccine developed in Bihar
D. MDT—99% coverage

5. SURFACE INFECTIONS

1. Regarding TRACHOMA:
I. A chronic infection of conjunctiva
II. An acute infection of cornea
III. A chronic infection of cornea
IV. Caused by chlamydia trachomatis
Select the true answer as per following code given below:
A. , III and IV
B. II and III only
C. I and IV
D. III and IV
E. I, II, III and IV All

2. The blinding lesions of trachoma includes:
A. Entropion
B. Trichiasis
C. Corneal ulcer
D. All of the above
E. Both A and C above

3. The criteria for diagnosing trachoma includes all, *except* for one:
A. Follicles on the upper tarsal conjunctiva
B. Madarosis

C. Typical conjunctival scarring (trichiasis, entropion)
D. Vascular pannus, most marked at the superior limbus

4. **Trachoma is estimated to be responsible for .... of visual impairment and blindness in India.**
A. 0.2%
B. 1%
C. 2%
D. 3.5%
E. 5.0%

5. **The classical endemic trachoma of developing countries is caused by chlamydia trachmatis of following immune types, *but* one:**
A. Type A
B. Type B
C. Type C
D. Type D

6. **In India, trachoma cases are estimated to be about:**
A. 20 million
B. 50 million
C. 75 million
D. 100 million
E. 120 million

7. **Most dangerous lesion of conjunctiva is caused by which organisms?**
A. Morax-axenfeld diplobacillus
B. Koch-weeks bacillus
C. Gonococcus
D. Chlamydia trachomatis
E. Any of these

8. **The I.P. of trachoma is:**
A. 1 to 3 days
B. 2 to 5 days
C. 5 to 12 days
D. 7 to 14 days
E. 9 to 27 days

9. **Highest prevalence of trachoma in childhood is observed in two to five years age group, which cannot be attributed to:**
A. Low immunity levels
B. Poor health consciousness of children of guardians
C. Closer contact with infected family members
D. Use of "Kajal or surama"
E. Predisposing factors operate more in them

10. **In under 10 years population the mass or blanket treatment for trachoma is advocated if the percentage of prevalence of moderate/severe trachoma is more than how much?**
A. 1 %
B. 2%
C. 3%
D. 4%
E. 5%

11. **The choice of antibiotic for local treatment of trachoma is:**
A. Penicillin
B. Tetracycline
C. Gentamicin
D. Erythromycin

12. **Tetracycline is the antibiotic of choice in trachoma, which is used as?**
A. 1% topically as ointment
B. 250 mg orally 10 days
C. 500 mg BD IM deep
D. 5% topically as ointment
E. 250 mg tds IM/IV for 7 days

13. **The trachoma control pogramme was launched in India in which year?**
A. 1960
B. 1961
C. 1963
D. 1973
E. 1977

14. **The HFA by 2000 AD has set a target of reducing the prevalence of blindness to ....:**
A. 0.1%
B. 1%
C. 0.2%

D. 0.3%
E. 0.5%

15. **In which communicable disease, even with treatment, the case fatality rate can be as high as 80 to 90%?**
A. Rabies
B. Tetanus
C. Cholera
D. Dengue
E. All of these

16. **Regarding tetanus, which is true?**
A. Lock-jaw
B. Risus sardonicus
C. Opisthotonus
D. Soil and dustborne disease
E. All of these

17. **The World Health Assembly resolved to eliminate neonatal tetanus by:**
A. 1992
B. 1993
C. 1994
D. 1995
E. 2000 AD

18. **Which disease is second only to measles among the six target diseases of the expanded programme of Immunization (EPI)?**
A. Tetanus
B. Pertussis
C. T.B.
D. Diphtheria
E. Poliomyelitis

19. **More than 50% of the total annual cases of neonatal tetanus occur in the month of:**
A. January, February, March
B. July, August, September
C. April, May, June
D. October, November, December

20. **Regarding tetanus, all are true statement, *save* for one:**
A. Clostridium tetani is a gram + ve, anaerobic, spore-bearing organisms having terminal spore giving it a drum-stick appearance
B. They germinate 'under aerobic condition and form a potent exotoxin
C. The natural habitat of organism is soil and dust
D. Agricultural workers are at special risk to tetanus

21. **Tetanus spores are highly resistant to following injurious agent, *save* for one:**
A. Boiling
B. Autoclaving for 15 mts at 120°C
C. Phenol/cresol only
D. Steam under pressure at 120°C for 20 mts or by gamma irradiation

22. **The tetanus bacilli are found in intestine of following:**
A. Horses
B. Goats and sheep
C. Cattle
D. Man
E. All of these

23. **Regarding TETANOSPASMIN, which is false?**
A. It is an insoluble toxin
B. Its toxicity is superseded by botulinum toxin
C. The lethal dose for a 70 kg man is about 0.1 mg
D. It is a soluble exotoxin
E. None of these

24. **The period of communicability in tetanus is:**
A. One week from 1st symptom
B. 10 days from 1st symptom
C. Upto one month after clinical attack
D. None of these

25. **The exotoxin of clostridium tetani does not act on:**
A. The motor end plates in skeletal system
B. The spinal cord
C. Muscles
D. Brain
E. The sympathetic system

26. In which of the following communicable disease herd immunity does not protect the individual?
A. Tetanus
B. Polio
C. Measles
D. Both B and C above
E. All of the above

27. The incidence of tetanus is much lower in urban than rural areas because:
I. Of close association with animals
II. More people live in rural areas
III. The main occupation is agriculture
IV. The health facilities are concentrated in urban area

Select the true answer as per code given below:
A. I and II
B. I and III
C. I, II and III
D. I, II, III and IV All

28. The I.P. for tetanus is:
A. 1 to 5 days
B. 2 to 6 days
C. 6 to 10 days
D. 11 to 18 days
E. 15 to 30 days

29. Infection is acquired by contamination of wounds with:
A. Tetanus bacilli
B. Tetanus spores
C. Both of the above
D. Neither A nor B above

30. Under the following conditions of transmission/exposure tetanus will not occur:
A. Contamination of wound
B. Contamination of infected eye
C. Ingestion of organism
D. All of the above
E. Both A and B above

31. A major and important cause of tetanus is:
A. Idiopathic
B. Puerperal
C. Tetanus neonatorum
D. Traumatic
E. Otogenic

32. Which is false regarding tetanus?
A. Tetanus follows abortion more frequently than a normal labour
B. Otogenic tetanus is basically a pediatric problem
C. A post abortal uterus is a favourable site for the germination of tetanus spores
D. All of these
E. None of these

33. Neonatal tetanus usually manifest about the:
A. Birth
B. 3rd day
C. 5th day
D. 7th day
E. 10th day

34. In which state in India, tetanus is called as "8th day disease"?
A. Assam
B. Bihar
C. Punjab
D. Delhi
E. Tamil Nadu

35. As per standard recommendations for tetanus nothing more than surgical toilet is required for wounds if:
A. Has had complete course of toxoid and booster in the past five years
B. A person has had complete course of toxoid and booster more than 10 years ago
C. Has had complete course of toxoid and booster 5 to 10 years ago
D. All of the above
E. Both B and C above

36. In all treatment of a case of tetanus bacilli vegetative form:
A. Tetanus spores
B. Tetanus bacilli vegetative form

C. Organisms causing secondary infection
D. All of the above
E. Both A and C above

37. A patient with lacerated wound after road traffic accident if reaches the hospital within .... hours, then he can be put on chemoprophylaxis for tetanus with penicillin.
A. Six hours
B. Twelve hours
C. 12 to 18 hours
D. 6 to 24 hours

38. The immunization of expectant mothers with tetanus toxoid should be so timed that the second dose is given one month after the 1st dose or should falls .... before expected date of delivery.
A. 7 days
B. 14 days
C. 21 days
D. 28 days

39. A protective level of antitoxin against tetanus is about:
A. 0.001 units/ml throughout life
B. 0.01 IU/ml serum throughout life
C. 0.1 ml/IU serum throughout life
D. None of these

40. Infants born to unimmunized mother should receive within 6 hours of birth .... of tetanus antitoxin for prevention of neonatal tetanus.
A. 250 IU
B. 350 IU
C. 500 IU
D. 750 IU
E. 1000 IU

41. Leprosy or Hansen's disease is clinically characterized by the following, *except*:
A. Hypopigmented patches
B. Partial or total loss of cutaneous sensation in the affected areas
C. Presence of thickened nerves
D. Presence of AFB in the skin or nasal smears
E. None of these

42. In leprosy, the earliest sensation to be affected is:
A. Fine touch
B. Temperature
C. Crude touch
D. Pressure
E. All of the above

43. Probably the oldest disease known to mankind is:
A. Tetanus
B. Leprosy
C. Cholera
D. Rabies
E. Trachoma

44. The word LEPER comes from a Greek word meaning:
A. Red
B. Brown
C. Scaly
D. Handicapped
E. White patches

45. Hansen of Norway discovered Mycobacterium leprae in which year?
A. 1887
B. 1876
C. 1889
D. 1873
E. 1943

46. The National Leprosy Control Programme was launched by Government of India in:
A. 1943
B. 1955
C. 1961
D. 1971
E. 1977

47. Uptill now following animal models are used for leprosy research, *except*:
A. American ant eaters (armadillos)

B. Footpads of mice
C. Nude mice
D. Guinea pigs
E. None of these

48. With the goal of arresting the leprosy by 2000 AD, the NLCP in India was redesignated as National Leprosy Eradication Programme in:
A. 1970
B. 1977
C. 1983
D. 1985
E. 1990

49. The estimates for 1996 indicates that there are about 1.3 million cases of leprosy in the world.
A. True
B. Partially true
C. False

50. India account for about .... of the leprosy cases in the world and has by far the greatest number of registered cases among individual nations.
A. 20.3%
B. 33.3%
C. 43.2%
D. 50.2%
E. 70.8%

51. In India, the state having least prevalence of leprosy is:
A. Punjab
B. Bihar
C. Haryana
D. J and K
E. M.P.

52. Maximum prevalence of leprosy in India reported from which states/UT?
A. Nagaland
B. Bihar
C. Tamil Nadu
D. Daman and Diu
E. Pondicherry

53. Currently large quantities of Myco. leprae are being produced by multiplication in the:
A. 9-branded armadillo
B. Nude mouse
C. Both of the above
D. None of the above

54. Natural infection with M. leprae are present in the following:
A. Armadillos
B. Mangabey monkeys
C. Chimpanzees
D. All of the above

55. Male preponderance of leprosy is observed in the following age group:
A. Under five
B. Reproductive age groups
C. Adults
D. Under fifteen

56. Concerning leprosy, all statements are true, *but* one:
A. Leprosy is a highly infectious disease but of low pathogenicity
B. The bacteriological load is highest in TT cases
C. M. leprae can remain viable in dried nasal secretions for atleast 9 days and in moist soil at room temperature for 46 days
D. The nose is the major portal of exit
E. M. leprae characteristically occur as globi and have an affinity for schwann cells and cells of RE system

57. In leprosy, a high prevalence of infection among children means that the disease is:
A. Active
B. Spreading
C. Dormant
D. Both A and B above
E. All of the above

58. In India, the youngest case of leprosy seen is of 2½ months old infant in:
A. North eastern state

B. South India
C. South eastern region
D. Western India
E. Central India

59. Regarding immunity leprosy, which is false?

A. CMI is responsible for resistance to infection with M. leprae
B. There is complete breakdown of CMI in LL
C. In LL cases lepromin test is strongly positive
D. Antibodies are more pronounced at the lepromatous end (IgG and IgM)
E. The anergy of LL is due to suppression of T-cell production of IL-2

60. Leprosy can be transmitted by:

A. Droplet
B. Breast milk
C. Contact
D. Insect vectors/Tattooing
E. All of the above

61. On the basis of immunity, which classification of leprosy has been devised?

A. Ridley-Jopling
B. Indian
C. Madrid
D. All of the above

62. Which classification system is most widely used in field leprosy programmes?

A. Indian
B. Madrid
C. Ridley-Jopling
D. Both A and B
E. All of the above

63. The "pure neuritic form" of leprosy has got place in which classification?

A. Ridley-Jopling
B. Indian
C. Madrid
D. All of the above
E. Both A and C

64. Following lesions in leprosy is bacteriologically negative, *but* one:

A. Pure neuritic type
B. TT type
C. Borderline type
D. Indeterminate

65. The term paucibacillary leprosy includes the following, *but* one:

A. Smear negative intermediate
B. BT
C. Pure neuritic
D. BL
E. TT

66. In leprosy, the signs of activity includes all, *but* one:

A. Thick tender nerve
B. Increase/decrease in number and size of patches
C. Bacterilogically positive patch/patches
D. Anesthetic patch
E. Oozing ulcer

67. In leprosy the disease is said to be inactive if a lepromatous case remains inactive for:

A. 6 months
B. 12 months
C. 24 months
D. 60 months

68. In leprosy the disease is said to be arrested in LL/BL cases if the case remains inactive for:

A. One year
B. Two years
C. Three years
D. Four years
E. Five years

69. In leprosy the disease is said to be inactive if the tuberculoid case remains inactive for:

A. 6 months
B. 9 months
C. 12 months
D. 18 months
E. 24 months

70. In leprosy the disease is said to be arrested if the TT case remains inactive for:
A. 42 months
B. 12 months
C. 24 months
D. 36 months
E. 60 months

71. Following is an important clinical sign of a static leprosy patch:
A. Loss of hair
B. Loss of toes
C. Wrinkling on the patch
D. All of the above

72. Lewis triple response consists of wheal, erythema and flare. In histamine test for leprosy, which of the following triple response is lost?
A. Wheal
B. Flare
C. Redness
D. All of the above
E. Both A and C above

73. Longest I.P. among the following, is of:
A. Leprosy
B. Malaria
C. Filaria
D. Hepatitis 'B'
E. All of the above

74. Of the following types of leprosy, which is the most severe?
A. TT
B. BL
C. BT
D. LL only

75. The most common mode of transmission of leprosy is:
A. Skin contact
B. Droplet
C. Vectors
D. Fomites
E. All of the above

76. Most sensitive index of transmission of leprosy is:
A. Incidence
B. Prevalence
C. Detection rate
D. Disability rate

77. Following are associated with social stigma, *except*:
A. Addiction
B. Leprosy
C. Hepatitis
D. Syphilis

78. True about tuberculoid leprosy is:
A. Spreads by air
B. Tuberculin positive
C. Symmetrical neuropathy
D. Diagnosed by skin biopsy
E. All of these

79. WHO recommends the following drugs in the treatment of multibacillary leprosy, *save* for one:
A. Ethionamide
B. Rifampicin
C. Clofazimine
D. Dapsone

80. Lepromine test is done to diagnose:
A. Local antibodies
B. Prognosis of disease
C. CMI
D. Diagnosis of disease
E. All of the above

81. The mean I.P. of leprosy is calculated from:
A. Harmonic means
B. Median
C. Mode
D. Geometric mean

82. Nerve biopsy is indicated in:
A. TT without skin lesion
B. Indeterminate type
C. LL only
D. TT with skin lesion
E. All of these

83. "Lepromin test" in indeterminate leprosy is:
A. Positive
B. Negative
C. Doubtful
D. None of these

84. Best diagnostic method for leprosy is:
A. Mitsuda reaction
B. Skinsmear
C. Culture
D. Droplet smear

85. Skin smear is negative in:
A. LL
B. BL
C. Neuritic type
D. Both A and B above

86. In the following test, negative result means antibody present:
A. Lepromin
B. Schick
C. Frei
D. Tuberculin
E. All of the above

87. To determine whether leprosy is still active:
A. Lepromin test
B. Presence of anesthetic patch
C. Culture of bacilli
D. Response to drugs

88. Bacteriological examination of Myco. leprae is essential for:
A. Monitoring the benefit of treatment
B. Identifying cases and carriers both
C. Classifying the disease
D. All of these

89. Following is true regarding bacterial index, *save* for one:
A. In paucibacillary cases the B_1 is less than 2 while in multibacillary more than 2
B. A minimum of seven sites should be examined
C. Negative means no bacilli found in 100 fields
D. It should be done at regular intervals
E. None of these

90. Mouse foot pad technique has been successfully used for:
A. Detecting drug resistance
B. Evaluating the potency of anti-leprosy drugs
C. Detecting the viability of the bacilli during treatment
D. All of the above

91. Mouse foot pad inoculation is 10 times more sensitive at detecting Myco. leprae than are slit-skin smears.
A. True
B. False

92. NOT true about lepromin test is:
A. 1st reported by K. Mitsuda (Japanese) in 1916
B. In fact a mini dose vaccine
C. Measures pre-existing CMI
D. Strongly positive in LL cases

93. "Lepromin-H" is found in:
A. Mitsuda lepromin
B. Dharmendra lepromin
C. Both of the above
D. None of the above

94. Dharmendra's antigen of leprosy is:
A. Integral
B. Bacillary
C. Defatted
D. All of the above
E. Both B and C above

95. Early lepromin positivity is a reaction of the following size or more in .... read after 48 hours.
A. 5 mm
B. 10 mm
C. 15 mm
D. 20 mm
E. 30 mm

96. Late lepromin positivity is a reaction of the following size or more of nodule in .... read in 21st day.

A. 5 mm
B. 7 mm
C. 10 mm
D. 12 mm
E. 15 mm

97. The dividing number of bateriological index between paucibacillary and multibacillary leprosy is:

A. 1
B. 2
C. 3
D. 4
E. 5

98. The degree of lepromin positivity and infectiousness of a leprosy case is:

A. Partially related
B. Directly proportional to each other
C. Inversely proportional to each other
D. Not related to each other

99. Consider the following statement:

I. The early lepromin reaction is also called as Fernandez reaction
II. The Dharmendra antigen is more potent in inducing early reaction
III. The late reaction is the classical Mitsuda reaction
IV. In case of Dharmendra antigen, the late reaction, is smaller
V. Lepromin 'A' the specific soluble antigen produces only early reaction

Choose the correct answer as per code given below:

A. I, II and III
B. I, II, III and IV
C. I, II, III, IV and V All
D. I, III and V

100. BCG vaccination is capable of converting the lepra reaction from negative to positive in a large proportion of individuals.

A. True
B. False

101. Which is not true regarding lepromin test?

A. The test has been generally accepted as a useful tool in evaluating the immune status of leprosy patients
B. It is a diagnostic test
C. The test is also of great value in estimating the prognosis in cases of leprosy of all types
D. This test is now being increasingly used in epidemiological studies combined with serological test (FLA-ABS)

102. Which of the following serological tests is widely used for identification of subclinical infection?

A. FLA-ABS
B. Monoclonal antibodies
C. SACT
D. ELISA

103. Which of the following serological tests of leprosy is based on a phenolic glycolipid (PGL) antigen?

A. FLA-ABS
B. Monoclonal antibodies
C. SACT
D. ELISA

104. The three main goals of leprosy control includes all, *but* one:

A. To interrupt transmission of infection
B. To reduce disease incidence
C. To treat patients in order to achieve their cure and if possible complete rehabilitation
D. To prevent the development of associated deformities
E. None of these

105. The best method of case detection when the prevalence of leprosy in a community is less than 1 per 1000 is:

A. Contact survey
B. Mass survey
C. Group survey
D. All of the above

106. Regarding mass surveys for leprosy, all are true, *save* for one:
A. Hyperendemic area areas where prevalence of leprosy is about 10 or more per 1000 population
B. A coverage of not less than 95% of the population should be obtained
C. Mass survey involves only leprosy case other diseases are discarded
D. Mass survey require high quality team work

107. Leprosy is an "iceberg" disease.
A. True
B. Partially true
C. False

108. The main objective of multidrug therapy (MDT) is:
A. To interrupt transmission of the infection in the community by sterilizing infectious patients as rapidly as possible with bactericidal drugs
B. To ensure early detection and T/t of cases to prevent deformities
C. To prevent drug resistance
D. All of these
E. Both A and B above

109. Consider the following statements:
I. A case of leprosy in a person showing clinical signs of leprosy with or without bacteriological confirmation of the diagnosis
II. In most leprosy clinics in India, paucibacillary cases make up more than 60% of the total leprosy patients
III. Adequate T/t implies the completion of a regimen of MDT within a reasonably short period of time
IV. In multidrug regimens, only bactericidal drugs are used

Choose the correct answer as per code given below:
A. I and II
B. I and III
C. I and IV
D. I, II and III
E. I, II, III and IV All

110. The only drug which is highly bactericidal against M. leprae is:
A. Rifampicin
B. Protionamide
C. Clofazimine
D. Dapsone only
E. Ethionamide

111. The dose of dapsone in treatment of leprosy is:
A. 1 mg/kg body weight
B. 0.5 mg/kg body weight
C. 2 mg/kg body weight
D. 1 to 2 mg/kg body weight

112. The common adverse effect of DDS (dapsone) includes:
I. Haemolytic anemia, methaemoglobinaemia, agranulocytosis
II. Hepatitis
III. Peripheral neuropathy
IV. Psychosis and lepra reaction

Select the true answer as per following code:
A. I and II
B. I, II, III and IV All
C. I, II and III
D. I and IV
E. II, III and IV

113. Regarding clofazimine, all are true, *but* one:
A. Originally synthesized for the T/t of T.B.
B. Have greater value in leprosy
C. It has got no role in suppressing lepra reactions
D. It causes darkish red discolouration to skin, mucosa, urine and sweat

114. The W.H.O. has recommended that ethionamide or protionamide should be used as the 3rd drug in the treatment of

multibacillary leprosy in those patients who find clofazimine unacceptable.

A. True
B. Partially true
C. False

115. Following are recognised new drugs for treatment of leprosy:

I. Ofloxacin
II. Minocycline
III. Rifabutin
IV. Clarithromycin

Choose the true answer as per code given below:

A. I and III
B. I, II and III
C. I, II, III and IV All
D. II and IV
E. I and IV

116. WHO regimen for multibacillary leprosy includes the following:

A. Rifampicin 450 mg once daily + Dapsone 100 mg daily + CLF 100 mg daily
B. RMP 600 mg once monthly + Dapsone 100 mg daily + CLF 300 mg once monthly supervised and 50 mg daily, self administered
C. RMP 600 mg daily + DDS 50 mg daily + CLF 100 mg daily
D. RMP 450 mg daily + DDS 50 mg daily + CLF 300 mg monthly

117. WHO regimen for paucibacillary leprosy includes:

A. RMP 600 mg once a month for 6 months + DDS 100 mg daily for 6 months
B. RPM 450 mg daily for 6 months + DDS 50 mg daily for 6 months
C. RPM 500 mg daily for 6 months + DDS 50 mg daily for 9 months
D. RPM 500 mg daily for 6 months + DDS 50 mg daily for 12 months

118. Government of India, working group (1982) on leprosy recommends the following multidrug regimen:

A. RPM 600 mg monthly supervised DDS 100 mg daily self-administered, CLF 300 mg monthly supervised
B. RPM 600 monthly supervised DDS 100 mg daily self-administered
C. RPM 600 mg monthly DDS 50 mg daily + CLF 300 mg monthly
D. RPM 600 mg and DDS 100 mg/days × 2 wks then DDS 100 mg/day and RPM 600 mg per month × 6 months (supervised) followed by CLF 50 mg/days DDS 100 mg per day × 2 years

119. Government of India (1982) recommended the following drug regimen for a paucibacillary leprosy case:

A. CLF 50 mg and DDS 50 mg daily non-supervised
B. Monthly 600 mg Rifampicin for six months
C. DDS 100 mg nonsupervised daily
D. RPM 600 mg once a month for 6 months and DDS 1 to 2 mg/kg body wt. daily unsupervised for six months

120. The conjugal leprosy rate is about:

A. 2%
B. 5%
C. 10%
D. 15%
E. 20%

121. Following is NOT an epidemiological reservoir of leprosy infection:

A. Indeterminate
B. Lepromatous with lesions
C. Early lepromatous
D. Tuberculoid in reaction
E. None of these

122. What % of leprosy cases heal spontaneously?

A. 40%
B. 50%
C. 60%
D. 65%
E. 70%

123. In which country BCG provide high degree of protection against leprosy?
A. India
B. Burma
C. Uganda
D. Papua New Guinea

124. "CANDIDATE" vaccine is developed against:
A. Leprosy
B. Rabies
C. Kala-azar
D. Malaria

125. One IM injection of "ACEDAPSONE" (a long acting repository sulphone) is given once every:
A. 3 weeks
B. 6 weeks
C. 8 weeks
D. 10 weeks
E. 20 weeks

126. Those patients of leprosy are not treated at an early stage develop deformity in order of approximately:
A. 15%
B. 25%
C. 30%
D. 40%
E. 100%

127. Following deformities do not seen in leprosy patients:
A. Gynaecomastia
B. Perforation of palate
C. Nodules on extensor of the forearm
D. Wrist drop/Foot drop
E. None of these

128. The 1st Leprosy Mission in India was founded by Baily at Chamba in which of the following year?
A. 1874
B. 1884
C. 1901
D. 1925
E. 1935

129. Which voluntary organisation operating against leprosy has taken over by the ICMR in 1975?
A. Hind Kusht Nivaran Sangh
B. JALMA
C. Damien Foundation
D. Gandhi Memorial Leprosy Foundation

130. The National Leprosy Control Programme initiated in the middle of 1954 was converted into an eradication programme in which year?
A. 1960
B. 1962
C. 1983
D. 1986
E. 1993

131. Which is not a bacterial STD?
A. Gonorrhoea
B. Genital chlamydial infection
C. Syphilis
D. Chancroid
E. None of these

132. Following are recognised classical venereal diseases:
I. Syphilis
II. Gonorrhoea
III. Chancroid
IV. LGV
V. Donovanosis

Select the true answer as per code given below:
A. I and II only
B. I, II and III
C. I, II, III and IV
D. I, II, III, IV and V All

133. Following are recognised protozoal STD's, *save* for one:
A. Entamoeba histolytica
B. Giardia lamblia
C. Candida albicans
D. Trichomonas vaginalis
E. None of these

134. Which is not regarded as a viral STD?
A. α-HSV-l and 2
B. HAV
C. HIV
D. HBV
E. HPV only

135. The age group which has the highest incidence of STDs is:
A. 15 to 19 years
B. 25 to 29 years
C. 20 to 24 years
D. 30 to 34 years
E. Above 35 years

136. An individual is considered as "repeater" if he/she contracts STD annually:
A. Once
B. Twice
C. Thrice
D. Five times
E. Ten times

137. An individual is termed as "repeater" if he contracts STD:
A. Once a month
B. Twice a month
C. Thrice a month
D. Four times

138. The incidence of STD is not directly proportional to:
A. Sex education
B. Women's education
C. Contraceptive methods
D. All of these

139. Endemic syphilis does not occur in:
A. Syria
B. Saudi Arabia
C. Americas
D. Africa
E. Australia

140. Which of the following statement is/are false?
A. Bejal is the local name for endemic syphilis in Syria
B. A single injection of Benzathine PG is the treatment of choice
C. An acute infectious disease caused by Treponema carateum is pinta
D. Yaws is a chronic contagious non-venereal disease caused by T. pertenue
E. Yaws is also known as pian, bubas or framboesia

141. Regarding YAWS, all, *but* one, are true:
A. It is exclusively confined to the belt between the tropic of capricorn and the tropic of cancer
B. It is endemic in India in A.P., M.P., Maharashtra, Orissa and Tamil Nadu
C. The reservoir of infection is the man
D. Caused by T. pertenue
E. The organisms survive for few days outside host tissue

142. NOT a usual finding in yaws is:
A. It is a crippling disease
B. I.P. 3 to 5 weeks
C. Transmitted only venereally
D. The early lesions are highly infectious

143. Regarding syphilis, which is false?
A. Spread by sexual contact
B. The site of inoculation is shown by an ulcer
C. Hard chancre
D. Painful ulcer
E. None of the above

144. Treponema carateum causes what?
A. Bejel
B. Pinta
C. Yaws
D. Syphilis

145. "Soft chancre" is due to:
A. T. pallidum
B. H. ducreyi
C. Both of the above
D. None of the above

146. "Chancroid" is caused by:
A. Virus
B. Bacteria

C. Fungus
D. Protozoon

147. The general prevalence of NGU is to the extent of:
A. 10%
B. 20%
C. 30%
D. 40%
E. 50%

148. The nonfatal, chronic, progressive bacterial STD is:
A. Gonorrhoea
B. Donovanosis
C. Chancroid
D. Syphilis

149. The exact I.P. of following STD is not known:
A. Donovanosis
B. Genital molluscum
C. Chancroid
D. All of the above

150. The case of STD on enquiry reveals names and address of persons moving in his sociosexual circle, who then are examined for STD. This method is termed as:
A. Screening
B. Contact tracing
C. Cluster testing
D. All of the above

151. Epidemiological treatment of contacts of STD cases is:
A. Immunoprophylaxis
B. Chemotherapy
C. Chemoprophylaxis
D. Epidemiological investigation
E. All of these

152. W.H.O. recommends total mass treatment for yaws if prevalence per 1000 population is more than:
A. 5% B. 10%
C. 15% D. 18%
E. 20%

153. W.H.O. recommends juvenile mass treatment of yaws if its prevalence in mesoendemic areas is in the range of:
A. 0 to 5%
B. 3 to 10%
C. 5 to 10%
D. 7 to 10%
E. 10 to 15%

154. "Slim disease" is the name given to:
A. AIDS
B. Syphilis
C. Malnutrition
D. Malaria

155. "AIDS virus" belongs to the group of:
A. Adeno
B. Retro
C. Slow
D. Rotavirus
E. None of the above

156. Worldwide, 75 to 85% of HIV infections in adults have been transmitted through unprotected sexual intercourse.
A. True
B. Partially true
C. False

157. The 1st case of AIDS was registered in India in which year?
A. 1981 B. 1982
C. 1985 D. 1986
E. 1988

158. Currently seropositivity for AIDS in India per 1000 population is:
A. 5.8 B. 9.6
C. 18.3 D. 20.0
E. 15.2

159. The major concentration of HIV infected individual in India is:
A. Bombay
B. Puna
C. Madras
D. Vellore
E. All of the above

160. A new highly AIDS infected area recently (1993) found in India is:
A. Assam
B. Goa
C. Manipur
D. Himachal Pradesh

161. Regarding the morphological characteristics of HIV, all correct, *except* for:
A. It is a protein capsule containing two short strands of genetic material RNA and enzymes
B. The virus is 1/10,000th of a mm in diameter
C. The virus does not penetrate the blood brain barrier (BBB)
D. The virus replicates in actively dividing T_4 lymphocytes
E. The virus has the unique ability to destroy human T_4 helper cells

162. The most recently recognised AIDS' virus in West Africa is called as:
A. HIV-l
B. HIV-2
C. HIV-3
D. HIV-4
E. HIV-5

163. HIV virus is relatively resistant to:
A. Acetone
B. β-propiolactone
C. Ether
D. UVL
E. Ethanol

164. Once person is infected with HIV, the virus remains in the body:
A. 1 year
B. 5 years
C. 10 years
D. 20 years
E. Life long

165. Regarding HIV, all are true statement, *save* for one:
A. The reservoir of infection is cases and carriers
B. The virus has been found in greatest concentration in blood, semen and CSF
C. Most cases have occurred among sexually active persons aged 20 to 49 years
D. Higher rate of HIV infection is found in prostitutes
E. None of these

166. Which of the following statements is/are true?
A. The CD_4^+ cells play a key role in regulating the immune response
B. HIV selectively infects T-helper cells apart from several other cells like B-cells, microphages, and nerve cells
C. A decreased ratio of T-helper to T-suppresser cells may be an indirect indicator of reduced cellular immunity
D. The most striking feature of the immune system of patients with AIDS is profound lymphopenia, with a total lymphocyte count often below 500 cmm
E. All of the above

167. In AIDS, the alteration in T-cell function is responsible for the:
A. Development of neoplasms
B. Development of opportunistic infections
C. Inability to mount a delayed type hypersensitivity response
D. All of these
E. Both A and C above

168. HIV infection most frequently transmitted through:
A. Sexual transmission
B. Blood contact
C. Maternal foetal transmission: mother to child transmission
D. All of these
E. Both B and C above

169. AIDS can be transmitted by following, *except* for:
A. Albumin
B. Whole blood
C. Platelets
D. Factor VII and IX

170. HIV antibodies usually take between .... to appear in the blood-stream though take longer.
A. 1 to 2 weeks
B. 2 to 4 weeks
C. 2 to 8 weeks
D. 2 to 12 weeks

171. Recognised C/M of AIDS related complex includes:
I. **Unexplained diarrhoea lasting longer than a month**
II. **Fatigue, malaise, loss of > 10% body weight**
III. **Fever, night sweats, oral thrush, generalised lymphadenopathy, splenomegaly**

Select the true answer as per following code:
A. I only
B. I, II and III All
C. II and III
D. I and III

172. Which of the following statements is/are false?
A. A person with ARC has illnesses caused by damage to the immune system but without the opportunistic infections and cancers related with AIDS
B. AIDS is the end stage of HIV infection
C. In Africa it is popularly known as slim disease
D. None of the above

173. T-helper cell count below 50 shows the following infections:
A. TB
B. Kaposi's sarcoma
C. CMV retinitis
D. Toxoplasma gondii

174. In HIV infection, the kaposi's sarcoma is seen in:
A. Sheen of tibia
B. Mouth
C. Gut
D. All of the above
E. Both B and C

175. Following infections are seen when T-helper cell count has dropped to around 100, *save* for one:
A. Candida oesophagitis
B. T.B.
C. T. gondii encephalitis
D. Cryptococcus meningitis and penicillosis
E. Pneumocystis pneumonia carinii

176. WHO clinical diagnosis of AIDS includes 2 major and 1 minor signs in an adult or adolescents. Following is the minor signs, *but* one:
A. Persistent cough for one month
B. Generalized pruritic matitis
C. Prolonged fever for month
D. History of herpes zoster
E. Generalised lymphadenopathy

177. For surveillance purpose for the diagnosis of AIDS which is sufficient?
A. Generalized kaposi sarcoma
B. Cryptococcal meningitis
C. Weight loss10%
D. Both A and B above
E. All of the above

178. Expanded WHO case definition for AIDS surveillance includes:
A. HIV serological test
B. T.B. and pneumonia
C. Invasive cervical cancer
D. Neurological impairment
E. All of these

179. World's AIDS Day is celebrated on:
A. 1st January
B. 1st February
C. 1st December
D. 7th April

180. The most specific test against AIDS antibodies is:
A. ELISA

B. Virus isolation
C. Western blot
D. All of these

181. Which tests against AIDS andibodies is based on detecting specific antibody to viral core protein (P_{24}) and envelop glycoprotein (gp41)?
A. ELISA
B. Western blot
C. Virus isolation
D. All of the above

182. The most widely lab markers to provide prognostic information and guide therapy decisions include:
A. Anaemia
B. Thrombocytopenia
C. The absolute CD_4 lymphocyte count
D. Leukopenia
E. All of these

183. People with AIDS usually have CD_4 cell count below:
A. 50
B. 100
C. 200
D. 300
E. 400

184. Regarding AIDS control, presently which is the most appropriate measures?
A. Health education
B. Antiretroviral treatment
C. Specific prophylaxis
D. Primary health care
E. All of these

185. Drugs used in AIDS patients are all, *but* one:
A. Zidovudine
B. Didanosine
C. Cytosine arabinoside
D. Zalcitabine
E. Stavudine

186. "Peripheral neuropathy" is the recognised side-effects of following drugs, *except*:
A. Zalcitabine
B. Zidovudine
C. Stavudine
D. Didanosine

187. The WHO has launched a "global programme on AIDS" on 1st February 1987 to provide global leadership and to support the development of national AIDS programmes.
A. True
B. False

188. Screening test for HIV infection is:
A. ELISA
B. Western blot
C. β_2-Microglobulin
D. HIV virus load tests

189. Confirmatory test for HIV infection is:
A. HIV viral load tests
B. ELISA
C. Western blot
D. P_{24} antigen

190. Most widely used predictor of HIV progression is:
A. CD_4 lymphocyte percentage
B. Absolute CD_4 lymphocyte count
C. HIV viral load tests
D. β_2-microglobulin

191. Which test indicates active HIV replication?
A. ELISA
B. Western blot
C. CD_4 lymphocyte%
D. P_{24} antigen

192. Following nucleoside analogs may cause peripheral neuropathy as side-effects of used in AIDS patients, *but* one:
A. Zidovudine
B. Zalcitabine
C. Stavudine
D. Lamivudine

193. Which nucleoside analog may cause myopathy?
A. Abacavir

B. Zidovudine
C. Zalcitabine
D. Didanosine

194. No specific monitoring is needed with use of which antiretroviral drugs?
A. Tenofovir
B. Abacavir
C. Stavudine
D. Amprenavir

195. Following is a antiretroviral nucleotide analog?
A. Tenofovir
B. Abacavir
C. Ritonavir
D. Indinavir

196. Following antiretroviral are protease inhibitors *but* one:
A. Saquinavir
B. Ritonavir
C. Nelfinavir
D. Tenofovir

197. Following antiretroviral drugs are non-nucleoside reverse transcriptase inhibitors (NNRTIs), *except* for:
A. Nevirapine
B. Amprenavir
C. Efavirenz
D. Delavirdine

198. The following treatment is recommended by the US centre for disease control and prevention for health care workers accidentally exposed to HIV (Post Exposure Prophylaxis—PEP):
A. Double combination of treatment with AZT (200 mg tds) plus lamivudine (3TC) (150 mg BD) for 4 weeks
B. If the "source" individual has advanced AIDS, the protease inhibitor nelfinavir (750 mg 3 times daily) should be added to the AZT/3TC regimen
C. If the "source" individual has failed on AZT/3TC therapy (e.g. no benefit or intolerance), stavudine (d4T) plus ddI should be used instead of AZT/3TC
D. All of the above

199. Primary prophylaxis against P. carinii pneumonia should be offered to patients with CD_4 count below:
A. 100 cells/μL
B. 150 cells/μL
C. 200 cells/μL
D. 300 cells/μL

200. Consider the following infection and its prophylaxis and treatment in AIDS patients:
I. Kaposi sarcoma—Interferon, chemotherapy or radiation
II. CMV retinitis—Ganciclovir
III. Cryptococcal meningitis—Fluconazole
IV. Esophageal/vaginal candidiasis—Ketoconazole
V. HSV infection/Herpes Zoster—Acyclovir or Foscarnet

Select the true answer from the code given below:
A. I, II and III
B. I, II, III, IV and V All
C. I, III and V
D. I, II, IV and V

201. In the heterosexual transmission (from infective to non-infective partner) of HIV:
A. There is a greater risk of transmission from man to a woman
B. There is a greater risk of transmission from woman to man
C. Risk is equal either ways
D. HIV infection is not transmissible by heterosexual act

202. Mortality for AIDS is almost:
A. 25%
B. 50%
C. 75 to 90%
D. 100%

6. EMERGING AND REEMERGING INFECTIOUS DISEASES

1. **"Emerging Infectious Disease Global Alert: Global Response" has been the theme of World Health Day in which year?**
   A. 1977
   B. 1982
   C. 1987
   D. 1995
   E. 1997
2. **The most dramatic example of new diseases is:**
   A. AIDS
   B. Yellow fever
   C. Cholera
   D. Dengue
   E. Ebola disease
3. **Ebola virus appeared for the 1st time in 1976 in:**
   A. Zaire
   B. Sudan
   C. Both of the above
   D. None of the above
4. **In USA, hantavirus pulmonary syndrome was 1st seen in the year:**
   A. 1991
   B. 1993
   C. 1995
   D. 1997
   E. 1998
5. **"Deer mice" is the recognised vector for:**
   A. Yellow fever
   B. Ebola virus
   C. HIV
   D. Hantavirus
6. **Asian hantaviruses causes the following:**
   A. Hemorrhagic fever
   B. Renal involvement
   C. Both of the above
   D. None of the above
7. **The strain of E. coli first reported in 1982 is:**
   A. 0157: H7 strain
   B. 0137: H3 strain
   C. 01558: H4 strain
   D. All of the above
8. **Major shifts in influenza virus occurs once every:**
   A. 5 years
   B. 10 years
   C. 15 years
   D. 20 years
   E. 50 years
9. **Syphilis is now emerging owing to:**
   A. Changes in lifestyle
   B. Behaviour
   C. Cultural or social values
   D. All of these
   E. Both A and C above
10. **Increased human mobility as an national/international travelling/tour has been associated with following diseases:**
    A. HIV infection
    B. STDs
    C. Both of the above
    D. Neither A nor B
11. **Major cause of infantile diarrhea worldwide is:**
    A. Guanarito virus
    B. Rotavirus
    C. Hantavirus
    D. HTLV-2
12. **HTLV-2 causes:**
    A. Aplastic crisis in chronic hemolytic anaemia
    B. Toxic shock syndrome
    C. Human ehrlichiosis
    D. Hairy cell leukaemia

13. **E. coli 0157 : H7 causes:**
    A. Toxic shock syndrome
    B. Haemolytic, uraemic syndrome
    C. Hemorrhagic colitis
    D. Both A and B above
    E. Both B and C above

14. **"Persistent diarrhoea" may be caused by:**
    A. Enterocytozoon bieneusi
    B. Cyclospora cayetanensis
    C. Cryptosporidium parvum
    D. Both A and B above
    E. All of these

15. **Hantavirus pulmonary syndrome is caused by:**
    A. Sin Nambre virus
    B. Guanarito virus
    C. Parvovirus B_{19}
    D. Hantaan virus
    E. Ebola virus

16. **In the year 1977 following organisms were discovered, *except* for:**
    A. Ebola virus
    B. Cryptosporidium parvum
    C. Campylobacter jejuni
    D. Hantaan virus
    E. Legionella pneumophila

17. **Helicobacter pylori may be related to:**
    A. Infantile diarrhoea
    B. Haemolytic anemia
    C. Peptic ulcer
    D. Toxic shock syndrome
    E. All of these

18. **Hemorrhagic fever with renal syndrome is caused by:**
    A. Hantaan virus
    B. HTLV-2
    C. Ebola virus
    D. Guanarito virus

19. **"Bartonella henselae" causes:**
    A. Cat-scratch disease
    B. Bacillary angiomatosis
    C. Both of the above
    D. None of the above

20. **Staphylococcus aureus may cause the following:**
    A. Acute and chronic diarrhoea
    B. Toxic shock syndrome
    C. Disseminated disease
    D. All of these
    E. Both A and C above

21. **"SABIA virus" causes:**
    A. Infantile diarrhoea
    B. Lyme disease
    C. T-cell lymphoma leukaemia
    D. Persistent diarrhoea
    E. Brazilian hemorrhagic fever

22. **"Ehrlichia chaffeensis" is a:**
    A. Parasite
    B. Virus
    C. Bacterium
    D. None of the above

23. **T-cell lymphoma-leukaemia is caused by:**
    A. HTLV-l
    B. HTLV-2
    C. HIV
    D. HHV-6
    E. Ebola virus

24. **Following organisms are recognised in the year 1991, *except:***
    A. Guanarito virus
    B. Hepatitis virus
    C. New species of babesia
    D. Encephalitozoon hallem
    E. None of the above

25. **Which organisms is associated with Kaposi's sarcoma in AIDS patients?**
    A. Human herpesvirus-1
    B. Human herpesvirus-2
    C. Human herpesvirus-6
    D. Human herpesvirus-8
    E. HTLV-2

26. **"Borrelia burgdoferi" causes what?**
    A. Hairy cell leukaemia
    B. Legionnaire's disease
    C. Lyme disease

D. Venezuelan hemorrhagic fever
E. All of these

27. Aplastic crises in chronic haemolytic anemia is due to:
A. Parvovirus B_{19}
B. HHV-6
C. HHV-8
D. HTLV-2
E. HTLV-I

28. Relaxation in immunization practices against which organisms causes resurgence of disease recently in USSR?
A. Tetanus
B. T.B.
C. Cholera
D. Diphtheria
E. All of these

29. "Mad Cow disease" is otherwise known as:
A. Bacillary angiomatosis
B. Bovine spongiform encephalopathy
C. Cat scratch disease
D. Legionnaire's disease

30. In variant Creutzfeldt-Jakob disease of human, which organ system is chiefly involved?
A. Heart
B. Lung
C. Brain
D. Kidney
E. Liver

31. A major cause of the urgent crisis in antimicrobial resistance is the uncontrolled and inappropriate use of antibiotic drugs, in both industrialized and developing countries.
A. True
B. False

32. Drug resistance is the result of:
A. Poor prescribing practices
B. Poor patients compliance with treatment
C. Both of the above
D. None of the above

33. Which of the following communicable disease presents a double resistance problem?
A. T.B.
B. Malaria
C. Plague
D. Cholera
E. Pneumonia

34. Staphylococci have developed resistance to all, *but* one:
A. Ampicillin
B. Cephalosporin
C. Tetracycline
D. Vancomycin

35. The drug recommended by WHO against pneumonia is:
A. Ampicillin
B. Gentamicin
C. Cotrimoxazole
D. Doxicycline

36. What % of antibiotic produced worldwide are used in animals?
A. 10%
B. 20%
C. 30%
D. 40%
E. 50%

37. Following human pathogen of animal origin are today highly resistant to antibiotics:
A. E. coli
B. Salmonella
C. Neisseria gonorrhea
D. Both A and B above
E. All of these

38. The natural history of disease is unknown in the following:
A. T.B.
B. Malaria
C. Cholera
D. Dengue
E. Ebola fever

39. Without effective antibiotic treatment, Typhoid fever kills almost what % of those infected ?

A. 5%
B. 10%
C. 25%
D. 50%
E. 70%

40. Among the most common disease causing bacteria is:

A. Staphylococcus
B. Bacillus species
C. Streptococcus
D. Pneumococcus
E. E. coli

41. The recognised strategy for controlling re-emerging diseases is through available following interventions:

A. Early diagnosis and prompt treatment
B. Vector control measures
C. DOTS
D. Drugs and vaccines
E. All of the above

Answers

1. RESPIRATORY INFECTIONS

1 D	2 A	3 C	4 B	5 C	6 D	7 E	8 C	9 D	10 E
11 A	12 C	13 B	14 C	15 C	16 E	17 A	18 E	19 C	20 E
21 A	22 B	23 E	24 A	25 B	26 C	27 D	28 E	29 A	30 D
31 B	32 A	33 C	34 D	35 E	36 A	37 C	38 A	39 D	40 A
41 B	42 C	43 D	44 A	45 C	46 B	47 C	48 A	49 B	50 D
51 B	52 C	53 D	54 A	55 C	56 A	57 C	58 A	59 B	60 C
61 C	62 D	63 A	64 C	65 B	66 A	67 C	68 D	69 E	70 B
71 B	72 A	73 C	74 A	75 E	76 E	77 C	78 A	79 E	80 C
81 A	82 C	83 B	84 D	85 C	86 A	87 B	88 A	89 D	90 E
91 B	92 E	93 C	94 B	95 E	96 D	97 A	98 B	99 C	100 D
101 A	102 B	103 C	104 D	105 D	106 A	107 C	108 D	109 A	110 B
111 A	112 B	113 E	114 C	115 D	116 C	117 D	118 A	119 D	120 E
121 C	122 D	123 A	124 A	125 E	126 C	127 B	128 A	129 C	130 A
131 B	132 C	133 B	134 C	135 A	136 D	137 A	138 B	139 A	140 B
141 A	142 C	143 D	144 E	145 D	146 C	147 A	148 E	149 D	150 B
151 D	152 A	153 C	154 B	155 C	156 D	157 A	158 B	159 E	160 B
161 A	162 C	163 D	164 A	165 B	166 A	167 B	168 C	169 A	170 B
171 C	172 D	173 A	174 B	175 C	176 A	177 D	178 B	179 E	180 B
181 C	182 D	183 A	184 B	185 C	186 C	187 B	188 A	189 C	190 D
191 E	192 B	193 A	194 D	195 E	196 C	197 E	198 C	199 E	200 C
201 A	202 B	203 D	204 C	205 D	206 A	207 C	208 A	209 A	210 D
211 C	212 D	213 E	214 B	215 A	216 B	217 D	218 C	219 E	220 D

221 D	222 C	223 B	224 A	225 D	226 B	227 D	228 B	229 C	230 D
231 A	232 C	233 C	234 D	235 A	236 B	237 B	238 B	239 A	240 D
241 C	242 D	243 B	244 C	245 C	246 D	247 A	248 C	249 C	250 C
251 D	252 B	253 C	254 A	255 B	256 D	257 C	258 C	259 B	260 A
261 A									

2. INTESTINAL INFECTIONS

1 A	2 A	3 C	4 D	5 B	6 C	7 D	8 A	9 B	10 A
11 E	12 B	13 C	14 B	15 A	16 C	17 B	18 A	19 C	20 B
21 D	22 C	23 B	24 D	25 C	26 D	27 A	28 B	29 B	30 C
31 B	32 A	33 C	34 D	35 C	36 E	37 B	38 A	39 E	40 B
41 A	42 C	43 D	44 E	45 C	46 E	47 A	48 B	49 D	50 E
51 D	52 E	53 D	54 A	55 D	56 B	57 C	58 C	59 A	60 B
61 E	62 A	63 B	64 C	65 D	66 E	67 A	68 A	69 D	70 D
71 A	72 C	73 A	74 A	75 A	76 E	77 A	78 B	79 C	80 A
81 E	82 B	83 C	84 D	85 A	86 C	87 E	88 D	89 C	90 B
91 A	92 D	93 D	94 C	95 B	96 A	97 B	98 A	99 C	100 B
101 E	102 B	103 D	104 C	105 E	106 B	107 A	108 B	109 E	110 B
111 B	112 C	113 B	114 A	115 D	116 C	117 B	118 D	119 C	120 B
121 A	122 C	123 D	124 B	125 E	126 E	127 A	128 B	129 A	130 D
131 A	132 B	133 C	134 D	135 B	136 E	137 B	138 A	139 B	140 D
141 D	142 A	143 A	144 B	145 C	146 B	147 A	148 D	149 C	150 C
151 A	152 C	153 D	154 E	155 C	156 B	157 D	158 C	159 A	160 B
161 E	162 D	163 A	164 C	165 B	166 D	167 A	168 A	169 E	170 C

171 B	172 C	173 A	174 E	175 D	176 B	177 C	178 B	179 E	180 B
181 A	182 C	183 D	184 D	185 B	186 C	187 D	188 B	189 A	190 B
191 C	192 D	193 E	194 C	195 D	196 A	197 D	198 E	199 D	200 C
201 A	202 C	203 B	204 B	205 A	206 C	207 D	208 B	209 A	210 B
211 C	212 B	213 A	214 C	215 B	216 A	217 D	218 A	219 C	220 D
221 A	222 B	223 D	224 C	225 B	226 D	227 A	228 B	229 D	230 B
231 D	232 A	233 D	234 A	235 B	236 A	237 B	238 A	239 D	240 A
241 A	242 B	243 C	244 A	245 C	246 B	247 C	248 A	249 C	250 A
251 B	252 A	253 A	254 B	255 C					

3. ARTHROPOD BORNE INFECTIONS

1 A	2 E	3 B	4 D	5 C	6 E	7 E	8 A	9 C	10 B
11 C	12 C	13 E	14 D	15 A	16 B	17 E	18 A	19 B	20 D
21 C	22 E	23 B	24 A	25 C	26 B	27 C	28 A	29 B	30 C
31 A	32 B	33 C	34 A	35 B	36 C	37 A	38 B	39 C	40 D
41 A	42 B	43 C	44 D	45 E	46 A	47 B	48 C	49 E	50 D
51 A	52 B	53 D	54 A	55 E	56 C	57 D	58 B	59 A	60 C
61 B	62 E	63 E	64 B	65 A	66 A	67 B	68 C	69 D	70 B
71 A	72 C	73 B	74 A	75 C	76 C	77 A	78 B	79 C	80 E
81 A	82 B	83 C	84 A	85 B	86 D	87 C	88 D	89 A	90 B
91 C	92 A	93 B	94 C	95 E	96 D	97 A	98 D	99 A	100 B
101 C	102 D	103 C	104 A	105 D	106 B	107 E	108 B	109 B	110 A
111 C	112 E	113 B	114 A	115 C	116 D	117 C	118 D	119 B	120 E
121 A	122 B	123 D	124 C	125 D	126 A	127 B	128 C	129 A	130 B

131 D	132 C	133 E	134 A	135 D	136 B	137 C	138 D	139 A	140 B
141 A	142 B	143 D	144 C	145 A	146 B	147 C	148 A	149 B	150 D
151 B	152 D	153 C	154 D	155 A	156 D	157 B	158 D	159 B	160 C
161 C									

4. ZOONOSES

1 A	2 B	3 D	4 C	5 A	6 B	7 A	8 D	9 B	10 D
11 E	12 C	13 A	14 A	15 B	16 D	17 C	18 E	19 C	20 A
21 A	22 B	23 E	24 B	25 B	26 C	27 B	28 A	29 B	30 D
31 A	32 C	33 A	34 D	35 E	36 B	37 C	38 A	39 B	40 D
41 C	42 B	43 D	44 A	45 B	46 D	47 C	48 D	49 B	50 C
51 A	52 E	53 C	54 B	55 A	56 C	57 E	58 C	59 B	60 C
61 D	62 B	63 A	64 C	65 C	66 A	67 C	68 A	69 B	70 D
71 C	72 D	73 E	74 B	75 D	76 C	77 D	78 E	79 B	80 C
81 A	82 E	83 B	84 C	85 A	86 C	87 B	88 C	89 D	90 B
91 D	92 E	93 A	94 B	95 D	96 C	97 D	98 A	99 B	100 A
101 B	102 A	103 B	104 C	105 E	106 A	107 A	108 C	109 B	110 B
111 A	112 C	113 D	114 E	115 A	116 B	117 C	118 D	119 E	120 E
121 B	122 E	123 A	124 C	125 B	126 A	127 B	128 C	129 D	130 A
131 A	132 B	133 C	134 D	135 B	136 E	137 A	138 A	139 D	140 A
141 B	142 A	143 C	144 A	145 C	146 A	147 D	148 E	149 C	150 B
151 D	152 B	153 A	154 B	155 C	156 D	157 C	158 D	159 A	160 B
161 C	162 A	163 B	164 A	165 B	166 C	167 D	168 B	169 C	170 A
171 E	172 A	173 B	174 C	175 A	176 B	177 C	178 A	179 E	180 B

181 D	182 E	183 B	184 A	185 C	186 D	187 B	188 E	189 A	190 B
191 C	192 A	193 B	194 C	195 C	196 D	197 A	198 E	199 A	200 B
201 D	202 E	203 E	204 D	205 B	206 A	207 C	208 B	209 A	210 D
211 C	212 A	213 E	214 A	215 C	216 B	217 A	218 C	219 D	220 E
221 C	222 A	223 B	224 A	225 B	226 C	227 A	228 B	229 C	230 D
231 C	232 A	233 B	234 D						

5. SURFACE INFECTIONS

1 A	2 B	3 B	4 A	5 D	6 E	7 C	8 C	9 A	10 E
11 B	12 A	13 C	14 D	15 B	16 E	17 D	18 A	19 B	20 B
21 D	22 —	23 A	24 D	25 C	26 A	27 B	28 C	29 B	30 C
31 D	32 E	33 D	34 C	35 A	36 B	37 A	38 C	39 B	40 D
41 E	42 A	43 B	44 C	45 D	46 B	47 D	48 C	49 A	50 B
51 C	52 B	53 C	54 D	55 C	56 B	57 D	58 B	59 C	60 E
61 A	62 D	63 B	64 C	65 D	66 E	67 B	68 C	69 A	70 B
71 C	72 B	73 A	74 D	75 B	76 A	77 C	78 B	79 A	80 B
81 C	82 A	83 C	84 B	85 C	86 A	87 B	88 A	89 E	90 D
91 A	92 D	93 C	94 C	95 B	96 A	97 B	98 D	99 C	100 A
101 B	102 A	103 D	104 E	105 A	106 C	107 A	108 D	109 E	110 A
111 D	112 B	113 C	114 A	115 C	116 B	117 A	118 D	119 D	120 B
121 A	122 E	123 C	124 A	125 D	126 B	127 C	128 A	129 B	130 C
131 E	132 D	133 C	134 B	135 C	136 C	137 A	138 D	139 C	140 C
141 B	142 C	143 D	144 B	145 B	146 B	147 D	148 B	149 A	150 C
151 B	152 B	153 C	154 A	155 B	156 A	157 D	158 C	159 E	160 B

161 C	162 B	163 D	164 E	165 E	166 E	167 D	168 A	169 A	170 D
171 B	172 D	173 C	174 E	175 B	176 C	177 D	178 E	179 C	180 C
181 B	182 C	183 C	184 A	185 C	186 B	187 A	188 A	189 C	190 B
191 D	192 A	193 B	194 B	195 A	196 D	197 B	198 D	199 C	200 B
201 A	202 D								

6. EMERGING AND REEMERGING INFECTIOUS DISEASES

1 E	2 A	3 C	4 B	5 D	6 C	7 A	8 D	9 D	10 C
11 B	12 D	13 E	14 D	15 A	16 B	17 C	18 A	19 C	20 B
21 E	22 C	23 A	24 B	25 D	26 C	27 A	28 D	29 B	30 C
31 A	32 C	33 B	34 D	35 C	36 E	37 D	38 E	39 B	40 C
41 E									

C•H•A•P•T•E•R SIX

Epidemiology of Chronic Non-communicable Diseases and Conditions

DIRECTION: Following MCQ's are provided with a few suggestive answers/completions. Only one answer is correct. You have to identify the *BEST* one in each case.

1. "An impairment of bodily structure and/or function that necessitates a modification of the patient's normal life, and has persisted over an extended period of time". This is the definition of chronic disease and condition given by EURO symposium in which of the following year?

A. 1947
B. 1957
C. 1967
D. 1987
E. 1977

2. Recognised characteristics of chronic disease include:

I. Are permanent
II. Leave residual disability
III. Are caused by non-reversible pathological alteration
IV. Require special training of the patient for rehabilitation
V. May be expected to require a long period of supervision, observation or care

Select the true answer as per code given below:

A. I, II and III
B. I, II, III and IV
C. I, II, III, IV and V All
D. I, III and V
E. I, II, IV and V

3. A disease is said to be chronic when it had a duration of at least:

A. One month
B. Three months
C. Four months
D. Six months

4. The leading cause of death in developed countries is:

A. CVS
B. Respiratory
C. Renal
D. Diabetes mellitus
E. All of these

5. Gaps in the natural history of chronic disease includes the following:

I. Absence of a known agent
II. Multifactorial causation
III. Long latent period
IV. Indefinite onset

Choose the correct answer as per following code given below:

A. I and II only
B. I, II and III
C. I, II, III and IV only

D. II, III and IV
E. I and IV only

6. **Following non-communicable disease 'risk factors' are responsible for a major share of adult non-communicable disease morbidity and premature mortality.**
A. Alcohol abuse and smoking only
B. Stress factors and lifestyle changes
C. Failure or inability to obtain preventive health services
D. Environmental risk factors
E. All of the above

7. **According to W.H.O. which is regarded as our modern "epidemic"?**
A. AIDS
B. Breast C_A
C. C_AC_X
D. Coronary heart disease
E. None of the above

8. **Following C/M is specific to coronary heart disease (CHD):**
A. Angina pectoris
B. Myocardial infarction
C. Cardiac failure
D. Irregularities of the heart
E. Sudden death

9. **The simplest measure of the burden of CHD is:**
A. Proportional mortality ratio
B. Loss of life expectancy
C. Prevalence rate
D. Case fatality rate
E. Age specific death rates

10. **The prevalence of CHD can be estimated from cross-sectional surveys using the following parameters:**
A. Serum enzymology
B. History of prolonged chest pain
C. ECG recording
D. Both B and C above
E. All of the above

11. **"The proportion of attacks of CHD that are fatal within 28 days of onset" is called as or defined as:**
A. Age specific death rate
B. Proportional mortality ratio
C. Case fatality rate
D. CHD incidence rate
E. All of the above

12. **"Cardiovascular survey methods" has been published by whom?**
A. R.J. Last
B. Rose and Blackburn
C. Hurst and Camay
D. R.J. Stanby

13. **In what % of all cardiac deaths mortality ensues within the 1st hour?**
A. 10 to 15%
B. 15 to 25%
C. 30 to 40%
D. About 55%
E. 70 to 80%

14. **The epidemics of CHD has first of all been noted in which countries?**
A. USA
B. Britain
C. Canada
D. Denmark
E. Ecquador

15. **The W.H.O. has recently completed a project called MONICA concerned with:**
A. Rheumatology
B. Cancers
C. CHD
D. Diabetes mellitus

16. **The highest coronary mortality is seen at present in the following countries, *save* for one:**
A. Finland
B. Italy
C. Scotland
D. Ireland
E. Sweden

17. Which is NOT a modifiable risk factors for CHD?
A. Stress
B. High blood pressure
C. Age and sex
D. Diabetes mellitus
E. Raised serum cholesterol

18. Which fraction of lipoprotein is most directly associated with coronary heart disease (CHD)?
A. VLDL
B. LDL
C. Chylomicrons
D. HDL only

19. "Intermittent claudication" is most strongly associated with:
A. VLDL
B. LDL
C. Chylomicrons
D. HDL only
E. All of these

20. Prevention of CHD is more likely when HDL only should be more than:
A. VLDL
B. IDL
C. HDL
D. LDL

21. "Apolopoprotein A1" is the major .... protein.
A. VLDL
B. IDL
C. HDL
D. LDL only

22. Apoliporprotein 'B' is the major.......... protein.
A. VLDL
B. IDL
C. Chylomicrons
D. HDL
E. LDL only

23. Consider the following statements:
I. Women using OCP have higher systolic but not diastolic blood pressure
II. The risk of CHD is 2 to 3 times higher in diabetics than in non-diabetics
III. Regular physical exercise decreases the level of HDL level
IV. High alcohol intake defined as 75 gm or more per day is an independent risk factor for CHD hypertension and other cardiovascular diseases

Choose the false answer as per code given below:
A. I and III only
B. I, II and III only
C. I, III and IV only
D. II and IV only
E. I, II, III and IV All

24. "PRUDENT DIET" means what?
A. Reduced salt intake
B. Regular physical activity and weight control
C. Avoidance of a high alcohol intake
D. Both A and C above
E. All of the above

25. Which of the following well-planned risk factor intervention trials have demonstrated that primary prevention can achieve substantial reduction in the incidence of coronary heart disease in Finland?
A. MRFIT
B. Stanford heart disease prevention programme
C. The North Kerelia project
D. All of these
E. Both A and B above

26. The most effective single means of intervention currently available in the

management of patients after a heart attack is:
A. Give β-blocker regularly
B. Cessation of smoking
C. Regular physical exercise
D. Avoidance of fatty food
E. All of the above

27. What % of all deaths ensues within 30 mts of onset of heart attack?
A. 10% **B.** 20%
C. 30% **D.** 40%
E. 50%

28. Which strategy has got the greatest potential is curbing the CHD?
A. Population strategy
B. High risk strategy
C. Secondary prevention
D. All of the above
E. Both B and C above

29. The major risk factors of CHD includes:
A. Raised serum cholesterol
B. Smoking only
C. Hypertension only
D. Sedentary habits only
E. All of the above

30. To prevent coronany attack or sudden death, a secondary prevention trials have been performed using the four main groups of drugs. The most promising results to date have come from which groups?
A. Anticoagulants
B. Lipid-lowering agents
C. Anti-thrombotic agents
D. Beta-blockers
E. All are equally potent

31. The WHO Expert Committee (1978) defined hypertension in adults as:
A. A systolic pressure equal to or greater than 140 mmHg and/or a diastolic pressure equal to or greater than 95 mmHg
B. A SBP equal to or > 160 mmHg and/or DBP equal to or > 95 mmHg
C. A SBP equal to or > 140 mmHg and/or DBP equal to or > 105 mmHg
D. A SBP equal to or > 160 mmHg and/or DBP equal to or > 105 mmHg

32. A WHO study group has recommended which position for measuring the blood pressure of an individual?
A. Supine
B. Standing
C. Sitting
D. Left lateral recumbent

33. Consider the following statements about blood pressure measurement:
I. Three sources of errors have been identified in the recording of blood pressure like observer errors, instrumental errors and subject-errors
II. If the cuff is too small and fails to encircle the arm then too high a reading will be obtained
III. The systolic and diastolic pressures should be measured at least 3 times over a period of atleast 3 minutes and the lowest reading recorded

Choose the wrong answer as per code given below:
A. I only
B. II only
C. I and II only
D. I, II and III All
E. None of these

34. High blood pressure is a major risk factor for:
A. Stroke
B. Coronary heart disease
C. Heart failure
D. Kidney failure
E. All of the above

35. Which of the following statement is/are false?
A. The higher the B.P. the greater the risk and lower the life expectancy

B. The bulk of mortality associated with hypertension is due to CVS disease
C. In Western nations it is mainly due to coronary heart disease
D. In Japan and Taiwan from stroke
E. None of the above

36. Which of the following statements is/are false about modifiable risk factors of hypertension?
A. The greater the weight gain, the greater the risk of blood pressure
B. Low Na^+ intake (salt) has been found to lower blood pressure
C. Potassium (K^+) antagonises the biological effects of Na^+ and thereby reduces the blood pressure
D. High intake of Ca^{++} and Mg^{++} raises blood pressure
E. Saturated fats raises blood pressure as well as serum cholesterol

37. A major reason for identifying and treating asymptomatic hypertension is:
A. To reduce the incidence of stroke
B. To reduce the kidney damage
C. To reduce the heart damage
D. To reduce liver damage
E. All of these

38. The main somatoneurological disorder in about 90% of patients of stroke is:
A. Coma
B. Hemiplegia
C. Paraplegia
D. Speech disturbances
E. All of the above

39. "Strokes in the young" can be seen in which countries of the world?
A. Japan
B. Taiwan
C. India
D. USA
E. UK only

40. "Arterial hypertension" is the major cause of:
A. Stroke
B. Heart failure
C. Kidney failure
D. Diabetes mellitus

41. "Juvenile mitral stenosis" means, the disease is seen below the age of:
A. 1 year
B. 5 years
C. 10 years
D. 16 years
E. 20 years

42. In India, it is estimated that over .... children are affected by RHD (Rheumatic heart disease):
A. 3 million
B. 6 million
C. 12 million
D. 15 million
E. 20 million

43. Which virus is associated with rheumatic fever causation?
A. Adenovirus
B. Bunyavirus
C. Coxsachie B-4
D. Rhinovirus

44. In RHD, the most common ECG finding is the:
A. Prolonged PR interval
B. 1st degree AV block
C. 2nd degree AV block
D. Pulsus bigeminus
E. Two of the above

45. Following C/M of rheumatic fever do not cause permanent residual damage, *but* one:
A. Polyarthritis
B. Subcutaneous nodules
C. Chorea
D. Carditis
E. Erythema marginatum

46. Which of the following minor manifestations are not included under revised

Jones criteria for diagnosing rheumatic fever?
A. Demonstration of ASO titre
B. Abnormal ESR
C. C-reactive protein
D. Leukocytosis
E. Prolonged PR interval

47. **The most common C/M of rheumatic fever is:**
A. Carditis
B. Polyarthritis
C. Chorea
D. Subcutaneous nodules

48. **Following C/M in a patient of RF seen during active acute phase, *except:***
A. Fever
B. Carditis
C. Subcutaneous nodules
D. Polyarthritis

49. **Following is mandatory to diagnose rheumatic fever:**
A. Polyarthritis
B. Chorea
C. Carditis
D. +ve ASO antibodies
E. All of these

50. **In the world arenas what % of death has been attributed to cancers?**
A. 2% B. 5%
C. 7.5% D. 10%
E. 12%

51. **For both developed and developing nations the most common cancer site in men is:**
A. Lung
B. Prostate
C. Oropharynx
D. Skin
E. All the above

52. **The incidence of lung C_A increase gradually since:**
A. 1930s
B. 1990s
C. 1940s
D. 1970s
E. 1960s

53. **Cancer was the 6th leading cause of death at the beginning of this century. Now it is 2nd leading cause of death owing to following reasons:**
A. Longer life expectancy
B. More accurate diagnostic methodology
C. Rise in cigarette smoking
D. All of these
E. Both A and B above

54. **The cervical C_A is high in which countries?**
A. Angola
B. Britain
C. Columbia
D. Denmark
E. Japan

55. **What % of all human cancers are attributable to environmental factors?**
A. 10%
B. 25%
C. 30 to 50%
D. 51 to 75%
E. 80 to 90%

56. **Tobacco is the major environmental cause of following cancers:**
I. C_A lung
II. C_A larynx
III. C_A mouth and pharynx
IV. C_A urinary bladder
V. C_A oesophagus
VI. C_A pancreas
Choose the correct answer as per code given below:
A. I, II, III and V only
B. I, II, III, IV and V only
C. I, II, III, IV, V and VI All
D. I, III and V

57. **What % of cancer deaths has been attributed to "ALCOHOL" use?**
A. 1% B. 3%
C. 5% D. 7%
E. 11% only

58. Regarding dietary factors and cancer which is false?

A. Smoked fish stomach C_A
B. Dietary fibres cause intestinal C_A
C. Beef consumption to bowel C_A
D. High fat diet to Breast C_A
E. None of these

59. Consider the following statement about viral aetiology of cancer:

I. EBV (Epstein-Barr Virus) is associated with 2 malignancy like Burkitt's lymphoma and Nasopharyngeal C_A
II. HPV is a chief suspect in CA cervix
III. Classical Kaposi's sarcoma is associated with a higher prevalence of antibodies to CMV
IV. HBV and HCV is causally related to hepatocellular CA

Choose the correct answer as per code given below:

A. I, II, III and IV All
B. I, II and IV
C. I, II and III
D. I and III only
E. II and IV only

60. The 1st C/M of AIDS epidemic to be recognised is:

A. NHL
B. Burkitt's lymphoma
C. Kaposi's sarcoma
D. All of the above
E. Both A and B above

61. Which parasitoses is associated with cancer in human?

A. Ascariasis
B. Naegleria fowleri
C. Onchocerciasis only
D. Schistosomiasis only
E. Two of the above

62. Which nation in the world has developed ambitious programme to eradicate tobacco smoking by the year 2000?

A. Argentina
B. Britain
C. USA
D. Japan
E. Norway only

63. Following are recognised PRECANCEROUS lesions, *save* for one:

A. Adenomata
B. Chronic gastritis/cervicitis
C. Cervical tears only
D. Intestinal polyposis only
E. None of these

64. "DANGER SIGNALS" of cancer includes all the following, *but* one:

A. A lump or hard area in breast
B. Unexplained fever
C. Unexplained loss of weight
D. Blood loss from any natural orifice

65. Primary prevention in cancer control include the following, *but* one:

A. Cancer screening
B. Control of tobacco and alcohol consumption
C. Cancer education
D. Treatment of precancerous lesions
E. Legislation

66. Population-based cancer registries have been established at the following cities in India under the National Cancer Registry Project of the ICMR, *but* one:

A. Mumbai
B. Bangalore
C. Calcutta
D. Chennai
E. None of the above

67. Effective screening programmes have been developed for:

A. Cervical C_A
B. Breast C_A
C. Oral C_A
D. All of these
E. Both A and C above

68. Radiation is NOT the chief hazard in breast C_A screening, *but* one:
A. BSE
B. Palpation by a physician
C. Mammography
D. Thermography
E. None of these

69. Which is NOT a constituent of Nass or Nasswar?
A. Tobacco
B. Betel quid
C. Ashes
D. Lime
E. Cottonseed oil

70. "Betel quid" consists of the following:
I. Betal leaf
II. Arecanut
III. Lime
IV. Tobacco

Choose the correct answer from the code given below:
A. I, II, III and IV All
B. I, II and III
C. I and IV only
D. I, III and IV only
E. I and III only

71. "Epidermoid C_A of hard palate" is common in India in:
A. Assam
B. Andhra Pradesh
C. Bihar
D. Delhi
E. J and K

72. Which is NOT true about carcinoma cervix?
A. CACX is more common in low socio-economic class
B. It is the 1st most common cancer among women worldwide
C. The 5 years survival rate is virtually 100% for carcinoma in situ
D. CACX is difficult to cure once symptoms develop and is fatal if left untreated

73. Incidence of Breast C_A is high in the following *but* one:
A. USA
B. Scotland
C. Japan
D. Australia
E. Canada

74. Regarding Breast C_A which is NOT correct?
A. The mean age of occurrence is about 42 in India
B. It is uncommon below the age of 35 years
C. Positive family history
D. Married women tend to have more breast tumours

75. "Early menarche and late menopause" is an established risk factors in which of the following tumours?
A. C_AC_X
B. C_A breast
C. C_A bladder
D. C_A lung
E. C_A pancreas

76. Consider the following statements about lung cancer:
I. Lung C_A is directly related to amount and duration of cigarette smoking
II. In India it accounts for 6.8% of all malignancies
III. It is the most common malignancy globally in both sexes combined
IV. "Passive smokers" are at increased risk for developing lung C_A

Choose the correct answer from the code given below:
A. I, II, III and IV All
B. I, II and III only
C. II, III and IV only
D. I and II only
E. I and III only

77. The most carcinogenic substance in tobacco smoke includes:
A. Nicotine

B. Tar
C. Carbonmonoxide
D. All of the above
E. Both A and C above

78. Factors implicated in causation of lung C_A includes the following:
I. Air pollution
II. Radioactivity
III. Chromates
IV. Occupational exposure to asbestos, arsenic and its compounds
V. Particles containing polycyclic aromatic hydrocarbons and certain nickel-bearing dusts

Select the true response from the code given below:
A. I, II and III
B. II, III and IV
C. II, III and V
D. I, II, III, IV and V All
E. I, II, IV and V

79. Causation of smoking in smokers leads to following "ABSTINENCE SYMPTOMS" *save* for one:
A. Sleeplessness
B. Dizziness
C. Craving for smoking
D. Constipation
E. Diarrhoea only

80. Regarding stomach cancer, which of the following is/are false?
A. It is the world's 2nd most common cancer
B. High risk areas include central and South America and Eastern Asia and Japan
C. Most gastric cancers are adenoacanthomas
D. Helicobacter pylori has been implicated in its causation
E. Most cases diagnosed when the disease is at an advanced stage

81. The most severe from of diabetes mellitus (DM) is:
A. IDDM
B. NIDDM
C. MRDM
D. IGT
E. GDM only

82. Regarding diabetes, which is NOT true?
A. It is the 4th leading cause of death in USA
B. An "iceberg" disease
C. Affecting 150 million people throughout the world
D. Severe hypoglycaemia is a significant cause of death in diabetes
E. IDDM is very uncommon in Chinese, Japanese and American Indians

83. Which of the following countries reported LEAST incidence of diabetes mortality?
A. Trinidad and Tobago
B. Japan
C. USA
D. Belgium
E. Greece

84. The major causes of prolonged ill health in diabetics includes the following, select the true one as per code given below:
I. Coronary heart disease
II. Glomerulosclerosis
III. Retinopathy
IV. Gangrene of a lower extremity
V. Neuropathy
VI. Stroke and cataract

Code:
A. I, II, III, IV, V and VI All
B. I, III and V only
C. I, II, IV, V and VI
D. II, III, V and VI

85. In India the overall prevalence rate for diabetes mellitus is:
A. 1.1%
B. 0.5%
C. 1.73%
D. 2.75%
E. 3.85%

86. IDDM is related to following HLA-genetic markers:

I. HLA-DR_3

II. HLA-DR_4

III. HLA-B_8

IV. HLA-B_{15}

Of these with which it is more powerfully associated:

A. I and III
B. I and II only
C. I, II and III
D. I, II, III and IV All
E. III and IV only

87. Which is NOT true regarding host factors in diabetes mellitus?

A. Malnutrition related D.M. affects large numbers of young people
B. In India males outnumbers females in respect of D.M.
C. The highest risk of IDDM is carried by individuals with both DR_3 and DR_4
D. NIDDM is strongly associated with HLA-B_8 and HLA-B_{15}
E. Obesity appears to play no role in IDDM pathogenesis

88. Following viral infection may cause D.M. *save* for one:

A. Rubeola
B. Mumps
C. Coxsackie B_4
D. Rubella
E. None of the above

89. Excessive intake of ALCOHOL may increase the risk of D.M. by:

A. Damaging pancreas
B. Damaging liver
C. Promoting obesity
D. All of the above
E. Both A and C above

90. Which of the following toxins selectively damages Red cells of pancreas?

A. Alloxan only
B. Valcor
C. Streptozotocin
D. Both A and B above
E. All of the above

91. Which of the following statements is/are false about D.M.?

A. Insulin deficiency is absolute in IDDM while partial in NIDDM
B. Sedentary lifestyle appears to be an important risk factor for the development of IDDM
C. Surgery trauma or stress may bring out the disease
D. It is now common in the lower social classes

92. Screening of following "high risk groups" in D.M. considered appropriate:

I. Those in the age group of 40 and above

II. Those with a F/H of D.M.

III. Women who show excess weight gain during pregnancy

IV. Obese person

V. Patients with premature atherosclerosis

Choose the true answer from the code given below:

A. I, II and III
B. I, II, III and IV
C. I, II, III, IV and V All
D. I, III and V
E. I, II and IV

93. The cornerstone of diagnosis of diabetes mellitus (D.M.) is:

A. Standard oral glucose test
B. Random blood sample
C. Urine test only
D. Glucose measurement of fasting
E. Postprandial glucose estimation

94. Which of the following is regarded as DIABETOGENIC DRUGS?

A. Antipshchotics
B. Barbiturates

C. Cannabis
D. Oral contraceptives

95. **Following high-risk strategy are applicable for NIDDM, *but* one:**
A. Smoking
B. High B.P.
C. Raised cholesterol
D. High triglyceride level
E. None of the above

96. **Primordial prevention has got definite role in:**
A. IDDM
B. NIDDM
C. IGT
D. All of these
E. Both A and B above

97. **Regarding glycosylated hemoglobin, which is incorrect?**
A. It should be estimated at monthly intervals
B. It provides a long-term index of glucose control
C. The rationale behind this test is that glucose in the blood is complexed to a certain fraction of Hb to an extent proportional to the blood glucose concentration
D. The % of glycated Hb reflects the mean blood glucose levels during the red cell life-time (previous 2 to 3 months)

98. **Consider the following statements about OBESITY and give answer correctly according to the code given below:**
I. Obesity may be defined as an abnormal growth of adipose tissue that causes either enlarged cell size or its number or combination of both
II. A BMI of 30 or more in males and 28.6 or more in females indicate obesity
III. Hyperplastic obesity in adults is extremely difficult to treat with conventional methods
IV. The accumulation of one Kg of fat corresponds to 7700 Kcals of energy
Code:
A. I, II and III
B. I, II, III and IV All
C. I, II and IV
D. I, III and IV

99. **Obesity can be seen in the following:**
A. Cushing's syndrome
B. G H deficiency
C. Both of the above
D. None of the above

100. **Human body consists of following components:**
I. The active mass (muscle, liver, hearts etc.)
II. The Adipose tissue
III. The ECF (blood, lymph etc.)
IV. The connective tissue (skin, bones etc.)
In obesity which of the above component gets increased at the expense of the other code:
A. I only
B. I and II only
C. I, II and III
D. II only
E. I, II, III and IV All

101. **In obesity water (H_2O) content of body .... increases.**
A. Often
B. Sometimes
C. Never
D. Always
E. Not documented

102. **"Quitelet's index" is also known as:**
A. Ponderal index
B. Body mass index
C. Corpulence index
D. Broca index
E. None of these

103. For assessment of obesity which index is widely used?
A. Quetelet's index
B. Broca index
C. Corpulence index
D. Both A and B above
E. All of the above

104. Regarding skin fold thickness for obesity assessment, true is:
A. It is a rapid and non-invasive method for assessing body fat
B. Harpenden skin calipers are used for this purpose
C. The measurement may be taken at all the 4 sites—triceps, biceps, subscapular and suprailiac region
D. The sum of measurements at all 4 sites should be < 40 mm in boys and < 50 mm in girls
E. All of the above

105. More accurate method of obesity can be done by measuring:
A. Body density
B. Total body water
C. Total body potassium
D. All of the above

106. Obesity is the positive risk factor in the development of the following:
A. Hypertension
B. D.M.
C. Gall bladder disease
D. Coronary heart diseases
E. All of the above

107. The WHO defined blindness as "visual acuity of < .... (snellen) or its equivalent".
A. 3/60
B. 2/60
C. 1/60
D. 6/18
E. 6/60

108. According to NPCB-WHO Survey (1986-89), the following Indian states have highest prevalence of blindness, *save* for one:
A. Andhra Pradesh
B. Bihar
C. Tamil Nadu
D. Rajasthan
E. Orissa

109. In India what % of blindness cases are attributable to injuries?
A. 0.5%
B. 1.0%
C. 1.2%
D. 2.1%
E. 2.95%

110. Most common cause of blindness in India is:
A. Vitamin-A deficiency
B. Glaucoma
C. Corneal opacity
D. Cataract
E. All of the above

111. DOCTORS are more prone to develop premature cataracts because they are more exposed to:
A. X-rays
B. UVR rays
C. Heat waves
D. All of these
E. Both A and C above

112. The goal of the national programmes for the control of blindness in India is to reduce blindness in the country to .... by 2000 AD.
A. 3.30%
B. 0.1%
C. 0.3%
D. 0.9%
E. 1.0%

113. The most frequent causes of blindness in developed nations include all, *except:*
A. Accident
B. Glaucoma
C. Diabetes

D. Trachoma
E. Vascular diseases

114. **Common causes of blindness in younger age groups include all, *but* one:**
A. Accidents
B. Conjunctivitis
C. Cataract
D. Diabetes
E. Glaucoma

115. **People working in factories, workshops and cottage industries are more prone to eye injuries owing to following reasons:**
A. Exposure to dust and air borne particles
B. Exposure to flying objects
C. Exposure to gases and fumes
D. Exposure to radiation etc.
E. All of the above

116. **What % of total blindness has been attributable to cataract in India?**
A. 60%
B. 66%
C. 70%
D. 81%
E. 90%

117. **Which of the following diseases of the eye needs tertiary care?**
A. Corneal grafting
B. Glaucoma
C. Cataract
D. Ocular trauma
E. All of the above

118. **Secondary eye care may be provided by all the following, *but* one:**
A. Primary health centre
B. Medical colleges
C. Mobile eye clinic
D. District hospitals only
E. None of these

119. **In India, National Institute for Blind is established at:**
A. Ahmedabad
B. Mumbai
C. Dehradun
D. Sitapur
E. Amritsar

120. **The goal of WHO and International Agency for Prevention of Blindness is to eliminate what % of the world's avoidable blindness by the year 2000 AD?**
A. 50%
B. 60%
C. 70%
D. 80%
E. 100%

121. **Accidents are responsible for approximately what % of all deaths in the world?**
A. 2%
B. 4%
C. 9.1%
D. 12%
E. 16%

122. **The term "KILLED" in road traffic accidents indicates death of an individual within how many days of trauma?**
A. One
B. Three
C. Seven
D. 15 days
E. 30 days

123. **The highest road accident rates (motor vehicles) in the world is reported from:**
A. U.S.A.
B. India
C. Canada
D. U.K.
E. Italy only

124. **The main factor involved in railway accidents is:**
A. Faulty track
B. Faulty equipment
C. Human failure
D. Sabotage
E. All of the above

125. Promotion of following safety measures reduces the risks of accidents:
A. Seat belts
B. Safety helmets
C. Leather clothing and boots
D. All of those
E. Both A and B above

126. Bearing safety helmets reduces the risk of fatal outcome in accidents by what percentage?
A. 10%
B. 20%
C. 30%
D. 40%
E. 50%

127. What % of severe road accidents has been attributable to alcohol consumption?
A. 10 to 20%
B. 20 to 40%
C. 30 to 50%
D. 40 to 60%

128. The risks of accident rises significantly between blood alcohol level:
A. 10 to 20 mg/100 ml
B. 20 to 30 mg/100 ml
C. 40 to 60 mg/100 ml
D. 50 to 80 mg/100 ml

129. Drugs should be strictly avoided owing to impair one's ability to drive safely includes the following *but* one:
A. Piroxicam
B. Barbiturates
C. Amphetamines
D. Cannabis

130. What % of GDP losses attributable to road accidents around the world?
A. 0 to 1%
B. 1 to 2%
C. 2 to 3%
D. 4 to 5%

131. In 2002 the global rate of deaths from road traffic injuries was about how much?
A. 10 per 100,000 people
B. 19 per 100,000 people
C. 30 per 100,000 people
D. 40 per 100,000 people

132. Injury is not a problem as a road traffic accident in which of the following nations?
A. DPR Korea
B. Nepal
C. Bhutan
D. Thailand

133. The main objective of Vision 2020 is to avoid:
A. Avoidable blindness
B. Childhood blindness
C. Corneal blindness
D. All of the above

134. In which nations screening by photo-fluoroscopy for stomach C_A has been in operation since 1960s?
A. USA
B. Japan
C. Canada
D. UK (Britain)

135. "Isolated systolic hypertension" is defined as a systolic B.P. of .... mm kg or more and a diastolic B.P. of < .... mm Hg.
A. 140, 90
B. 160, 100
C. 180, 105
D. 200, 110

136. In India "Jai Vigyan Mission Mode Project" on community control of which disease has been implemented?
A. Hypertension
B. CAD
C. RF and RHD
D. Diabetes mellitus

137. "CAREMOMAS" arises from epithelial linings of:
A. GIT tract
B. Uterus
C. Skin
D. All of the above

138. Following cancers may be associated with top three (1, 2, 3) causes of death from cancer, *but* one:
A. C_A lung
B. C_A breast
C. C_A stomach
D. C_A liver

139. "Cancer of affluent societies" includes the following, *except:*
A. Hepatic C_A
B. C_A breast
C. C_A lung
D. C_A colorectum
E. C_A prostate

140. The term "tracking" of blood pressure refers to:
A. 24 hours BP monitoring
B. BP control with nifedipine
C. Identifying children at risk of developing hypertension at future date
D. Pictorial representation of BP

141. For every 100,000 population, the highest prevalence of blindness in the world is seen in:
A. South Asia
B. Sub-Sahara Africa
C. Latin America
D. Eastern Europe

142. Taking the definition of blindness as visual acquity < 3/60 in the better eye, the number of blind person per 100,000 population in India is estimated to be:
A. 500
B. 600
C. 700
D. 1000

143. Prevalence of RHD in childdren in India:
A. 3/1000
B. 6/1000
C. 8/1000
D. 10/100

144. The most sensitive and specific screening test to detect breast C_A is:
A. Regular X-ray
B. Self breast examination
C. Regular biopsy
D. Mammography

145. According to WHO, blindness is defined as a visual acuity of the better eye, less than:
A. 3/60
B. 4/60
C. 5/60
D. 6/60

146. Several studies have shown that 85% of cases of lung cancer are due to cigarette smoking. It is a measure of:
A. Attributable risk
B. Relative risk
C. Absolute risk
D. Incidence rate

147. Following is most strongly associated with coronary heart disease?
A. VLDL
B. Apolipoproteins
C. HDL
D. Total lipoproteins

148. Under NPCPNB, a child in the age group of 6 to 11 months is given a mega dose of Vitamin A equal to:
A. 50,000 IU
B. 1 lakh IU
C. 1.5 lakh IU
D. 2 lakh IU

Answers

1 B	2 C	3 B	4 A	5 C	6 E	7 D	8 B	9 A	10 D
11 C	12 B	13 D	14 A	15 C	16 B	17 C	18 B	19 A	20 D
21 C	22 E	23 A	24 D	25 C	26 B	27 C	28 A	29 E	30 D
31 B	32 C	33 E	34 E	35 E	36 D	37 A	38 B	39 C	40 A
41 E	42 B	43 C	44 B	45 D	46 A	47 B	48 C	49 D	50 E
51 A	52 A	53 D	54 C	55 E	56 C	57 B	58 E	59 A	60 C
61 D	62 E	63 E	64 B	65 A	66 C	67 D	68 C	69 B	70 A
71 B	72 B	73 C	74 D	75 B	76 A	77 B	78 D	79 E	80 C
81 A	82 D	83 B	84 A	85 E	86 B	87 D	88 A	89 D	90 E
91 B	92 C	93 A	94 D	95 E	96 B	97 A	98 B	99 C	100 D
101 C	102 B	103 D	104 E	105 D	106 E	107 A	108 B	109 C	110 D
111 D	112 C	113 D	114 B	115 E	116 D	117 A	118 B	119 C	120 A
121 C	122 E	123 A	124 C	125 D	126 D	127 C	128 D	129 A	130 B
131 B	132 A	133 D	134 B	135 A	136 C	137 D	138 B	139 A	140 C
141 B	142 C	143 A	144 D	145 A	146 A	147 B	148 B		

C•H•A•P•T•E•R **SEVEN**

PSM in Obstetrics, Paediatrics and Geriatrics

DIRECTION: Following MCQ's are provided with a few suggestive answers/completions. Only one answer is correct. You have to identify the *BEST* one in each case.

1. **In developing countries % of mother and children overall is:**
   A. 50%
   B. 60%
   C. 65%
   D. 70%
   E. 75%

2. **In India, women of child-bearing age (15 to 44) constitute about:**
   A. 19%
   B. 22%
   C. 25%
   D. 15%
   E. 27%

3. **In India, % of children under 15 years of age is:**
   A. 35%
   B. 40%
   C. 42%
   D. 45%

4. **Statement (S): Mother and child must be considered as one unit.**

   Reason (R): Because in the care cycle of women, there are few occasions where service to the child is not simultaneously called for.

   Select the true answer as per code given below:
   A. Both (S) and (R) are true but unrelated to cause and affect
   B. (S) is true, (R) is false
   C. (R) is true, (S) is false
   D. Both (S) and (R) are true and are related to cause and effect
   E. Both (S) and (R) are false

5. **The period of development of foetus in mother is about:**
   A. 265 days
   B. 270 days
   C. 280 days
   D. 300 days

6. **The 1st clinical subject to link itself to preventive medicine is:**
   A. Medicine
   B. Paediatrics
   C. Obstetrics
   D. Pathology

7. **The stages of maternity cycle includes the following:**
   I. Fertilization
   II. Antenatal or prenatal period
   III. Intranatal period

IV. Post-natal period
V. Interconceptional period

Select the true answer as per code given below:
A. I, II and III
B. I, II, III and IV
C. I, II, III, IV and V All
D. I, III and V

8. **"Embryo" is the term for concepts material after:**
A. 0 to 7 days
B. 0 to 14 days
C. 0 to 3 days
D. 14 days to 9 weeks
E. 14 days to 6 weeks

9. **From the period 9th week upto birth the product of conception is called as:**
A. Foetus
B. Embryo
C. Ovum only
D. Full term birth
E. Premature infant

10. **A premature infant is that infant who is born from:**
A. 0 to 14 days
B. 28 to 37 weeks
C. 9th weeks to birth
D. 14 days to 9 weeks

11. **Currently, the main health problems affecting the health of the mother and the child in India and other developing countries is:**
A. Malnutrition
B. Infection
C. Unregulated fertility
D. All of the above
E. Both A and B above

12. **Maternal infections may cause following adverse effects:**
I. Foetal growth retardation.
II. Low birth weight
III. Embryopathy
IV. Abortion
V. Puerperal sepsis

Select the true answers as per code given below:
A. I, II and III
B. I, II, III and IV
C. I, II, III, IV and V All
D. I, III and V

13. **What % of women in rural areas suffer at least one bout of urinary tract (UTI)?**
A. 5%
B. 10%
C. 15%
D. 20%
E. 25%

14. **Statement (S): Indirect notation interventions have still under ramifications.**
Reason (R): Because they are not specifically related to nutrition.
Select the true answer as per code given below:
A. Both (S) and (R) are true, and are related to cause and effect
B. Both (S) and (R) are true, but are not related to cause and effect
C. (S) is true, (R) are false
D. (R) is true, (S) is false
E. Both (S) and (R) are false

15. **Upto 1996, IMR is least in which nations of the world?**
A. UK
B. Japan
C. USA
D. Switzerland
E. India

16. **Crude birth rate is highest in which country?**
A. India
B. Bangladesh
C. Pakistan
D. China

17. Upto 1996, IMR is highest in which country?
A. Thailand
B. Bangladesh
C. Pakistan
D. China

18. Under five mortality rate per 1000 live births (1996) is highest in which country of the world?
A. Bangladesh
B. India
C. Pakistan
D. Singapore

19. In India, CBR (1993) ....., IMR (1996) ....., under five mortality rate (1996) ..... is:
A. 10, 4, 6
B. 40, 78, 104
C. 29, 75, 99
D. 19, 35, 43

20. The ultimate objective of MCH services is:
A. Reduction of maternal, parental, childhood morbidity
B. Promotion of reproductive health
C. Promotion of the physical and psychological development of the child and adolescent within the family
D. Life-long health
E. All of these

21. Antenatal care means:
A. Care of women during pregnancy
B. Care of women during 1st trimester of gestation
C. Care of women during 2nd trimester of gestation
D. Care of women during 3rd trimester of gestation

22. Minimum number of antenatal visits during pregnancy is:
A. One
B. Two
C. Three
D. Four
E. Five

23. All are important antenatal investigation, *except:*
A. X-ray chest
B. Hb estimation
C. Serological tests
D. Blood grouping and Rh determination

24. Recognised high risk antenatal cases include:
I. Elderly primi
II. Short statured primi
III. Preeclampsia
IV. Malpresentation
V. Anaemia

Choose the correct answer from the code given below:
A. I, III and V
B. I, II, III, IV and V All
C. I, II and III
D. I, II, III and IV

25. On an average, a normal healthy woman gains:
A. 8 kg
B. 10 kg
C. 12 kg
D. 14 kg
E. 16 kg

26. Strike the false statement regarding personal hygiene in pregnancy:
A. Smoking should be cut down to minimum
B. Should bath everyday and wear clean clothes
C. Constipation should be avoided by regular intake of green leafy vegetables
D. 8 hours sleep is necessary 2 hours rest after lunch
E. Sexual intercourse should be allowed especially during last trimester

27. The most source of radiation during pregnancy is:
A. Skull X-ray
B. Chest X-ray
C. X-ray of neck region

D. Abdominal X-ray
E. All of the above

28. Following drugs adversely affect the foetus if taken by mother during pregnancy, *save* for one:
A. Thalidomide only
B. L.S.D.
C. Corticosteroids only
D. Streptomycin/Tetracycline
E. Penicillin

29. Recognised warning signs in pregnancy includes the following:
I. Swelling of the feet
II. Headache and blurring of vision
III. Bleeding and discharge P/V
IV. Fits only

Choose the correct answer as per code given below:
A. I and II only
B. I, II and III
C. I, II, III and IV All
D. II, III and IV

30. What type of anemia commonly encountered in pregnancy in India?
A. Iron deficiency
B. Folate deficiency
C. Both of the above
D. None of these

31. Regarding active immunization against tetanus to all expectant mothers, which is false?
A. Two doses of TT should be given those not immunized
B. Those earlier immunized should not be given any dose
C. The 1st dose at 16 to 20 weeks
D. The 2nd dose 20 to 24 weeks

32. Consider the following statement:
I. The presence of albumin in urine and an increase in blood pressure indicates toxaemias of pregnancy
II. Women who smoke during pregnancy give birth to babies which are an average weigh 170 gm less at term than the babies of non-smokers
III. The Government of India recommended 60 mg of elemental iron and 500 mcg of folic acid daily to pregnant
IV. Pregnancies in women with primary and secondary syphilis often and in spontaneous abortion

Select the true answer from the code given below:
A. I and II
B. I, II and III
C. I, II, III and IV All
D. I, III and IV

33. Alcohol consumption (moderate/heavy) during pregnancy may cause the following:
A. Spontaneous abortion
B. Foetal alcohol syndrome
C. IUGR
D. Developmental delay
E. All of the above

34. The use of THALIDOMIDE during pregnancy has been proved to be most serious:
A. 1 to 3 weeks of IUL
B. 4 to 8 weeks of IUL
C. 9 to 12 weeks of IUL
D. 2 to 4 months of IUL
E. 3 to 6 months of intrauterine life

35. When the mother is suffering from syphilis, infection of the foetus does not ensue before the .... of pregnancy.
A. 1st month
B. 2nd month
C. 3rd month
D. 4th month

36. The risk of all degrees of malformation may remain in the region of what % upto 20th weeks of IUL following germ and measles infection?
A. 5%

B. 10%
C. 20%
D. 30%
E. 35%

37. In a Rh negative mother, following Rh +ve gestation to prevent sensitization during the 1st pregnancy the Rh anti D Ig should preferably be given at what weeks of gestation?

A. 20 weeks
B. 24 weeks
C. 28 weeks
D. 32 weeks
E. 36 weeks

38. HIV infection may pass from an infected mother to her foetus:

A. Through the placenta
B. During delivery
C. Breast feeding
D. All of these
E. Both A and B

39. Recognised advantages of domiciliary deliveries include all the following, *but* one:

A. The chances of cross infection are generally fewer
B. The mother may have less medical and nursing supervision
C. The mother delivers in the familiar surroundings
D. The mother is able to keep an eye upon her children and domestic affairs

40. Who is regarded as a "pivot" of domiciliary care?

A. Female health worker
B. Trained dais
C. Midwife nurse
D. Female health assistant

41. Following is/are "danger signals" during labour:

I. Good pains for an hour after rupture of membranes
II. Prolapse of the cord or hand
III. Meconium stained liquor or a slow irregular or excessively fast FHS (foetal heart sound)
IV. A placenta not separated within half an hour after delivery

Choose the true answer as per code given below:

A. I and II only
B. I, II, III and IV All
C. I, II and III
D. II, III and IV

42. Recognised advantages of "Rooming in" includes:

A. To know her baby
B. Better for breast feeding
C. Allays the fear about misplaced baby in central nursery
D. Builds up self-confidence
E. All of the above

43. Consider the following statements:

I. Keeping the baby's crib by the side of the mother's bed is called "rooming-in"
II. Bleeding from vagina anytime from 6 hours, after delivery to the end of the puerperium (6 weeks) is called secondary haemorrhage
III. Thrombophlebitis is an infection of the veins of the legs, frequently associated with varicose veins

Choose the correct answer as per following code:

A. I, II and III All
B. I and II only
C. I and III
D. II and III

44. The common condition found on examination during the late postnatal period includes:

I. Subinvolution of uterus
II. Retroverted uterus
III. Prolapse of uterus
IV. Cervicitis

Select the true answer as per code given below:

A. I and IV
B. I, II and III
C. I, II, III and IV All
D. II, III and IV

45. Postpartum sterilization is generally recommended on which day after delivery?

A. 1st
B. 2nd
C. 3rd
D. 4th
E. 5th day

46. Statement (S): The childhood period is also a vital period.

Reason (R): Because, they are valuable to disease death and disability, owing to their age, sex, place of living, socioeconomic class and a host of other variables.

Select the true answer as per following code:

A. Both (S) and (R) are true and are related to each other
B. Both (S) and (R) are true but are unrelated to each other
C. (S) is true, (R) is false
D. (R) is true, (S) is false
E. Both (S) and (R) are false

47. Maximum output breast milk occurs at months of lactation?

A. 0-2
B. 2-3
C. 3-4
D. 5-6
E. 6-7 months

48. In India, INFANTS (0 to 1 year) constitute what % of the total population?

A. 1%
B. 1.92%
C. 2.92%
D. 3.29%
E. 4.19%

49. If "Neonatal period" means first 28 days of life, then what is "post neonatal period"?

A. 7 months of IUL to 1st 6 months after birth
B. After first 4 weeks of life to 1st 3 months of birth
C. After 28 days to 1st 4 years of life
D. 28th day to 1 year of life

50. To date the main purpose of antenatal care is:

A. "Foetus at risk"
B. Prevention of MMR
C. Perinatal mortality
D. Perinatal morbidity

51. The number of children born each year in the entire world arena is:

A. 100 million
B. 140 million
C. 180 million
D. 240 million
E. 500 million

52. What % of total infant mortality ensues in the 1st month of life?

A. 10%
B. 25%
C. 35%
D. 50%
E. 60%

53. Many low cost measures are available for saving life of million of children includes all, *but* one:

A. Immunization
B. Birth spacing
C. Bottle feeding
D. Growth monitoring and improved weaning
E. ORS

54. The most crucial period in the life of an infant is:

A. 1st week of life
B. 2nd week of life
C. 3rd week of life

D. 4th week of life
E. 5th week of life

55. Recognised objectives of early neonatal care includes:

I. Establishments and maintenance of cardiorespiratory functions
II. Maintenance of temperature
III. Avoidance of infection
IV. Establishment of satisfactory feeding regimen
V. Early detection and treatment of congenital and acquired disorders.

Choose the correct answer as per following code:

A. I, II and III only
B. I, III and V only
C. I, II, III and IV only
D. I, II, III, IV and V All
E. II, III, IV only

56. In the "APGAR SCORE" system, the total score is:

A. Zero
B. 5
C. 10
D. 12
E. 14

57. A child is born with slow heart rate, absent respiratory effort, flaccid muscle tone, grimace and body pink and blue extremities. What is its Apgar score?

A. Zero
B. Only one
C. Two
D. Three
E. Five

58. What is the Apgar score of a child who has over 100 heart beat, good crying active movements, grimace and completely pink colour?

A. Three
B. Four
C. Five
D. Seven
E. Nine

59. What provides an immediate estimate of the physical condition of the body?

A. Apgar score
B. Body temperature
C. Muscle
D. Body colour
E. Reflex response

60. The most common organism implicated in cases of ophthalmia neonatorum is:

A. N. gonorrhoea
B. Chlamydia trachomatis
C. Candida albicans
D. Staph aureus

61. Statements (S): The most serious cause of conjunctivitis of the newborn is infection with gonococcus.

Reason (R): Because it can rapidly cause blindness.

Select the true response as per code given below:

A. Both (S) and (R) are true, and are related to each other
B. Both (S) and (R) are true but are unrelated to each other
C. (S) is true, (R) is false
D. (R) is true, (S) is false
E. Both (S) and (R) are false

62. Consider the following statements:

I. A newborn has little thermal control and can lose body heat quickly
II. Most of the heat loss occurs through evaporation of the amniotic fluid from the body of the wet child
III. About 75% of the heat loss can occur from the head
IV. Preterm and LBW babies lose heat more slowly

Choose the correct answer as per following code:

A. I and II only
B. I and III only
C. I, II and III only
D. I, II, III and IV All
E. II, III and IV only

63. The 1st milk (COLOSTRUM) is the most suitable food for baby during early life because:

A. It contains a high concentration of protein
B. It is rich in anti infective factors
C. It protects the body against respiratory and diarrhoeal disease
D. All of these
E. Both A and B above

64. Which examination of the neonates should be preferably done by paediatrician?

A. 1st
B. 2nd
C. 3rd
D. 4th
E. 5th

65. Consider the following statements:

I. In Africa, neonatal infection is particularly common
II. Transplacental contamination is one of the important cause of infection in newborns
III. Neonatal tetanus can be prevented by vaccination of pregnant women
IV. The frequency of congenital syphilis is on decrease in some large African cities

Choose the correct answer as per code given below:

A. I, II and III
B. II and IV only
C. I and III only
D. I, II, III and IV All

66. The risk of transmission of HBV to neonates to how much when the mother has HBS+HBe antigen +ve?

A. 20%
B. 30%
C. 50%
D. 75%
E. 90%

67. Infected neonates with HBV are tend to develop which of the following during adulthood?

A. Chronic active hepatitis
B. Cirrhosis of liver
C. Hepatoma
D. All of these
E. Both A and B above

68. What % of babies born to HIV positive (+ve) mothers get infected with AIDS virus?

A. 10%
B. 20%
C. 30%
D. 50%
E. 100%

69. Following child birth, the most preferable time for recording birth weight is:

A. 1st hour
B. 3rd hour
C. 6 hours
D. 12 hours

70. The birth length or height should be recorded how many days of child birth?

A. One
B. Two
C. Three
D. Four
E. Five days

71. Regarding phenylketonuria (PKU) all are true, *save* for one:

A. Incidence 1 in 10,000 to 20,000
B. Deficient enzyme is phenylalanine hydroxylase
C. Mental retardation and seizures
D. Blood tyrosine markedly increased
E. Guthrie test is the good screening test

72. The most common disorder that is screened today is:

A. Neonatal hypothyroidism
B. Maple syrup urine disease
C. Galactosaemia
D. Phenylketonuria only

73. The basic criteria for identifying "at risk" infants includes all, *but* one:
A. Twins
B. Breast feeding
C. Children with PEM, diarrhea
D. Weight below 70% of the expected weight
E. Failure to gain weight during three successive months

74. The single most important determinant of infant's cleanses of survival, healthy growth and development is:
A. Apgar score
B. Head size determination
C. Birth weight
D. Breast feeding
E. All of the above

75. In India, majority of low birth weight infants are due to the following:
A. Premature delivery
B. Foetal growth retardation
C. Both of the above
D. None of the above

76. The WHO target is reduction in the incidence of LBW to less than how much by 2000 AD?
A. 10%
B. 15%
C. 20%
D. 25%
E. 33%

77. The reported incidence of LBW infants (1990) is least in which countries?
A. India
B. Bangladesh
C. China
D. Holland

78. The reported incidence of LBW infants (1990) is greatest in which nations of the world?
A. Srilanka
B. Thailand
C. Bangladesh
D. China

79. What percentage of infants who weigh less than 2.5 kg at birth represent all live births in India?
A. 10%
B. 22%
C. 30%
D. 33%
E. 43%

80. Consider the following statement about LBW:
I. LBW is the single most important factor determining the survival chances of the child
II. The IMR is about 20 times more for all LBW babies than for other babies of optimum weight
III. LBW babies carry more risk of developing protein energy malnutrition and infection (recurrent)
IV. There is a strong and significant positive correlation between maternal nuritional status and the length of pregnancy and birth weight
Choose the correct answer as per following code:
A. I, II and III only
B. I, II, III and IV All
C. I and IV only
D. I and II only
E. II, III and IV only

81. The following risk factor has to be reduced to prevent LBW babies:
A. Mother's malnutrition
B. Heavy workload
C. Disease and infections
D. High blood pressure
E. All of the above

82. Recognised direct intervention measures to prevent LBW babies includes the following *save* for one:
A. Avoidance smoking
B. Controlling infections
C. Increasing food intake
D. Early detection and treatment of medical disorders

83. **The leading causes of death in LBW babies include:**
I. **Atelectasis**
II. **Malformation**
III. **Pulmonary hemorrhage**
IV. **Intracranial bleeding secondary to anoxia or birth trauma**
V. **Pneumonia and other infections**

Choose the true answer as per following code:
A. I, IV and V only
B. I, II, III, IV and V All
C. I, III and V
D. III, IV and V only
E. I, II and IV only

84. **Which of the following statement is/are false?**
A. Breast milk is the ideal food for infant upto 4 to 5 months after birth
B. Breast milk contains 1.2 gm% protein
C. The energy value of human milk is 70 kcals/100 ml
D. Prolonged breast feeding is not beneficial for infant
E. None of the above

85. **Recognised advantages of breast feeding includes the following, *but* one:**
A. Lactoferrin provide protection against diarrhoeal diseases and necrotizing enterocolitis
B. It retards development of jaws and teeth
C. It protects babies from tendency to obesity
D. Lactation prevents mother to become pregnant
E. It is easily digested and utilized by both the normal and premature infants

86. **Consider the following statements about artificial feeding:**
I. **Infants require 150 ml of mild (100 kcals) per kg of body weight per day**
II. **About 8 to 10% of calories are given as protein**
III. **The carbohydrate, intake should be 10 gm/kg of body weight daily**
IV. **After 4 months of age, undiluted boiled and cooled milk should be given**
V. **During illness (fever) the calories need should preferably be decreased to reduce solute load**

Choose the correct answer as per following code:
A. I, II and III only
B. II, III and V only
C. I, II, III and IV
D. I, II, III, IV and V All
E. I, II and V only

87. **Which of the following constituents is absent in breast milk while comparing with the cow's milk?**
A. β-lactoglobulin
B. Lactalbumin
C. Lactose
D. Linoleic acid
E. Iron only

88. **Artificial feeding is a hazardous procedure in poor homes because of the dangers of:**
A. Contamination
B. Overdilution of the feed
C. Both of the above
D. None of the above

89. **Regarding artificial feeding which is true?**
A. Whole milk should be given 1 month onwards
B. Whole milk should be given 2 months onwards
C. Whole milk should be given 3 months onwards
D. Whole milk should be given 4 months onwards
E. Whole milk should be given 5 months onwards

90. **WEANING should be started around:**
A. 1 to 2 months of age
B. 2 to 3 months of age

C. 3 to 4 months of age
D. 4 to 5 months of age

91. Growth rate is maximum during:
A. Foetal life
B. 1st year of life
C. Puberty
D. Both B and C above
E. All of the above

92. Growth and development in infants may be hampered by the following, *save* for one:
A. Rubella
B. Measles
C. Roundworm infestations
D. Diarrhoeal diseases
E. None of these

93. Consider the following statement:
I. Measurement of weight and rate of gain in weight are the best single parameters for assessing physical growth
II. On an average healthy baby double their birth weight by 5 months, treble by 1 year and quadruple by the end of 2 years of life
III. During the 1st year of life weight increases by 7 kg
IV. In different parts of India the average weight is between 2.7 and 2.9 kg
Select the true answer as per code given below:
A. I, II and III only
B. I, II, III and IV All
C. I and II only
D. I and III only
E. I and IV only

94. The length of baby at birth is:
A. 40 cm
B. 45 cm
C. 50 cm
D. 55 cm
E. 30 cm

95. The gain in length during the 1st year of life is:
A. 10 cm
B. 15 cm
C. 20 cm
D. 25 cm
E. 75 cm

96. Statement (S): Health is a stable measurement of growth as opposed to body weight.
Reason (R): Because weight reflects only the present health status of the child, height indicates the events in the past also.
Select the correct response as per following code:
A. Both (S) and (R) are true but are not related to each other
B. Both (S) and (R) are true and are related to each other
C. (S) is true, (R) is false
D. (R) is true, (S) is false
E. Both (S) and (R) are false

97. A child on the 75th centile of both his height and weight is:
A. Overweight
B. Underweight
C. Normal
D. Neither overweight nor underweight

98. Low weight for height is also known as:
A. Nutritional wasting
B. Emaciation
C. Acute malnutrition
D. Both A and B above
E. All of the above

99. A baby looks at mother and smiles by:
A. 6 to 8 weeks
B. 4 weeks
C. 1 to 3 weeks
D. 8 to 12 weeks

100. A baby recognises mother by:
A. 6 to 8 weeks
B. 3 months

C. 4 to 5 months
D. 6 to 7 months
E. 8 to 10 months

101. A baby begins to reach out for objects is:
A. 6 to 8 weeks
B. 2 months
C. 3 months
D. 4 to 5 months

102. A baby sits without support by:
A. 6 to 8 weeks
B. 3 months
C. 4 months
D. 5 months
E. 6 to 8 months

103. A baby transfers objects hand to hand by:
A. 1 to 2 months
B. 3 months
C. 4 months
D. 6 to 8 months
E. 9 to 10 months

104. A child becomes "dry by day" by:
A. 6 months
B. 12 months
C. 18 months
D. 24 months
E. 36 months

105. At birth, the head circumference is about:
A. 30 cm
B. 34 cm
C. 40 cm
D. 45 cm
E. 50 cm

106. The "head and chest circumference" become equal by:
A. 6 to 9 months
B. 6 to 8 weeks
C. 3 to 6 months
D. One year
E. 2 years

107. The growth or "road-to-health" chart was first designed by:
A. Dean Jones
B. David Morley
C. Charles Mackay
D. Perkins
E. John Snow

108. Statement (S): While assessing growth, the weight-for-age chart has been taken into consideration.

Reason (R): Because weight is the most sensitive measure of growth, and any deviation from "NORMAL" can be assessed easily by comparison with that of reference curves.

Select the correct response as per following code:
A. Both (S) and (R) are true and are related to each other
B. Both (S) and (R) are true but are not related to each other
C. (S) ture, (R) false
D. (R) true, (S) false
E. Both (S) and (R) are false

109. Regarding WHO growth chart, which is true?
A. It has only two reference curves
B. The upper reference curve represents the median (50th percentile) for girls
C. The space between the two growth curves has been called the road-to-health
D. Flattening or falling of the child's weight curve is the earliest sign of protein energy malnutrition
E. All of the above

110. In a reference curve, the 3rd percentile corresponds approximately to how much standard deviations below the median of the weight-for-age reference value?
A. One S.D.
B. Two S.D.
C. Three S.D.

D. Four S.D.
E. Five standard deviation

111. In India, how many growth chart are in use?
A. Nine
B. Nineteen
C. Twentynine
D. Thirtynine
E. Fourtynine only

112. What % of total population in India has been formed by preschool age children?
A. 12%
B. 15%
C. 7%
D. 9%
E. 5.6%

113. What % of total death in India has been shared by preschool age children?
A. 5%
B. 9%
C. 11.2%
D. 15%
E. 25%

114. The diarrhoeal diseases accounts for what % of under five mortality during 1996 in the developing world?
A. 10% B. 13%
C. 18% D. 19%

115. The international union for child welfare has estimated that behavioural problems in children in India is about:
A. 1 million
B. 1.5 million
C. 2.5 million
D. 5 million
E. 7.5 million

116. Which article of Indian Constitution prohibits the employment of children below age 14 in factories?
A. Article 24
B. Article 39
C. Article 45
D. Article 42

117. The aims and objectives of under-fives clinic is embodied in its emblem, that denotes the following:
I. Care in illness
II. Adequate nutrition
III. Immunization
IV. Family planning
V. Health education

Select the true response from the code given below:
A. I, II and IV only
B. I, II and III only
C. I, II, III, IV and V All
D. I, II and V only
E. I, II, III and V only

118. Which article of Indian Constitution provides free and compulsory education for all children until they complete the age of 14 years?
A. Article 14
B. Article 24
C. Article 39
D. Article 42
E. Article 45 only

119. United Nations (UN) declaration of rights of a child do not include:
A. Right for adoption
B. Right for free education
C. Right to a name and nationality
D. Right to enjoy the benefits of social security

120. The uppermost line of the "road to health card" is equivalent to:
A. 50% of Harvard standard
B. 50th percentile of Harvard standard
C. 3rd percentile of Harvard standard
D. 80% of Harvard standard

121. Symbol for under five clinics includes a big triangle having double borderline, inside which lies a small inverted triangle. The double line of the symbol indicates what?
A. Care in illness

B. Growth monitoring
C. Health education
D. Family planning

122. November 14th is observed as universal Children's Day which was started by:
A. The international union for child welfare
B. UNICEF
C. WHO
D. Both A and B above
E. All of the above

123. In which year, the Government of India adopted a national policy for children?
A. Jan 1972
B. Aug 1974
C. May 1976
D. July 1974

124. MCH groups (children under the age 5 years and women in the reproductive age groups (15-44 years) comprises about what % of total population in India?
A. 22%
B. 27%
C. 31.6%
D. 35%
E. 42%

125. Recognised components of MCH care includes:
I. Maternal health
II. Family planning
III. Child health
IV. School health
V. Handicapped children
VI. Care of the children in special settings like day care centres

Choose the true answer as per code given below:
A. I, II, III, IV, V and IV All
B. I, II and III
C. I, II, III and IV
D. I, II, V and VI

126. Recently following field workers has been included under MCH care, *save* for one:
A. MPWs
B. Health visitors
C. Balsevikas
D. Dais (TBA)
E. Anganwadi workers

127. Following are National Health Policy MCH goals by 2000 AD, *except* for one:
A. IMR = < 60
B. Perinatal mortality rate = 35
C. Child mortality rate (0 to 4 years) = 20
D. MMR = 2

128. Under the National Health Policy, following MCH goals are covered by 2000 AD, *save* for:
A. Immunization infant = 100
B. Antenatal care = 100
C. Immunization pregnant ladies = 100
D. Deliveries by trained dai = 100

129. The peripheral outposts of the delivery of MCH/FP services includes the following:
A. PHC
B. Subcentre
C. Additional PHC
D. Anganwadi kendras
E. All of these

130. The principal worker in ICDS project is:
A. Health worker female
B. Trained dais
C. Midwifes
D. Anganwadi worker
E. Auxilliary nurse

131. How many anganwadi workers are working under one ICDS project?
A. 10
B. 50
C. 100
D. 200
E. 1000

132. The CSSM (child survival and safe motherhood) programme was launched on:
A. 20 April, 1990
B. 21 August 1991

C. 22 May, 1992
D. 22 August, 1992
E. 23 December, 1993

133. Out of 17 goals of National Health Policy (1983) how many programme has to be achieved by CSSM programme?
A. Two
B. Three
C. Five
D. Seven
E. Nine

134. "Non-formal education" is a component of:
A. School health programme
B. ICDS scheme
C. Rural education
D. Mid-day meal programme

135. Social safety net has the following features:
I. The Department of Family Welfare has identified 90 poor performing districts characterised by high birth rates, high IMR and very low levels of institutional deliveries
II. Out of 90 districts 83 are located in Bihar, MP, Rajasthan and UP
III. In each district 10 PHCs will get 1 million rupees to build well equipped labour room, operation theatre and 6 bedded observation ward
IV. Two quarters for LHV and ANM
V. One ambulance per block even ANM if already available
VI. One generator to ensure continuous electric supply
Choose the correct answer as per code given below:
A. I, II, III, IV and VI only
B. I, II, III, IV, V and VI All
C. I, III and V only
D. I, II, III and V only
E. I, III and V only

136. "BFHI" stands for:
A. Bihar Family Health Institution
B. Bengal Family Health Institution
C. British Family Health Institution
D. Baby Friendly Hospital Initiative

137. Which is NOT true regarding BFHI?
A. It is created and promoted by WHO and UNICEF
B. The global BFHI has listed five steps which the hospital must fulfill
C. It has proved highly successful in encouraging proper infant feeding practices starting at birth
D. It is supported in India by major professional medical and nursing bodies
E. Exclusive breast feeding should be promoted till 4 to 6 months of age

138. Following deaths are classified as maternal death, *except:*
A. During 1st month following delivery
B. During labour
C. During 3rd month of lactation
D. During abortion

139. In India (1990), maternal mortality ratio is:
A. 460/100,000 live births
B. 5/100,000 live births
C. 80/100,000 live births
D. 8/1000 live births

140. MMR in India is estimated to be:
A. 0.5/1000 live births
B. 3.4/1000 live births
C. 3.2/1000 live births
D. 8/1000 live births

141. The major cause MMR (1993) in India is:
A. Infection
B. Toxemia of pregnancy
C. Hemorrhage
D. Malnutrition
E. All of the above

142. Following are leading cause of MMR in India *save* for one:
A. Puerperal sepsis
B. Bleeding
C. Anaemia
D. None of these

143. Recognised obstetric causes of MMR in India includes all the following, *but* one:
A. Anemia
B. Hemorrhage
C. Infection
D. Toxemia of pregnancy
E. Obstructed labour

144. A village with a population of 10,000 has a birth rate of 36/4000 population. In one year there have been 5 maternal deaths. The MMR in this village is:
A. 0.5
B. 5
C. 13.8
D. 14.5

145. The perinatal mortality rate (PMR) in India (1995) is:
A. 5 B. 10
C. 20 D. 36
E. 46

146. The national goal is to achieve a PMR between ..... and ..... by the year 2000.
A. 10 and 20
B. 15 and 25
C. 20 and 30
D. 30 and 35

147. The denominator for calculating IMR is:
A. Number of live births in one year
B. No. of infants
C. Mid year population
D. No. of live births + still births in one year

148. The denominator for calculating post neonatal mortality rate (PNMR) is:
A. No. of live births + still births in one year
B. No. of live births in one year
C. No. of neonates
D. Mid year population

149. Most sensitive indicator of health and level of living of people in a community is:
A. MMR
B. PMR
C. IMR
D. NMR
E. None of the above

150. In a health subcentre area with a population of 10,000 there were 300 live births, 6 babies died within a week, 10 died between the 28th day and one year what will be the IMR?
A. 48 B. 78
C. 107 D. 130
E. 150

151. Currently highest IMR (1993) has been reported from which state in India?
A. Bihar
B. M.P.
C. U.P.
D. Rajasthan
E. Orissa

152. The IMR in Kerala in 1993 is:
A. 13 B. 17
C. 23 D. 27
E. 33

153. The IMR of India in 1996 is:
A. 60 B. 74
C. 80 D. 84
E. 90

154. Average calorie intake per day (k cal) in 1988-90 is highest in which of the following Indian states?
A. Andhra Pradesh
B. Tamil Nadu
C. M.P. only
D. Tamil Nadu
E. Karnataka

155. Kerala has managed to surpass all the Indian states in the following aspects *save* for one:
A. Lowest IMR
B. Lowest birth rate
C. Highest literacy rate
D. Highest per capita income

156. What % of infants deaths are attributed to neonatal death?
A. 20%
B. 30%
C. 50%
D. 60%
E. Only 10%

157. The single most important determinant of infant mortality is:
A. Birth weight
B. Age of the mother
C. Birth order
D. Birth spacing
E. Family size

158. Numerator for neonatal mortality is:
A. All infants death under one year
B. All infant deaths upto 28 days
C. All infants less than or equal to 7 days
D. All infant deaths between 28 days to one year

159. The numerator for calculating post-neonatal mortality rate is:
A. Total deaths of infants from 28th day to 1 year age
B. Total deaths of infants from 0 to 1 year age
C. Total deaths of infants from 0 to 1 month age
D. Total deaths of infants from 0 to 7 days age

160. Most common cause of post neonatal mortality is:
A. Malnutrition
B. Birth injury
C. Infection
D. Congenital anomalies
E. All of these

161. Following rate includes still births in numerator:
A. Infant mortality rate
B. Post neonatal mortality
C. PMR
D. NMR only

162. The most sensitive indicator of obstetrics and gynecology services is:
A. IMR
B. NRR
C. CDR
D. PMR
E. All of these

163. Consider the following statements regarding mortality pattern in Indian infants/children:
I. Fatality in 0-1 year age group accounts for 24.1% of all deaths in India
II. About 50% of infant death ensues within the first 4 weeks (neonatal period) of life (birth)
III. The risk of death is greatest during the 1st 24 to 48 hours of birth
IV. In India after the age of one months female deaths are invariably higher than male deaths

Choose the correct answer as per code given below:
A. I, II and III only
B. I, II, III and IV All
C. I and IV
D. II, III and IV

164. Regarding factors affecting infant mortality all are true, *save* for one:
A. An increase in birth wt. would lower the perinatal and neonatal mortality
B. The fate of the 5th and later children is always worse than the fate of the 3rd child
C. Infant mortality is directly proportional to high fertility
D. Wider spacing of birth enhances infant mortality

165. Which of the following Indian states is now on the verge to achieving zero population growth?
A. Kerala
B. Tamil Nadu

C. Karnataka
D. J and K
E. Nagaland

166. The most effective measure for lowering infant mortality is:
A. To immunize the child in proper way
B. To leave brutal habits and customs
C. To promote breast feeding
D. To make the mother well educated

167. In India, under five mortality rate in year (1996) is:
A. 9 per 1000 live births
B. 99 per 1000 live births
C. 19 per 1000 live births
D. 90 per 1000 live births

168. The global average for under five mortality in 1996 is:
A. 9 per 1000 live births
B. 19 per 1000 live births
C. 81 per 1000 live births
D. 90 per 1000 live births

169. UNICEF consider what as the best single indicator of social development and well being rather than GNP per capita is:
A. IMR
B. 1 to 4 years mortality rate
C. MMR only
D. Under 5 mortality rate
E. Child survival index

170. Which Indian states has lowest 1-4 years mortality rate?
A. Tamil Nadu
B. Bihar
C. M.P.
D. U.P.
E. Assam

171. The leading causes of death in 1 to 4 years age group in developing countries include:
I. Diarrhoeal disease
II. Respiratory infections
III. Malnutrition
IV. Infectious diseases
V. Accidents
Choose the correct answer as per following code:
A. I only
B. I and II only
C. I, II and III only
D. I, II, III and IV only
E. I, II, III, IV and V All

172. A child survival rate per 1000 births can be simply calculated by .... the under five mortality rate from 1000.
A. Multiplying
B. Adding
C. Substracting
D. Dividing
E. None of these

173. In India (1996), child survival rate is:
A. 75
B. 79
C. 80
D. 90.1
E. 99.1

174. The worldwide incidence of congenital disorders is estimated at .... per 1000 live births (1989).
A. 6 to 8
B. 16 to 18
C. 3 to 7
D. 20 to 50
E. 30 to 70

175. The most common congenital malformations are of the:
A. CVS
B. CNS
C. Pulmonary system
D. Mouth and palate
E. Both A and B

176. Which of the following statement is/are true?
A. Congenital malformation means merely structural defects at birth
B. Congenital anomaly means all biochemical structural and functional disorders
C. In India 2.5% of newborns have a birth defects

D. Congenital malformations rank as the 3rd most frequent cause of perinatal mortality in India
E. All of the above

177. The highest frequency of neural tube defects is not observed in which Indian states?
A. Punjab
B. West Bengal
C. Rajasthan
D. Delhi
E. Tamil Nadu

178. "Club foot" is the most common congenital malformation in the following Indian zone *save* for one:
A. Southern
B. Eastern
C. Northern
D. Western

179. Following are recognised genetic diseases due to chromosomal anomaly, *but* one:
A. Tay sachs disease
B. Turner syndrome
C. Klinefelter syndrome
D. Down's syndrome

180. A single gene dominant disorder is:
A. Hemophilia
B. Huntington's chorea
C. Thalassemia
D. Sickle cell disease
E. All of the above

181. Following diagnostic tools are available for prenatal diagnosis of genetic diseases, *but* one:
A. Alpha-fetoprotein
B. Ultrasound
C. Amniocentesis
D. Chorionic villi sampling
E. None of these

182. In India for the 1st time medical examination of school children was carried out in which year and where?
A. Patna (1900)
B. Baroda (1909)
C. Calcutta (1909)
D. Delhi (1925)
E. Ernakulam (1910)

183. Recognised objectives of school health services is:
A. The promotion of positive health
B. The prevention of diseases as well as early diagnosis and treatment and follow up of defects
C. Awakening health consciousness in children
D. The provision of healthful environment
E. All of the above

184. In India, the school health committee was established in which year?
A. 1960
B. 1961
C. 1962
D. 1963

185. In India, school health committee recommended medical examination of children at the time of entry and thereafter every:
A. One year
B. Two years
C. Three years
D. Four years
E. Five years

186. In School, Desks should be of:
A. Minus type
B. Plus type
C. Quadrangular
D. Epibolic
E. Any of the above

187. Per capita space for students in a classroom should not be less than:
A. 5 sq. ft
B. 10 sq. ft
C. 15 sq. ft
D. 20 sq. ft

188. Consider the following statement:
I. No class room should accommodate more than 40 students

II. In school combined door and window area should be atleast 25% of floor space
III. Class rooms should have sufficient natural light preferably from the left side
IV. In school one urinal for 60 students and one latrine for 100 students

Select the correct answer as per following code:

A. I, II and III only
B. I, II and IV only
C. I, II, III and IV All
D. II, III and IV only
E. I, III and IV only

189. The key person for health education in school is:

A. Doctor
B. Health assistant
C. Public health nurse
D. Teacher

190. The health of the school child is the responsibility of:

A. Parents only
B. Teachers
C. Community
D. Health administrators
E. All the above

191. Nearly .... million of the world's population are estimated to be mentally retarded.

A. 83 **B.** 103
C. 123 **D.** 143
E. 163

192. In India about .... of child population in 1 to 14 years age group is affected by in developmental delays.

A. 1% **B.** 2%
C. 3% **D.** 4%
E. 5%

193. Loss of phalanges in leprosy patients is termed as:

A. Handicap
B. Impairment
C. Disability
D. All of these

194. The inability to walk without support is termed as:

A. Impairment
B. Handicap
C. Disability
D. Physically unfit
E. All of the above

195. "Blindness" is a/an:

A. Intrinsic handicap
B. Extrinsic handicap
C. Impairment
D. Disability

196. A machinist who sits idle after loss of left hand in an accident is called as:

A. Physically unfit
B. Temporarily impaired
C. Handicapped
D. Disabled

197. What % of India's population are said to be suffering from some kind of mental disability?

A. 1% **B.** 2%
C. 3% **D.** 4%
E. 5%

198. Genetic causes of mental retardation includes the following, *but* one:

A. Neural tube defects
B. Microcephaly only
C. Congenital hypothyroidism
D. PKU only
E. Klinefelter's syndrome

199. Following perinatal factors may cause mental retardation, *save* for one:

A. Hypoxia
B. Birth injuries
C. Head injuries
D. Cerebral palsy
E. None of these

200. Which of the following conditions is NOT associated with mental retardation?
A. Protein energy malnutrition
B. Endemic goiter
C. Consanguineous marriages
D. Turner's syndrome
E. Pregnancy after 40 years of age

201. Which is NOT included under WHO classic fixation of mental retardation?
A. Normal—71 to 100
B. Mild MR—50 to 70
C. Moderate MR—35 to 49
D. Severe MR—20 to 34
E. Profound mental retardation—IQ under 20

202. Consider the following statements:
I. The optimum maternal age for producing normal babies is between 20 and 30 years
II. In India, the main cause of diability is polio
III. Proper nutrition of pregnant mother is essential to prevent mental handicap

Select the true answer as per code given below:
A. I and III
B. I, II and III All
C. I and II
D. I only

203. Aids and appliances upto Rs. 3600 provided to people with disabilities free if the monthly income is upto how much?
A. 1200
B. 2500
C. 3000
D. 3600
E. 4200

204. Following behaviour problems in children are antisocial in nature, *save* for one:
A. Stealing
B. Masturbation
C. Gambling only
D. Cruelty
E. Sexual offenses only

205. Which is NOT a personality disorder?
A. Temper-tantrums
B. Timidity
C. Depression
D. Day-dreaming
E. Hysterical manifestations

206. A child with school phobia, failure, and backwardness in studies has:
A. Personality defect
B. Juvenile delinquency
C. Habit defect
D. Educational difficulties

207. The term "Juvenile" means:
A. A boy who has not attained the age of 16 years
B. A girl who has not attained the age of 18 years
C. Both of the above
D. Neither A nor B

208. Following are true about juvenile delinquency *except* for one:
A. The highest incidence is found in children aged 15 and above
B. The incidence among boys is 4 to 5 times more than among girls
C. The xyz men suffer from severe disturbance of the whole personality
D. None of these

209. Following most closely resembles juvenile delinquency:
A. Destructiveness
B. Bedwetting
C. School failure
D. Speech problem

210. Who are used in the production and marketing of cocaine and the trafficking of cannabis and heroine?
A. Child labour
B. Street children
C. Child abuse

D. Battered baby only
E. All of these

211. According to the recent global estimates the number of street children is about:
A. 1 million
B. 10 million
C. 100 million
D. 150 million
E. 500 million

212. CRY—means child relief and you have been set up in India by whom?
A. Mother Terressa
B. Rippan Kapoor
C. Sonia Gandhi
D. All of the above

213. Regarding child labour in India which is false?
A. India fosters the largest number of child labour in the world
B. It contributes 20% of India's GNP
C. According to National Sample Survey 25 million child workers are in the age group of 5 to 15 years
D. J and K has the higher percentage of child labour

214. Which Act was enacted forbidding the practice of child marriages?
A. Sharda Act (1929)
B. Sonia Act 1987
C. Child Marriage Restraint Act (1978)
D. All of the above

215. The 1st child guidance clinic was started in 1909 in which city?
A. Delhi
B. London
C. Chicago
D. Dehradoon

216. The main service of child guidance clinic is:
A. Management of orphans
B. Psychotherapy
C. Career counselling
D. Any of the above

217. Currently, the most important scheme in the field of child welfare is:
A. ICCW
B. CARE
C. ICDS
D. BALWADIS

218. ICDS scheme was initiated by Government of India in:
A. 1971
B. 1973
C. 1974
D. 1975

219. Under ICDS scheme NON FORMAL EDUCATION is given to:
A. Children upto 6 years
B. Pregnant mothers
C. Nursing mothers in rural urban and tribal areas
D. Both B and C above
E. All of these

220. Each CDPO is an incharge of:
A. Four supervisors
B. 100 AW workers
C. Both of the above
D. Neither

221. The multipurpose agent of ICDS is:
A. AWW
B. Supervisors
C. CDPO
E. B and C above
D. All of the above

222. At present how many ICDS projects are operational in India?
A. 500
B. 1000
C. 2000
D. 5320
E. 10,320

223. Two World Bank assisted ICDS projects cover the following states in India, *but* one:
A. A.P.
B. Bihar

C. U.P.
D. M.P.
E. Orissa

224. Recognised indicators of ICDS programme includes the following, *save* for one:
A. Increased birth weight
B. Reduced MMR
C. Reduced malnutrition
D. Increased immunization
E. Reduced infant and child mortality rate

225. Who said, "You donot heal old age. You protect it; you promote it, you extend it"?
A. Ronald Ross
B. James Lind
C. Sir James Sterling Ross
D. David Cooper

226. In England about 12% of people are over the age of 65 years as against what % is living in India?
A. 1%
B. 2%
C. 3%
D. 3.8%
E. 4.5%

227. According to 1981 census what % of total population were above the age of 60 years in India?
A. 5%
B. 6.5%
C. 7.8%
D. 9.2%
E. 11%

228. Following may wrinkle the soul, *but* one:
A. Years
B. Worry
C. Fear and doubt
D. Anxiety and self-distrust
E. None of the above

229. Following disabilities are considered to be due to incident on aging, *but* one:
A. Senile cataract glaucoma and nerve deafness only
B. Bony changes affecting mobility
C. Emphysema
D. Changes in mental outlook
E. None of these

230. Following diseases are more frequent among the older people than in the younger one includes:
I. Degenerative diseases of heart and blood vessel
II. Diabetes mellitus
III. Diseases of locomotor system
IV. Genitourinary system
Choose the correct answer as per code given below:
A. I, II, III and IV All
B. I, II and IV
C. I, II and III
D. II, III and IV

231. In India, the most common cause of morbidity and mortality above 60 years of age is:
A. Asthma and bronchitis
B. Paralysis
C. Cancer
D. Anaemia
E. T.B. lung

232. The "triple evils" of aged includes all, *except:*
A. Awareness
B. Poverty
C. Loneliness
D. Ill-health
E. None of these

233. Recognised examples of conditions potentially amenable to primary prevention in older persons includes the following, *save* for one:
A. Myocardial infarction
B. Screening for diabetes
C. Osteoporosis prevention
D. Stroke prevention
E. Nutritionally induced anemia

234. Crude birth rate per 1000 population (2002) in India is:
A. 21
B. 23
C. 24
D. 22

235. IMR (2002) in India is:
A. 50
B. 70
C. 60
D. 67

236. Under five mortality rate per 1000 live birth (2002) in India is:
A. 107
B. 93
C. 39
D. 42

237. Under five mortality (2002) is least common seen in which nations of the world?
A. Singapore
B. Japan
C. Switzerland
D. USA

238. Homes where children are placed under the care of doctors and psychiatrists are called:
A. Foster homes
B. Remand homes
C. Borstals
D. Child guidance clinics

239. Infants constitute what % of population?
A. 1%
B. 2%
C. 3%
D. 4%

240. Regarding child guidance clinic, which is false?
A. It is intended for service to the children in orphanages
B. 1st started in Chicago (USA)
C. It is basically meant for children who do not fully adjust to their environment
D. Originally designed to deal with juvenile delinquency

241. Child guidance clinic is helpful for:
A. Bedwetting problem
B. Impaired hearing
C. Eye squint
D. Cerebral palsy

242. Absolute growth is maximally seen in:
A. 0 to 1 year age group
B. 1 to 4 years
C. 5 to 10 years
D. 14 to 16 years

243. "Road to health card" top line is:
A. 33rd percentile
B. 50th percentile
C. 80th percentile
D. 97th percentile

244. According to school health services recommendations, as school should have:
A. 1 urinal/60 children and 1 privy for 100 children
B. 1 urinal/80 children and 1 privy for 150 children
C. 1 urinal/100 children and 1 privy for 100 children
D. 1 urinal/100 children and 1 privy for 200 children

245. A 14-year-old boy having lost his father a year ago, is caught shoplifting. The boy will be sent to:
A. An orphanage
B. An anganwadi
C. A remand home
D. Prison

246. As per WHO classification, a case of severe mental retardation has I.Q. of:
A. 50 to 70
B. Below 20
C. 35 to 49
D. 20 to 34

247. Homes where children are placed under the care of doctors and psychiatrists are called:

A. Remand homes
B. Foster homes
C. Child guidance clinics
D. Borstals

248. Regarding baby-friendly UNICEF plan, all are true, *except:*

A. Feeding started within 4 hours of birth
B. Mother and child are left together 24 hours a day
C. Feeding on demand
D. No food/water given other than breast milk

249. Deficit in weight for height in a 3 years old child indicates:

A. Underweight
B. Acute malnutrition
C. Chronic malnutrition
D. Concomitant acute and chronic malnutrition

250. The extra energy allowances needed per day during pregnancy is:

A. 150 Kcals
B. 200 Kcals
C. 300 Kcals
D. 550 Kcals

Answers

1 D	2 A	3 B	4 D	5 C	6 B	7 C	8 D	9 A	10 B
11 D	12 C	13 E	14 A	15 B	16 C	17 B	18 A	19 C	20 D
21 A	22 C	23 A	24 B	25 C	26 E	27 D	28 E	29 C	30 C
31 B	32 C	33 E	34 B	35 D	36 C	37 C	38 D	39 B	40 A
41 B	42 E	43 A	44 C	45 B	46 A	47 D	48 C	49 D	50 A
51 B	52 D	53 C	54 A	55 D	56 C	57 D	58 E	59 A	60 B
61 A	62 C	63 D	64 B	65 A	66 E	67 D	68 C	69 A	70 C
71 D	72 A	73 B	74 C	75 B	76 A	77 D	78 C	79 D	80 B
81 E	82 A	83 B	84 D	85 B	86 C	87 A	88 C	89 C	90 D
91 E	92 A	93 B	94 C	95 D	96 B	97 D	98 E	99 A	100 C
101 D	102 E	103 D	104 D	105 B	106 A	107 B	108 A	109 E	110 B
111 E	112 A	113 C	114 D	115 B	116 A	117 C	118 E	119 A	120 B
121 C	122 D	123 B	124 C	125 A	126 B	127 C	128 A	129 B	130 D
131 C	132 D	133 E	134 B	135 A	136 D	137 B	138 C	139 A	140 B
141 C	142 D	143 A	144 C	145 E	146 A	147 B	148 B	149 C	150 D
151 E	152 A	153 B	154 C	155 D	156 C	157 A	158 B	159 A	160 C
161 B	162 D	163 B	164 D	165 B	166 C	167 B	168 C	169 D	170 A
171 B	172 C	173 D	174 E	175 E	176 E	177 B	178 C	179 A	180 B
181 E	182 B	183 E	184 A	185 D	186 A	187 B	188 C	189 D	190 E
191 A	192 C	193 B	194 C	195 A	196 C	197 B	198 A	199 C	200 D
201 A	202 B	203 A	204 B	205 C	206 D	207 C	208 D	209 A	210 B
211 C	212 B	213 C	214 A	215 C	216 B	217 C	218 D	219 E	220 C
221 A	222 D	223 C	224 B	225 C	226 D	227 B	228 A	229 E	230 A
231 B	232 A	233 C	234 C	235 D	236 B	237 A	238 B	239 C	240 A
241 A	242 B	243 B	244 A	245 C	246 D	247 A	248 A	249 B	250 C

C•H•A•P•T•E•R **EIGHT**

Environment and Health

DIRECTION: Following MCQ's are provided with a few suggestive answers/completions. Only one answer is correct. You have to identify the *BEST* one in each case.

1. What % of Indian population has access to safe water (1994-1995)?

A. 69.6% **B.** 71%
C. 80% **D.** 85%
E. 88%

2. Which of the following South-East Asian nations has LEAST access to adequate sanitation (1994-1995)?

A. India
B. Indonesia
C. Maldives
D. Myanmar
E. Srilanka

3. Which South-East Asian nations has BEST sanitation facilities to people?

A. Srilanka
B. Thailand
C. Indonesia
D. Bangladesh
E. Myanmar

4. Which South-East Asian countries has got best access to population to safe water?

A. Thailand
B. Bangladesh
C. India
D. Maldives
E. Srilanka

5. "The control of all those factors in man's physical environment which exercise or may exercise a deleterious effect on his physical development, health and survival." This is the definition of "environmental sanitation" given by:

A. WHO
B. National Sanitation Foundation of the U.S.A.
C. UN conference of sanitation
D. Sulabh International-India (Bihar)
E. None of these

6. "ARFICA 2000" a new venture aimed at providing:

A. Food for all African countries
B. Universal coverage of water supply and sanitation
C. Universal coverage for food supply
D. Water supply and sanitation to Africans

7. The global WHO/UNEP network for air and water quality monitoring are operational in more than .... countries.

A. 20 **B.** 40
C. 60 **D.** 30
E. 10 only

8. Surface and ground water quality are monitored in how many cities worldwide?

A. 50
B. 150
C. 250
D. 350
E. 550 cities

9. The UN General Assembly launched the international drinking water supply and sanitation decade as:

A. 1950-1959
B. 1961-1970
C. 1971-1980
D. 1981-1990
E. 1991-2000 AD

10. Recognised criteria for safe and wholesome water includes:

I. Free from pathogenic agents
II. Free from harmful chemical substances
III. Pleasant to taste
IV. Free from colour and odour
V. Usable for domestic purposes

Choose the correct answer as per code given below:

A. I, II, III, IV and V All
B. I, II and III only
C. I, II, III and IV only
D. I, II, III and V
E. I, III and V only

11. Which of the following statement is NOT true?

A. The basic physiological requirements for drinking from pathogenic water have been estimated at about 2 litres per head per day
B. A daily supply of 150-200 litre per capita is considered an adequate supply to meet the needs for all domestic purposes
C. In India 40 litres of water per day is the set target to be achieved by the end of the 8th five year plan
D. The safe yield is generally defined as the yield that is adequate 95% of the year
E. None of these

12. Regarding "RAIN", all statements are true, *save* for one:

A. Rain is the prime source of all water
B. It is the purest water in nature
C. It has got no corrosive action on lead pipes as it is very soft water
D. Physically it is clear, bright and sparkling
E. Chemically very soft containing only traces of dissolved solids (0.0005%)

13. The place in the world, which depend solely upon rain as a source of water supply is:

A. Argentina
B. Gibralter
C. Greenland
D. Denmark
E. Ethiopia

14. Following cities derive their water supply from impounding reservoirs, *except:*

A. Nagpur
B. Mumbai
C. Chandigarh
D. Chennai only
E. None of these

15. Following cities receive its water supply through rivers:

A. Allahabad
B. Delhi
C. Calcutta
D. All of these
E. Both A and B above

16. The percentage of salt in sea water is:

A. 1%
B. 2.5%
C. 3.5%
D. 4.5%
E. 5.0%

17. The cheapest and most practical means of providing water to small communities is:

A. Ground water
B. Impounding reservoir

C. Rivers
D. Tanks only

18. Recognised advantages of GROUND WATER includes all, *but* one:
A. It is likely to be free from pathogenic agents
B. It usually requires no treatment
C. The supply is likely to be certain even during dry season
D. It has high mineral contents
E. It is less subject to contamination than surface water

19. The usual ground water sources include the following, *except* for one:
A. Tanks
B. Shallow wells
C. Springs only
D. Deep wells
E. None of these

20. Statement (S): Ground water is superior to surface water.
Reason (R): Because the ground itself provides an effective filtering medium.
Select the true response from the code given below:
A. Both (S) and (R) are true, and are related to cause and effect
B. Both (S) and (R) are true, but are not related to cause and effect
C. (S) true, (R) false
D. (R) true, (S) false
E. Both (S) and (R) are false

21. Regarding shallow well:
I. Taps the water from above the 1st impervious layer
II. Much hard water
III. Often grossly contaminated
IV. Usually goes dry in summer
Choose the correct response from the following code:
A. I and II only
B. I, II and III
C. I, III and IV only
D. I, II, III and IV All
E. I and IV only

22. All the following are true about deep wells, *save* for one:
A. Taps the water from below the 1st impervious layer
B. Taps very soft water
C. Taps pure water
D. Provides a source of constant supply
E. None of these

23. Which of the following statements is/are false regarding wells?
A. In India most wells are of shallow variety
B. Dug wells are by far the most common type in India
C. Artesian wells are a kind of deep wells in which the water rises above the level of ground water, because it is held under pressure between the two impervious layers
D. Guineaworm disease is quite a public health problem in areas where step wells are in use
E. None of the above

24. To avoid bacterial contamination, the well should be located not less than .... from likely sources of contamination.
A. 15 meters
B. 20 feet
C. 50 feet
D. Both A and C
E. 25 meters

25. Which city in India derives its entire water supply from tube wells?
A. Jammu
B. Mumbai
C. Chandigarh
D. Delhi
E. Ernakulam

26. Man-made sources of water pollution includes the following:
I. Sewage
II. Industrial and trade waste

III. Agricultural pollutants
IV. Radioactive substances

Select the true answer from the code given below:

A. I and III only
B. I, II, III and IV All
C. I, II and III only
D. I and II only
E. I, III and IV only

27. **Recognised indicators of water pollution includes the following, *but* one:**
A. Amount of total suspended solids
B. Biochemical O_2 demand (BOD) at 20°C
C. Concentration of chlorides, nitrogen and phosphorous
D. Presence of dissolved oxygen
E. None of these

28. **Following water-borne diseases is NOT due to presence of an aquatic host:**
A. Schistosomiasis
B. Guineaworm disease
C. Weils disease only
D. Fish tapeworm disease
E. None of these

29. **Following water-borne diseases are NOT due to viral aetiology:**
A. HAV infection
B. HBV infection
C. Rotavirus diarrhoea in infants
D. Poliomyelitis only
E. Hepatitis 'E' virus infection

30. **In India, WATER ACT (Prevention and Control of Pollution) was passed in:**
A. 1954
B. 1964
C. 1974
D. 1984
E. 1994

31. **There is an inverse relationship between hardness of water (drinking) and:**
A. Cardiovascular disease
B. Obesity
C. Pulmonary congestion
D. Diabetes mellitus
E. All of the above

32. **Storing river water in reservoir before filtration leads to all, *but* one:**
A. Settling of suspended impurities
B. Decrease in nitrate content
C. Oxidation of organic matter by aerobic bacteria
D. Decrease in bacterial count
E. None of these

33. **The % of bacteria removed by filtration process is:**
A. 30%
B. 50%
C. 60%
D. 70 to 80%
E. 98 to 99%

34. **Regarding slow sand or biological filters, all are true, *save* for one:**
A. It was 1st used for water treatment in 1804 in Scotland and after that in London
B. The most important part of the filter is the sand bed
C. The vital layer is the "heart" of the slow sand filter
D. The sand bed presents a vast surface area
E. None of these

35. **The vital layer in a slow sand filter acts by the following:**
A. Removes organic matter
B. Holds back bacteria
C. Oxidises ammoniacal N_2 into NO_3
D. All of these
E. Both A and C above

36. **Action of slow sand filter depends upon:**
A. Schmutzdecke
B. Vital layer
C. Zoogleal layer
D. Biological layer
E. Any of the above

37. The following steps are involved in the purification of water by rapid sand filters:

I. Coagulation
II. Filtration
III. Rapid remixing
IV. Sedimentation
V. Flocculation

Choose the correct sequence as per code given below:

A. I, III, V, IV and II
B. I, II, III, IV and V
C. II, I, III, V and IV
D. III, II, I, IV and V
E. I, V, IV, III and II

38. In which year, the 1st rapid sand filters were installed in USA?

A. 1804
B. 1865
C. 1885
D. 1895
E. 1905

39. Rapid sand filters need frequent washing daily or weekly, depending upon the loss of head. The whole process of washing takes about how much time?

A. 1-5 hours
B. 15 mts
C. 2 hours
D. 3 hours
E. 150 mts only

40. Recognised advantages of a rapid sand filter over the slow sand filter includes the following *save* for one:

A. No preliminary storage is needed
B. The washing of the filter is easy
C. More flexibility in operation
D. The filter beds occupy more space
E. Filtration is rapid 40 to 50 times that of a slow sand filter

41. Which of the following is killed efficiently by simple chlorination?

A. Viral hepatitis
B. Helminthic ova
C. Polio virus
D. Typhoid bacilli
E. All of the above

42. Chlorination of water helps in the following:

A. Oxidation of Fe, Mn and H_2S
B. Destroys some taste and odour producing agents
C. Controls algae and slim organisms
D. Aids coagulation
E. All of these

43. Statement (S): Chlorine acts best as a disinfectant when the pH of water is around seven (R).

Reason (R) Because of preponderance of hypochlorous acid (HOCl).

A. Both (S) and (R) are true and are related to cause and effect
B. Both (S) and (R) are true but are not related to cause and effect
C. (S) is true, (R) is false
D. (R) is true, (S) is false
E. Both (S) and (R) are false

44. The action of chlorine for disinfection of water depends upon the following:

A. pH only
B. Time
C. Temperature
D. All of these
E. Both B and C above

45. Chlorine gas is the 1st choice for disinfecting large bodies of water, because:

A. It is cheap
B. Quick in action
C. Efficient
D. Easy to apply
E. All of the above

46. A device used for measuring, regulating and administering gaseous chlorine to water supplies is:

A. Horrocks apparatus
B. Paterson's chloronome
C. Pasteur apparatus

D. Katadyn apparatus
E. All of the above

47. Orthotolidine test (OT) was developed in which year?
A. 1918
B. 1928
C. 1939
D. 1948
E. 1958

48. OT test determines both free and combine chlorine in water, but for the detection of free chlorine the reagent must give positive test within:
A. 1 secs.
B. 5 secs.
C. 10 secs.
D. 10 mts.
E. 15 to 20 mts.

49. When OT is added to water containing chlorine, it turns:
A. Red
B. Purple
C. Green
D. Yellow
E. Blue

50. OT produces yellow colour with the following:
A. Chlorine only
B. Nitrites
C. Iron
D. Manganese
E. All of these

51. Orthotoludine arsenite test (OTA) gives yellow colour only with:
A. Chlorine
B. Nitrites
C. Iron
D. Manganese
E. All of the above

52. Regarding OZONATION—All are true, *save* for one:
A. Unstable gas
B. It is a powerful reducing agent
C. Strong virucidal
D. Eliminates undesirable odour, taste and colour
E. It removes all chlorine from water

53. More than 1000 municipal water treatment plant, around the world are using ozone (O_3) the oldest of which plant is installed in where and when?
A. India (1900)
B. Britain (1901)
C. France (1906)
D. U.S.A. (1908)

54. The ozone dosage required for potable water treatment varies from:
A. 0.1 to 0.2 mg per litre
B. 0.1 to 0.5 mg per litre
C. 0.1 to 0.8 mg per litre
D. 0.1 to 1.0 mg per litre
E. 0.2 to 1.5 mg per litre

55. The residual germicidal effect for disinfection of water is present in:
A. Ozonation
B. UV-irradiation
C. Chlorination
D. All of these

56. Boiling for what time periods kills all bacteria, spores, cysts and ova and yields sterilized water?
A. 1 to 2 mts.
B. 3 to 5 mts.
C. 5 to 10 mts.
D. 20 to 30 mts.

57. A freshly prepared bleaching powder contains what % of available chlorine?
A. 33% B. 44%
C. 55% D. 66%
E. 77%

58. High test hypochlorite (HTH) or perchloran is a calcium compound having what % of available chlorine?
A. 50% B. 60%
C. 70% D. 80%
E. Both B and C above

59. A chlorine tab. developed by NEERI, Nagpur of 0.5 mg is quite sufficient to disinfect how much quantity of water?
A. 1 litre
B. 5 litre
C. 10 litre
D. 20 litre
E. 50 litre

60. Most effective and cheapest method of disinfecting wells is by:
A. Potassium permangnate
B. Bleaching powder
C. Chlorine gas
D. Iodine

61. Following are done during chlorination of well, *but* one:
A. Estimation of volume
B. Estimation of chlorine demand of water
C. Put bleaching powder directly into the well
D. Contact period of 1 hour

62. Horrock's apparatus is used to calculate the dose of:
A. Iodine
B. Perchloran
C. Cb gas
D. Bleaching powder
E. $KMNO_4$

63. Roughly 2.5 gm of good quality bleaching powder ($CaOCl_2$) is needed to disinfect how much quantity of water?
A. 100 litres
B. 200 litres
C. 500 litres
D. 750 litres
E. 1000 litres

64. Water with turbidity of how much nephelometric turbidity units (NTU) is usually acceptable to consumer?
A. 1.5 NTU
B. 2.5 NTU
C. 5.0 NTU
D. 7.5 NTU
E. 10.0 NTU

65. The maximum permissible level of chloride in water is:
A. 200 mg/L
B. 400 mg/L
C. 600 mg/L
D. 800 mg/L
E. 1000 mg/L

66. Following are standards for water quality, *save* for one:
A. Chloride – 200 mg/dl
B. Nitrite = 1.2 g/L
C. Hardness < 300 mg/dL
D. Nitrate – < 1 mg/L
E. None of these

67. Regarding quality of drinking water, which of the following is true?
A. The acceptable pH drinking water is between 6.5 and 8.5
B. The drinking water should be colour free
C. Ideally, drinking water should not contain any microbes known to be pathogenic
D. All of these
E. Both B and C above

68. Presence of which microbes in water is regarded as important confirmatory evidence of recent faecal pollution of water?
A. E. coli
B. Klebsiella aerogenes
C. Faecal streptococci
D. Cl. perfringens

69. Consider the following statements:
I. The presence of spores of cl. perfringens in drinking water without coliform group suggests that faecal contamination occurred at some remote time
II. Drinking water should be free from any viruses infectious for man
III. Drinking water should not contain any pathogenic protozoa

IV. A single mature larva or fertilized egg can cause infection and such infective stages should be absent from drinking water

Select the wrong answer from the code given below:

A. I only
B. I and II only
C. I, II and III
D. I, II, III and IV All
E. None of these

70. Which of the following statements is/are true about lead?

A. Placental transfer of lead occurs in humans as early as 12th week of gestation and continues throughout development
B. Lead is a general toxicant that accumulates in the skeleton
C. Lead also interferes with calcium metabolism, both directly and by interfering with Vit. D. metabolism
D. All of the above
E. Both A and C above

71. Renal tumours have been induced in experimental animals exposed to high concentrations of .... in diets.

A. Mercury
B. Lead
C. Cadmium
D. All of the above
E. Both A and C above

72. Which organ system is the chief target organ for inorganic mercury?

A. Kidney
B. Brain
C. Adrenal gland
D. Thyroid gland

73. The enzyme GLUTATHIONE PEROXIDASE contains:

A. Antimony
B. Molybdenum
C. Selenium
D. Nickel

74. Tolerable daily intake (TDI) can be calculated by following formula:

A. $TDI = \frac{\text{NOAEL or LOAEL}}{\text{UF}}$
B. $TDI = \frac{\text{LOAEL}}{\text{NOAEL}} \times 100$
C. $TDI = \frac{\text{NOAEL}}{\text{LOAEL}} \times 100$
D. $TDI = \frac{\text{UF}}{\text{NOAEL}} \times \text{LOAEL}$

75. E. coli is almost the only organisms (coliform) which is capable of producing gas from lactose at:

A. 37°C
B. 40°C
C. 44°C
D. 48°C
E. 52°C

76. Presumptive test for faecal pollution of water involve utilization of:

A. Typhoid bacilli count
B. Methylene blue test
C. Turbidity
D. Gas formation in fermentation tubes of lactose bilesalt broth

77. Permanent hardness of water is due to all, *but* one:

A. $CaCO_3$
B. $CaSO_4$
C. $MgSO_4$
D. Chlorides nitrates

78. Drinking water should contain level of hardness (mEq./L):

A. < 1 m Eq/L
B. 1 to 3 m Eq/L
C. 3 to 6 m Eq/L
D. > 6 m Eq/L

79. Softening of water is recommended when the hardness exceeds:

A. 0.5 m Eq/L
B. 1 m Eq/L

C. 2 m Eq/L
D. 3 m Eq/L

80. Temporary hardness of water can be abolished by all, *save* for one:
A. Boiling
B. Addition of lime
C. Addition of sodium carbonate
D. Permutit process
E. Base exchange process

81. Regarding fluoridation of water, which is true?
A. The main source of fluorine is drinking water
B. Deficiency of fluorine in drinking water is associated with dental caries
C. Excess of fluorine in drinking water causes dental and skeletal fluorosis
D. All of these
E. Both A and B above

82. The most widely used method of pool disinfection is:
A. Chlorination
B. Ozonization
C. V.V. irradiation
D. Any of these

83. The national water supply and sanitation programme was launched in:
A. 1947
B. 1954
C. 1964
D. 1974
E. 1986

84. Horrock's apparatus is used to measure the dose of:
A. Perchloran
B. $KMNO_4$
C. Bleaching powder
D. Chlorine gas

85. An average person at rest gives off .... of CO_2 per hour:
A. 0.1 c.ft.
B. 0.3 c.ft.
C. 0.5 c.ft
D. 0.7 c.ft.
E. 1.0 c.ft.

86. A man at rest gives off approximately .... per hour.
A. 50 BTU
B. 100 BTU
C. 200 BTU
D. 300 BTU
E. 400 BTU

87. In Calcutta Black Hole experience 146 prisoners were put in a room of 18 × 14 × 10 with only 2 small windows. Only 23 persons survived deaths were due to:
A. Increased CO_2
B. ↑ed temperature and humidity
C. Lack of Sunlight
D. ↓ed O_2

88. The cause of discomfort in an over-crowded, poorly ventilated room are all, *but* one:
A. In CO_2
B. In temperature
C. In humidity
D. In air change

89. Mc Ardle's maximum allowable sweat rate is:
A. 1 L/12 hours
B. 4 L/1 hours
C. 4.5 L/4 hours
D. 4.5 L/8 hours

90. Corrected effective temperature in comfortable zone is:
A. 69 to 76°F
B. 77 to 80°F
C. 81 to 82°F
D. 83 + °F

91. Major air pollutions throughout the urban areas is:
A. Industries
B. Passive smoking
C. Motor vehicles
D. Burning coal

92. Which of the following statement is/are false about meteorological factors?

A. 1st 30 km holds the major portion of the atmospheric gases
B. Man is most directly concerned with only the 8 to 10 km of the atmosphere
C. The vertical diffusion of pollutants depends upon the temperature gradient
D. If the topography is dominated by mountains (or tall buildings) the winds become weak and calm and pollutants tend to concentrate in the breathing zone
E. None of these

93. The "temperature inversion" is a threat to human health is more frequent in:

A. Spring
B. Winter
C. Summer
D. All of the above
E. Both A and C above

94. Consider the following statements:

I. CO is one of the most common and widely distributed air pollutants
II. Incomplete combustion of carbon containing materials produces carbon monoxide gas
III. The combination of smoke and fog is called "smog"
IV. 80 to 90% of lead in ambient air derives from the combustion of leaded petrol

Choose the correct answer as per following code given below:

A. I and IV only
B. I, II and III
C. I, II, III and IV All
D. I and II only
E. I and III only

95. Which of the following statements is/are true?

A. The level of atmospheric pollution at anyone time depends upon meteorological factors e.g. topography, air movement and climate
B. Manmade sources of hydrocarbons include incineration, combustion of coal, wood, processing and use of petroleum
C. O_3 is one of the strongest oxidising agents
D. All of the above

96. Tobacco contains:

A. Cadmium
B. CO_2
C. Lead
D. SO_2
E. All of these

97. The best known PAH (polynuclear aromatic hydrocarbons) is:

A. PaP **B.** BaP
C. CaP **D.** MaP
E. NaP

98. In India the BaP exposure averaged about .... during cooking with biomass fuels.

A. 1 μ/m^3
B. 3 μ/m^3
C. 4 μ/m^3
D. 6 μ/m^3
E. 12 μ/m^3

99. Modern low tar cigarettes give:

A. 10 ng BaP
B. 18 ng BaP
C. 22 ng BaP
D. 35 ng BaP

100. Which pollutant is produced by gas cookers?

A. SO_2
B. CO_2 only
C. NO_2
D. CO only
E. None of the above

101. The best indicators of air pollution is/are:

A. SO_2
B. Smoke
C. Suspended particles
D. All of the above
E. Both B and C above

102. Soiling index is an indicator of:
A. Water pollution
B. Air Pollution
C. Sound pollution
D. Excreta pollution

103. Electric arch UVL sources produces what?
A. Asbestos
B. Radon
C. CO gas
D. Ozone
E. All of the above

104. Automobile exhaust are the recognised sources of following air pollutants, *save* for one:
A. SO_2
B. Lead
C. O_3
D. Oxides of N_2
E. Hydrocarbons

105. The Government of India has enacted the Air (Prevention and Control of Pollution) Act in which year?
A. 1971
B. 1981
C. 1991
D. 1992
E. 1996

106. It is recommended that in living rooms, there should be how many air changes in one hour?
A. Only one
B. Nil
C. Two to three
D. Four to six

107. The optimum floor space requirements per person vary from:
A. 10 to 20 sq. ft.
B. 30 to 50 sq. ft.
C. 50 to 75 sq. ft.
D. 50 to 100 sq. ft.

108. When the wind blows through a room, it is called:
A. Perflation
B. Aspiration
C. Cross-ventilation
D. Diffusion

109. Air conditioning means simultaneous control of:
A. Temperature
B. Humidity
C. Air movement
D. All of the above

110. Lux is:
A. Flow of light
B. Amount of light reaching surfaces
C. Brightness of point source
D. Amount of light remitted by surfaces

111. Brightness of point source is measured in:
A. Lux
B. Lambert
C. Candle power
D. Lumen

112. The day light factor in living rooms is at least:
A. 1% B. 3%
C. 5% D. 8%
E. 10%

113. Accumulation of dust on the bulbs reduces illumination by how much?
A. 10%
B. 20%
C. 30 to 40%
D. 50%
E. Just 1%

114. The illumination power of full moonlight night is:
A. 0.1 lux
B. 1 lux
C. 2 lux
D. 3 lux
E. 5 lux

115. The bright sunshine generates:
A. 1000 lux
B. 10,000 lux

C. 50,000 lux
D. 1,00,000 lux

116. Casual reading requires illumination of:
A. 50 lux
B. 100 lux
C. 150 lux
D. 200 lux
E. 400 lux

117. Biologic effects of light includes:
A. Bilirubin degradation
B. Stimulation of melanin synthesis
C. Activation of precursors of Vitamin 'D'
D. Adrenocortical secretion
E. All of the above

118. "Century of Noise" is the nickname given to which century?
A. 20th
B. 19th
C. 18th
D. 17th century

119. The acceptable noise levels for living room is:
A. 25 dBA
B. 40 dBA
C. 60 dBA
D. 20 dBA

120. A psycho-acoustic index of loudness is known as:
A. Hertz
B. Bell
C. Phone
D. Shone

121. The sound level of vacuum cleaner is:
A. 10 dB
B. 73 dB
C. 50 dB
D. 76 dB
E. 0 dB

122. Auditory fatigue is greatest at:
A. 500 Hz
B. 1000 Hz
C. 2000 Hz
D. 3000 Hz
E. 4000 Hz

123. Repeated and continuous exposure of noise around .... dB may result in a permanent hearing loss?)
A. 100
B. 200
C. 300
D. 400
E. 500

124. Noise causes: all, *but* one:
A. Miosis
B. Mydriasis
C. Affects colour perception
D. Reduce night vision

125. Following physiological changes occur due to noise, *save* for:
A. ↑ in B.P.
B. ↑ in I.C.P.
C. ↓ in sweating
D. ↑ in heart rate and breathing

126. It is estimated that man derives about how much radiation per annum from terrestrial radiation?
A. 10 mrad
B. 20 mrad
C. 30 mrad
D. 40 mrad
E. 50 mrad

127. In India, which state is exposed to highest terrestrial radiation?
A. Kerala
B. Bihar
C. M.P.
D. Maharashtra
E. Goa

128. The skin dose to the patient from a single X-ray film varies roughly from:
A. 0.02 to 1 rad
B. 0.02 1 rad
C. 0.02 to 2 rad
D. 0.02 to 3 rad

129. The half life of Sr 90 is about 28 years and that of CS 137 is:
A. 3 years
B. 13 years
C. 30 years
D. 50 years

130. A lead apron of 30 mm thickness cannot be penetrated by all, *except:*
A. X-rays
B. γ-rays
C. Cosmic rays
D. Electrons
E. Protons

131. The Bq (becqueral) is approximately equal to:
A. 2.7 picocuries
B. 7.2 picocuries
C. 17.2 picocuries
D. 27 picocuries

132. The amount of radioactive energy absorbed per gram of tissue or any material:
A. Rad
B. Becqueral
C. Roentgen
D. Rem

133. One sievert is equal to how many rems?
A. 10 rems
B. 20 rems
C. 100 rems
D. 500 rems
E. 1000 rems

134. The amount of radiation received from outer space and background radiation has been estimated to be .... a year.
A. 1 rad
B. 0.1 rad
C. 5 rad
D. 10 rad
E. 3 rad

135. In routine fluoroscopy, a dose of .... is delivered to a part of the body in about one minute:
A. 1 rad
B. 2 rad
C. 3 rad
D. 4 rad
E. 5 rad

136. It has been recommended that the genetic dose to the whole population from all sources additional to the natural background radiation, should not exceed .... over a period of 30 years.
A. 1 rem
B. 2 rems
C. 3 rems
D. 4 rems
E. 5 rems

137. The pressure increases at the rate of "one atmosphere" for each .... depth below sea level.
A. 11 feet
B. 22 feet
C. 33 feet
D. 44 feet
E. 55 feet

138. Which barometer is widely used by the Indian Meteorological Department for measuring the atmospheric pressure?
A. Kew Pattern barometer
B. Fortin's barometer
C. Barogragh
D. All of these
E. Both B and C above

139. The word "KATA" is a Greek word meaning:
A. Up
B. Down
C. Horizontal
D. Red colour

140. The "magenta" colour Kata thermometer is called as:
A. The Standard Kata
B. The High Temperature Kata
C. The Extra High Temperature Kata
D. All of the above

141. The most widely used instrument for measuring humidity is:
A. Assman psychrometer
B. Dry and wet bulb hygrometer
C. Sling psychrometer
D. All of these
E. Both A and C above

142. The rain gauge prescribed by the Government of India for the use at rainfall measuring stations in India is known as the:
A. Assman
B. Symon's rain gauge
C. Both
D. Neither

143. "Borehole latrine" was 1st introduced by the Rockefeller foundation during .... in campaigns of hookworm control:
A. 1930's
B. 1940's
C. 1950's
D. 1960's
E. 1970's

144. The only practical method for determining the organic load is:
A. Suspended solids
B. BOD
C. COD
D. All of the above

145. A sewage is said to be strong if the amount of suspended solids is:
A. 150 mg/l
B. 250 mg/l
C. 350 mg/l
D. 500 mg/l

146. The heart of the activated sludge process is the:
A. Aeration tank
B. Trickling filter
C. Grit chamber
D. All of the above

147. Following diseases are transmitted by sandfly, *but* one:
A. Kala-azar
B. Yaws
C. Oriental sore
D. Sandfly fever
E. Oraya fever

148. "Onchocerciasis" is transmitted by following vector:
A. Sandfly
B. Housefly
C. Blackfly
D. Tsetse fly

149. "Plague bacilli in rat flea" is an example of:
A. Propagative
B. Cyclopropagative
C. Cyclodevelopmental
D. All of the above

150. Guineaworm embryo in cyclops is:
A. Biological transmission
B. Propagative
C. Cyclodevelopment
D. All of the above

151. Normally the adult mosquito lives for about:
A. One week
B. Two weeks
C. Three weeks
D. Four weeks
E. Five weeks

152. Culex are the common "nuisance mosquitoes".
A. True
B. False

153. "Tiger mosquitoes" are the name given to:
A. Anopheles
B. Culex
C. Aedes
D. Mansonia

154. The vector for "VIRAL ARTHRITIS" includes:
A. Anopheles
B. Mansonia

C. Aedes
D. Culex

155. Biological control of mosquitoes involve:
A. Gambusia afflnis
B. Lebister reticulates
C. Barbados millions
D. Both A and B above
E. All of these

156. The number of holes in one square inch of mosquito net is usually:
A. 50
B. 75
C. 100
D. 150
E. 200

157. The size of mosquito net should not exceed 0.0475 inch in any diameter.
A. True
B. False

158. The outstanding all purpose repellent is:
A. Abate
B. OMS-33
C. Diethyltoluamide
D. Lindane only

159. "VOMIT DROP" is a characteristic feature of:
A. Mosquitoes
B. Housefly
C. Reduvid bug
D. Sandflies

160. "Sandfly fever" is carried by:
A. Phlebotomus argentipes
B. Phlebotomus papatasii
C. Phlebotomus sergenti
D. S. punjabensis
E. All of these

161. Lice are vectors of the following diseases:
A. Epidemic typhus
B. Relapsing fever
C. Trench fever
D. Dermatitis
E. All of the above

162. Hard ticks transmit the following diseases, *save* for one:
A. KFD
B. RMSF
C. Human Babesiosis
D. Tularaemia

163. "KFD in India" is transmitted by:
A. Soft tick
B. Hard tick
C. Sand flea
D. Trombiculid mites

164. The life span of "Trombiculid mites" is:
A. 3 months
B. 6 months
C. 9 months
D. 12 months
E. 15 months

165. The average life of cyclops is about:
A. 1 month
B. 2 months
C. 3 months
D. 4 months
E. 6 months

166. DDT was 1st synthesised by a German chemist Zielder (1874).
A. True
B. False

167. As a dust, DDT is used in 5 to 10% strength for the control of:
A. Lice
B. Fleas
C. Ticks
D. Bugs
E. All of these

168. The insecticidal properties of DDT was discovered by a Swiss scientist, Paul Muller (1939).
A. True
B. False

169. "Lindane" contains, what % of 'y' isomer of BHC?
A. 33%

B. 50%
C. 66%
D. 99%
E. 100%

170. Following are recognised fumigants, *save* for one:
A. HCN
B. CH_3Br
C. NaF
D. SO_2
E. CS_2 only

171. Following are NOT an organophosphorus insecticides:
A. Chlorthion
B. Ronnel
C. Naled
D. Kepone
E. Gardona

172. Which is NOT a stomach poison?
A. Paris green
B. Pyrolan
C. NaF
D. All of the above
E. Both A and C above

173. “Abate” is:
A. OMS-l
B. OMS-2
C. OMS-43
D. OMS-214
E. OMS-786

174. Which insecticide is recommended against anophelines those have developed resistance against both DDT and Dieldrin?
A. Propoxur
B. Resmethrin
C. Pothrin
D. All of the above

175. Cyanogas has been extensively used in India for the fumigation of rat burrows.
A. True
B. False

176. Venturimeter is used for:
A. Measuring bed strength in slow sand filter
B. Measuring dissolving capacity of gas
C. Measuring air velocity
D. All of these

177. A person working in hot environment who consumes more water without salt is likely to develop a condition called:
A. Heat stoke
B. Heat cramps
C. Heat exhaustion
D. All of the above

178. Vital layer in slow sand filter is seen in:
A. Near filter
B. Top of water
C. On the sand bed
D. None of the above

179. Paris green is a:
A. Fumigant
B. Repellant
C. Contact poison
D. Stomach poison

180. Dose of DDT used in residual spray is:
A. 1 to $2/gm^2$
B. 2 to $3/gm^2$
C. 3 to $4/gm^2$
D. 4 to $5/gm^2$

181. A naturally occurring radioactive substance in the body in small quantities is:
A. K-40
B. Ra^{226}
C. Bi60
D. I^{131}

Answers

1 D	2 A	3 B	4 D	5 A	6 B	7 C	8 D	9 D	10 A
11 E	12 C	13 B	14 C	15 D	16 C	17 A	18 D	19 A	20 A
21 C	22 B	23 E	24 D	25 C	26 B	27 D	28 C	29 B	30 C
31 A	32 B	33 E	34 E	35 D	36 E	37 A	38 C	39 B	40 D
41 D	42 E	43 A	44 D	45 E	46 B	47 A	48 C	49 D	50 E
51 A	52 B	53 C	54 E	55 C	56 C	57 A	58 E	59 D	60 B
61 C	62 D	63 E	64 C	65 C	66 B	67 D	68 C	69 E	70 D
71 B	72 A	73 C	74 A	75 C	76 D	77 A	78 B	79 D	80 E
81 D	82 A	83 B	84 C	85 D	86 E	87 B	88 A	89 C	90 B
91 C	92 E	93 B	94 C	95 D	96 A	97 B	98 C	99 A	100 C
101 D	102 B	103 D	104 A	105 B	106 C	107 D	108 A	109 D	110 B
111 C	112 D	113 C	114 A	115 D	116 B	117 E	118 A	119 B	120 C
121 D	122 E	123 A	124 B	125 C	126 E	127 A	128 D	129 C	130 B
131 D	132 A	133 C	134 B	135 D	136 E	137 C	138 A	139 B	140 C
141 B	142 B	143 A	144 C	145 D	146 A	147 B	148 C	149 A	150 C
151 B	152 A	153 C	154 B	155 E	156 D	157 A	158 C	159 B	160 D
161 E	162 A	163 B	164 B	165 C	166 A	167 E	168 A	169 D	170 C
171 D	172 B	173 E	174 A	175 A	176 A	177 B	178 C	179 D	180 A
181 A									

C•H•A•P•T•E•R NINE

Occupational Health

DIRECTION: Following MCQ's are provided with a few suggestive answers/completions. Only one answer is correct. You have to identify the ***BEST*** one in each case.

1. The term ERGONOMICS is derived from which of the following language?
A. Greek
B. Singhalese
C. Chinese
D. Hebrews
E. Roman only

2. "Ergonomics" means what?
A. Study of machinery
B. To place the right man in the right job
C. To keep the industries clear
D. A machine that measure power

3. The common physical hazard in most industries is:
A. Humidity
B. Noise
C. Heat
D. Ionizing radiation
E. All of these

4. Indirect effects of heat exposure includes all, *but* one:
A. Decreased efficiency
B. Increased fatigue
C. Enhanced accident rates
D. Heat exhaustion
E. None of these

5. Consider the following statements:
I. The direct effects of heat exposure are burns, heat exhaustion, heat stroke and heat cramps
II. Radiation heat is the main problem in foundry, glass and steel industries
III. Heat stagnation is the principal problem in jute and cotton textile industry
IV. The Indian Factories Act has not laid down any specific temperature standard
Choose the correct answer as per code given below:
A. I, II and III only
B. I, III and IV
C. I and II only
D. I and III only
E. I, II, III and IV All

6. The KOLAR GOLD MINES of Mysore which is the 2nd deepest mine of the world (11000 feet), temperature as .... has been recorded.
A. 125°F
B. 100°F
C. 150°F

D. 175°F
E. 250°F

7. **Important hazard associated with cold work includes:**
   I. Chilblains
   II. General hypothermia
   III. Immersion foot
   IV. Frostbite
   V. Erythrocyanosis

   Select the true answer as per following code:
   A. I, III and IV
   B. I, II, III, IV and V All
   C. I, II and III
   D. I, II, III and IV
   E. I, IV and V

8. **Which is NOT an acute effects of poor illumination?**
   A. Intensity and frequency range
   B. Duration of exposure
   C. Individual susceptibility
   D. All of these
   E. Both A and C above

9. **The degree of injury from exposure to noise depends upon:**
   A. Intensity and frequency range
   B. Duration of exposure
   C. Individual susceptibility
   D. All of these
   E. Both A and C above

10. **In "Arc welding", occupational exposure to .... ensues.**
    A. Infra red radiation
    B. Ultraviolet radiation
    C. Ionizing radiation
    D. X-rays exposure
    E. Any of the above

11. **The International Commission of Radiological Protection has set the maximum permissible level of occupational exposure .... per year to the whole body.**
    A. One rem
    B. Two rem
    C. Three rem
    D. Four rem
    E. Five rem

12. **Following chemicals are absorbed through the skin and cause systemic effects:**
    A. TNT
    B. Aniline
    C. Both of the above
    D. Neither A nor B above

13. **Who 1st draw attention in India to the prevalence of occupational dermatitis due to machine oil, rubber, X-rays, caustic soda and lime?**
    A. Lal and Kumar
    B. Prasad and Singh
    C. Hassan and Fernandes
    D. Rao and Banerji

14. **"Respirable dust" is more dangerous as they settle in the lungs causes pneumoconiosis usually of what size?**
    A. 0.1 μ
    B. < 5 μ
    C. 1 μ
    D. 10 μ
    E. 150 μ

15. **The most common dust diseases in India is:**
    A. Silicosis
    B. Anthracosis
    C. Both of these
    D. Neither A nor B above

16. **What % of accident in industry are said to be due to mechanical causes?**
    A. 1% only
    B. 3% only
    C. 7% only
    D. 10%
    E. 18%

17. **Heat exhaustion is seen in:**
    A. Farms

B. Textile industry
C. Lead factory
D. Bulb factory
E. All of the above

18. Following are recognised occupational cancers, *but* one:
A. C_A gall bladder
B. C_A urinary bladder
C. C_A skin
D. C_A lungs

19. All are recognised examples of "Asphyxiating gases", *save* for one:
A. CO gas
B. SO_2 gas
C. Trichloroethylene
D. Cyanide gas
E. Cl_2 gas

20. Which dusts in air predisposes to Tuberculosis?
A. Asbestos
B. Zinc
C. Carbon
D. Silica
E. None of the above

21. Which of the following occupation is most likely to be associated with leptospiral infections?
A. Poultry dressers
B. School personnel
C. Physicians
D. Salesman

22. Which of the following bacterial diseases may be encountered as an occupational hazard?
A. Anthrax
B. Brucellosis
C. Tetanus
D. Both A and B above
E. All of these

23. A patient with headache, nausea, vomiting, fatigue, jaundice, hepatomegaly and oliguria may have an occupational disease caused by:
A. Aluminium
B. Benzene
C. CCl_4
D. Lead (Pb)
E. Mercury (Hg)

24. The 1st pathogenic bacillus to be seen under the microscope was:
A. Anthrax
B. Brucella
C. Tetanus
D. Tuberculosis
E. Cholera

25. "Shaving brushes" have been incriminated in the transmission of:
A. Anthracosis
B. Anthrax
C. Brucellosis
D. Leprosy
E. None of these

26. Dust within the size range of .... predisposes pneumoconiosis.
A. 0.1 to 7 µ
B. 0.2 to 7 µ
C. 0.5 to 3 µ
D. 0.5 to 6 µ
E. 1 to 7 µ

27. Which type of pneumoconiosis was 1st of all reported in India from Kolar Gold Mines?
A. Asbestosis
B. Byssinosis
C. Anthracosis
D. Silicosis
E. Siderosis

28. A patient is presenting to you with irritant cough, dyspnoea on exertion and chest pain. O/E his total lung capacity is impaired. TLC and DLC within normal limit with slight lymphocytosis, ESR is

slightly raised, X-ray chart reveals, "Snow-storm-appearance". Most likely he suffers from:

A. Silicosis
B. Brucellosis
C. Asbestosis
D. Anthracosis
E. Two of the above

29. What causes "brown lung"?

A. Silicon dioxide
B. Cotton dust
C. Coal particles
D. Bagassosis

30. "Caisson's disease" is the result of:

A. Pneumoperitoneum
B. O_2 bubbles in soft tissue
C. N_2 bubbles in soft tissue
D. CO_2 saturation in blood
E. Subcutaneous emphysema

31. Acclimatization to higher altitude results in:

A. Decrease in RBC
B. Decrease in cardiac output
C. Respiratory acidosis
D. Respiratory alkalosis
E. All of the above

32. Byssinosis is seen in:

A. Textile industry
B. Grain fields
C. Sugarcane
D. Metal factories

33. Baggasse control is accomplished by keeping the moisture content above 20% and spraying the bagasse with:

A. 1% acetic acid
B. 2% propionic acid
C. 3% citric acid
D. 4% tartaric acid

34. Consider the following statements regarding asbestosis:

I. 90% of world's production of asbestos is of the serpentine variety
II. In India asbestos is mined in Andhra, Bihar, Karnataka and Rajasthan
III. Major asbestos producing nations in world are USSR, Canada, USA and South Africa
IV. Asbestos enters the body by ingestion

Select the true answer as per code given below:

A. I and IV only
B. I and II only
C. I, II and III only
D. II, III and IV
E. I, II, III and IV All

35. Asbestos dusts predisposes to the following cancers, *but* one:

A. C_AGIT
B. C_A bronchus
C. Mesothelioma of pleura or peritoneum
D. C_A urinary bladder
E. None of these

36. An X-ray chart shows a ground-glass appearance in the lower 2/3rds of the lung fields in cases of:

A. Asbestosis
B. Byssinosis
C. Bagassosis
D. Silicosis
E. All of the above

37. "Asbestos bodies" are:

A. Asbestos fibres coated with fibroblasts
B. Asbestos fibres only
C. Asbestos fibres coated with fibrin
D. Asbestos fibres + albumin coating

38. Statement (S): Lead is used widely in a variety of industries.
Reasons (R): Because it mixes with other metals easily to form alloys.

Select the correct answer as per code given below:

A. Both (S) and (R) are true and are related to cause and effect

B. Both (S) and (R) are true but are not related to cause and effect

C. (S) is true, (R) is false

D. (R) is true, (S) is false

E. Both (S) and (R) are false

39. Amenorrhoea and sterility may occur in females as a result of occupational exposure to:

A. Mercury

B. Lead

C. CO gas

D. Zinc

E. Chromium

40. Following occupations enumerated below is due to lead, *save* for:

A. Metal refiners

B. Paint makers

C. Colour makers

D. Pottery

E. Cable makers

41. All are the common S/S of lead poisoning, *except* for one:

A. Foot drop

B. Sensory changes

C. Stippling and punctate basophilia

D. Spongy gums

E. Teeth mottling

42. Toxic effect of "Organic lead" compounds are all, *but* one:

A. Insomnia

B. Headache

C. Wrist drop and foot drop only

D. Mental confusion only

E. Delerium only

43. Toxic effects of "inorganic lead" compounds are all, *save* for one:

A. Abdominal colic

B. Blue line on gums

C. Loss of appetite

D. Delerium only

E. Punctate basophilia only

44. All are standard lab tests to diagnose lead poisoning, *except* for one:

A. TLC and DLC of WBC

B. Basophilic stippling of RBC

C. CPU in urine

D. Lead in blood and urine

E. ALAU in urine

45. Consider the following statements about lead:

I. Organic lead (tetraethyl lead) is only absorbed through skin

II. The body store of lead in the average adult is about 150 to 400 mg

III. The blood lead level in adult averages 25 μg/100 ml

IV. Normal adults ingest about 0.2 to 0.3 mg of lead per day from food and beverages

V. 90% of ingested lead is excreted in the faeces

Select the true answer as per code given below:

A. I, II and III only

B. I, II and IV

C. I, III and V

D. I, II, III and IV

E. I, II, III, IV and V All

46. "Obstinate constipation" may occur due to poisoning with:

A. Alcohol

B. Inorganic lead

C. Organic lead

D. Calcium

E. Ether

47. In lead poisoning, a blood level of .... is associated with clinical symptoms.

A. 30 μg/100 ml

B. 40 μg/100 ml

C. 50 μg/100 ml
D. 70 μg/100 ml

48. Lead poisoning is a notifiable and compensatable disease in India:
A. Since 1924
B. Since 1943
C. Since 1944
D. Since 1954
E. Since 1964

49. About 75% of occupational cancers are:
A. Bladder C_A
B. Bone C_A
C. Skin C_A
D. Lung C_A

50. Workers working in uranium mines are particularly susceptible to:
A. Skin C_A
B. Lung C_A
C. Bladder C_A
D. Leukaemia
E. All of the above

51. Occupational exposure to which of the following cause leukaemia?
A. Benzol
B. X-rays
C. Radioactive substances
D. All of the above
E. Both B and C above

52. Following are possible bladder carcinogen:
I. β-naphthylamines
II. Benzidine
III. Paramino-diphenyl
IV. Auramine and magenta

Choose the correct answer from the code given below:
A. I and II only
B. I, II and III
C. I, II, III and IV All
D. I, II and IV
E. II, III and IV only

53. Percival Pott (1775) draw attention to cancer of which in chimney sweeps?
A. C_A scrotum
B. C_A bladder
C. C_A intestine
D. C_A rectum

54. Skins cancer may result from:
A. Radium burns
B. Pigmented moles
C. Scars of old burns
D. Arsenical keratosis
E. All of the above

55. The most common occupational disease is:
A. Asbestosis
B. Silicosis
C. Plumbism
D. Dermatosis
E. Cancer

56. Prodromal symptoms of acute radiation syndrome, include:
A. Anorexia
B. Prostration
C. Nausea and vomiting
D. Fatigue and sweating
E. All of the above

57. Tissues of high sensitivity to tumour induction by ionizing radiation:
A. Skin
B. Bone marrow
C. Bone
D. GIT
E. CNS only

58. Principal findings during overt stage (2 to 6 weeks) of acute radiation syndrome include:
A. Infection
B. Fever
C. Motor disorders
D. Purpura
E. All of these

59. In India, the highest accident rate is reported from:
A. Mines
B. Railways
C. Factories
D. Docks and ports
E. All of these

60. It was estimated that nearly .... man days are lost yearly in India owing to accidents.
A. 1 million
B. 2 millions
C. 3 millions
D. 4 millions
E. 5 millions

61. Medical thermography is based on the principal of man emitting:
A. X-rays
B. β-rays
C. UVL rays
D. Infra red radiation
E. None of the above

62. "Phossy jaw" is associated with which industry?
A. Mica
B. Match
C. Steel
D. Gold
E. Uranium

63. About how much % of the days lost were found to be due to occupational accidents?
A. 1%
B. 3%
C. 5%
D. 7%
E. 10%

64. The primary value of a preemployment physical examination is:
A. To prevent law suits
B. To test physical endurance
C. To detect cancer
D. To determine manual dexterity
E. None of these

65. "Industrial hygiene" is a responsibility of the:
A. Employer
B. Workers
C. Community health administration
D. All of these
E. Both A and B above

66. Which of the following probably contributed most to the development of industrial hygiene as an applied science?
A. W.H.O.
B. I.L.O.
C. Workmen's Compensation Act
D. Accident insurance

67. Persons suffering from which of the following diseases should not be employed in lead utilizing industry?
A. Anaemia
B. Hypertension
C. Nephritis
D. Peptic ulcer
E. All of these

68. Ordinarily workers are examined:
A. Once in a year
B. Per month
C. Six monthly
D. Every fortnightly

69. Radium, lead and toxic dyes workers should preferably be screened once:
A. Daily
B. Monthly
C. Quarterly
D. Six monthly
E. Yearly

70. Persons handling "dichromates" should be examined:
A. Annually
B. Monthly
C. Fortnightly

D. Weekly
E. Daily

71. In the Mines Act, how many diseases are notifiable?
A. Three
B. Five
C. Eight
D. Twenty-two
E. Only one

72. Factories Act (1978) prohibits employment of children below ....
A. 10 years
B. 12 years
C. 14 years
D. 16 years
E. 18 years

73. In Dock Regulations Act, how many diseases are listed?
A. Three
B. Five
C. Only one
D. Eight
E. Ten only

74. The ESI Act was passed in which of the following year?
A. 1948
B. 1949
C. 1950 and 1951
D. 1953

75. Who is the chairman of E.S.I. Corporation?
A. Union Health Minister
B. Union Labour Minister
C. Director General ESI
D. Director General of Health Services
E. Any of the above

76. In the Factories Act (1948), the total number of hours of work in a week including overtime shall not exceed:
A. 48 hours
B. 52 hours
C. 60 hours
D. 64 hours
E. 75 hours

77. Following causes the most lost work days:
A. Allergic disorders
B. Bone and joint disease
C. Nutritional disease
D. Circulatory disorders
E. All are equally prone

78. Under E.S.I. Act, employees getting daily wages of below are exempted from payment of contribution:
A. Rs. 15
B. Rs. 25
C. Rs. 30
D. Rs. 40
E. Rs. 50 only

79. Benefits to employees under ESI Act includes the following:
A. Medical sickness and maternity benefit
B. Disablement, Dependent's
C. Funeral expenses
D. Rehabilitation allowance
E. All of the above

80. An Insurance Medical Practitioner is allowed a maximum of how many family units?
A. 100
B. 200
C. 350
D. 500
E. 750 family units

81. The existing doctor-population ratio under the ESI scheme is:
A. 1 : 368
B. 1 : 585
C. 1 : 1500
D. 1 : 3500

82. The sickness benefit is payable for a maximum period of .... in any continuous period of 365 days, the daily rate

being about 7/12 of the average daily wages:
A. 30 days
B. 40 days
C. 50 days
D. 75 days
E. 91 days

83. Diseases for which extended sickness benefit is payable for 309 days includes the following:
A. Tuberculosis
B. Psychoses
C. Chronic CCF
D. Hemiplegia
E. All of the above

84. Regarding maternity benefit under E.S.I. Act, all are true, *but* one:
A. Safe confinement (12 weeks)
B. Miscarriage (6 weeks)
C. Sickness due to confinement (30 days)
D. The benefit is allowed at half wages

85. The amount payable as cash towards funeral benefits is upto how much?
A. Rs. 250
B. Rs. 500
C. Rs. 1000
D. Rs. 1500
E. Rs. 2000

86. Dependent's benefit under ESI covers children upto what ages?
A. 12 years
B. 14 years
C. 16 years
D. 18 years
E. 21 years only

87. The Directorate General, Factory inspection and Advisory Service was set up in which year?
A. 1945
B. 1947
C. 1950
D. 1952
E. 1962

88. The premium of the "Community based Universal Health Insurance Scheme" launched during 2003-04 ranges from:
A. Re. 1 per day poor and individual to Rs. 3 per day for a family of 7
B. Re. 1 per day poor and individual to Rs. 2 per day for a family of 7
C. Rs. 2 per day poor and individual to Rs. 2 per day for a family of 7
D. None of these

Answers

1 A	2 B	3 C	4 D	5 E	6 C	7 B	8 A	9 D	10 B
11 E	12 C	13 D	14 B	15 C	16 D	17 B	18 A	19 C	20 D
21 A	22 E	23 C	24 A	25 B	26 C	27 D	28 A	29 B	30 C
31 D	32 A	33 B	34 C	35 D	36 A	37 C	38 A	39 B	40 D
41 B	42 C	43 D	44 A	45 E	46 B	47 D	48 A	49 C	50 B
51 D	52 C	53 A	54 E	55 D	56 E	57 B	58 E	59 A	60 C
61 D	62 B	63 E	64 E	65 D	66 C	67 E	68 A	69 B	70 E
71 A	72 C	73 D	74 A	75 B	76 C	77 D	78 A	79 E	80 E
81 B	82 E	83 E	84 D	85 C	86 D	87 A	88 B		

C•H•A•P•T•E•R **TEN**

Genetics Health

DIRECTION: Following MCQ's are provided with a few suggestive answers/completions. Only one answer is correct. You have to identify the *BEST* one in each case.

1. **Two basic principles genetics was laid down by:**
   A. Aristotle
   B. Mendel
   C. Galton
   D. Hippocrates
   E. Both B and C above

2. **According to many authors, genetically conditioned disease or disease with a clear genetic component account for what % of all cases being treated by the health services?**
   A. < 1% only
   B. 5 to 15%
   C. 20 to 30% only
   D. 25 to 40%

3. **In which year Tjio and Levan surprised the scientific world by demonstrating only 46 chromosome in human Karyotype instead of 48 as previously reported?**
   A. 1901
   B. 1956
   C. 1966
   D. 1976
   E. 1936

4. **Which of the following statemente(s) is/are false?**
   A. Each pair of chromosome is homologous
   B. The chromosomes vary in length, the longest being about 5 times as long as the smallest
   C. The autosome are numbered according to their length, the 1st pair being the longest and the last pair shortest
   D. None of these
   E. Both B and C above

5. **The autosomes have been classified and divided on the basis of length and certain morphological similarities into how many groups?**
   A. Two
   B. Five
   C. Seven
   D. Twenty-two

6. **The "short acrocentric" are found in:**
   A. Group 6 to 12
   B. Group 13 to 15
   C. Group 16 to 18 only
   D. Group 19 to 29
   E. Group 21 to 22 only

7. The most convenient stage of cell division for the examination of somatic chromosomes is:
A. Metaphase
B. Anaphase
C. Telophase
D. Interphase

8. The systematic arrangement of the entire chromosome complement of the cell is called the:
A. Genotype
B. Phenotype
C. Karyotype
D. Mitotic figure

9. Colchicine inactivates the spindle apparatus and stops mitosis at:
A. Prophase
B. Metaphase
C. Anaphase
D. Telophase

10. The main chemical constituent of a chromosome is:
A. Genes
B. Protein
C. Ribosenucleic acid
D. DNA

11. The human mitotic chromosomes have a form similar to an:
A. X
B. Y
C. L
D. M
E. Any of the above

12. The largest chromosome measures about how much?
A. 3 μ
B. 7 μ
C. 10 μ
D. 15 μ
E. 21 μ

13. Following tissues are used to study chromosomes:
A. Buccal smears
B. Peripheral blood
C. Bone marrow
D. Skin only
E. All of these

14. The 1st meiotic division leading to the development of an ovum or spermatid is often called:
A. Reduction division
B. Mitosis
C. Amitosis
D. Prophase II
E. None of these

15. A gene is said to be dominant when it manifests its effect in the:
A. Heterozygous
B. Homozygous only
C. Both of the above
D. Neither of the above

16. Consider the following statements about genes:
I. Genes are the units of heredity
II. We inherit about 15,000 genes from the father and 15,000 from the mother
III. The locus for ABO blood group is in chomosome 9
IV. The Y chromosome contains genes that determine the normal development of testes

Choose the true answer as per code given below:
A. I and II
B. I, II and III
C. I, II, III and IV All
D. I, III and IV only

17. The human 'X' chromosome carries the genes governing:
A. Haemophilia
B. Glucose-6-phosphate dehydrogenase
C. Muscular dystrophy
D. Red green colour blindness
E. All of the above

18. In the ABO blood system, the possible genotypes are the following, *save* for one:
A. ABO only
B. AA and AB
C. AO and BO
D. BB and OO

19. Following are phenotypical expression of a particular genetic constitution:
I. Colour
II. Form
III. Size
IV. Stature of individuals

Choose the true answer as per code given below:
A. I and IV only
B. II and III only
C. I, II and III
D. I, II, III and IV All

20. The incidence of chromosomal abnormalities is .... per 1000 live births.
A. 1.2
B. 2.1
C. 3.2
D. 4.2
E. 5.6

21. A human tetraploid cell has got .... chromosomes.
A. 23 only
B. 46 only
C. 92 only
D. 69 only
E. 184 only

22. The most common cause of trisomy is:
A. Failure of homologous chromosomes to go to opposite poles during meiosis
B. Failure of homologous chromosomes to go to opposite poles during mitosis
C. Translocation
D. Mosaic formation
E. Failure of egg cleavage

23. Monosomy is the:
A. Mosaic formation
B. Loss of a chromosome
C. Addition of an extra chromosome
D. None of these

24. Isochromosomes are:
A. Translocation chromosomes
B. X-chromosome
C. Mosaic chromosomes
D. None of these

25. The result of nondisjunction occurring in mitotic divisions after fertilization is called:
A. Mosaicism
B. Isomerase inversion
C. Translocation
D. Trisomy state
E. Late replication

26. Agents capable of causing chromosomal breakage include the following, *but* one:
A. Nitrogen mustard
B. Measles virus
C. X-ray
D. Ultraviolet rays
E. None of these

27. Which of the following numerical aberrations of chromosome number represents aneuploidy?
A. Haploidy
B. Hypoploidy
C. Triploidy
D. Diploidy

28. If a fragment of one chromosome becomes attached to the broken end of another, the process is called:
A. Translocation
B. Inversion
C. Tetraploidy
D. Deletion
E. Hyperploidy

29. The genetic mechanism that most frequently causes aneuploidy is:
A. Inversion
B. Nondisjunction

C. Crossing-over
D. Deletion
E. Translocation

30. An individual with a karyotype of XY, XO and XYY would be expected to have how many sex chromatin bodies?
A. One
B. Two
C. Three
D. Four
E. NIL

31. Individual with karyotype of XX, XXY, and XXYY would be expected to have .... sex chromatin bodies.
A. One
B. Two
C. Three
D. Four
E. Virtually NIL

32. Gynaecomastia, aspermatogenesis with eunochoidism and increased excretion of FSH best describes:
A. Turner's syndrome
B. Familial dysautonomia
C. Klinefelter's syndrome
D. Down's syndrome

33. The basis of the abnormal sex chromosomal finding in Klinefelter's syndrome seems to be:
A. X/Y + translocation
B. Deletion of Y chromosomes
C. Meiotic nondisjunction of the Y chromosomes
D. Meiotic nondisjunction of the X chromosome

34. The most likely reason for the extra chromosome in Down's syndrome is:
A. Anaphase lag
B. Translocation
C. Nondisjunction
D. Oogenesis
E. Fragmentation

35. A patient with Down's syndrome due to reciprocal translocation would be expected to have how many chromosomes?
A. 45
B. 46
C. 47
D. 48
E. None of the above

36. Turner's syndrome is characterised by all the following, *except* for one:
A. Infantilism
B. Webbed neck
C. COA only
D. Cubitus valgus
E. Cubitus varus only

37. All the following are associated with Mongolism, *save* for one:
A. Short stature
B. Pelvic kidney
C. Congenital heart disease
D. Deformed ears
E. Slant of the eyes

38. Which of the following eye signs is NOT usually associated with Down's syndrome?
A. Absence of refractive errors
B. Epicanthal fold
C. Brushfield spots
D. Cataracts
E. Oblique palpebral fissures

39. The D_1 trisomy syndromes in characterized by all the following, *save* for one:
A. Apparent mental retardation
B. Abnormal helices
C. Normal palmar creases
D. Apparent deafness
E. Microphthalmos and/or colobomata

40. Only .... pairs of the human chromosome are homologous.
A. 12
B. 22
C. 23

D. 44
E. 46 only

41. Regarding Klinefelter's syndrome. All are true, *save* for one:
A. It is common sex chromosome aneuploidy
B. The most common karyotype is XXY pattern
C. The growth of hair on face, axillae and pubes are very exuberant
D. Incidence is 1: 1000 per live male births

42. Probably the most common chromosome disorder in humans is:
A. Turner's syndrome
B. Klinefelter's syndrome
C. Superfemales
D. Down's syndrome

43. The most likely genetic mechanism causing Turner's syndrome is:
A. Inversion
B. Nondisjunction
C. Isochromosome
D. Deletion only
E. Translocation

44. NOT a usual finding in Turner's syndrome:
A. Short stature
B. Pulmonary stenosis
C. 45XO karyotype
D. Primary amenorrhoea
E. No mental retardation

45. Mongolism was 1st described by.......... in 1866.
A. Mendel
B. Browne
C. Langdon Down
D. Degrnchi
E. Emil Fischer

46. The outstanding example of sex linked inheritance is:
A. Total colour blindness
B. Hemophilia
C. Cri-du-chat syndrome
D. Blood grouping

47. An individual who is homozygous for a pathological trait marries a heterozygous genotype for the same trait .... will appear normal of all the offspring.
A. 1/4th
B. 1/3rd
C. 1/2 only
D. 3/4th
E. None

48. Of the offsprings of two individuals with an abnormal recessive gene .... of these will have an abnormal genotype.
A. 1/4th
B. 1/2
C. 3/4th
D. All of the above
E. None

49. A heterozygous individual with an abnormal recessive gene marries another heterogygous individual with the same abnormal recessive gene. Of the offspring .... will display the abnormality.
A. 1/3rd
B. 1/4th
C. 112 only
D. All of the above
E. None

50. A man with hemophilia marries a non-transmitter female; off spring of this union would show a ratio of:
A. All with hemophilia
B. All males with hemophilia, all females normal
C. All females are carriers, all males normal
D. All males are carriers, all females normal
E. All offspring are normal genotypically

51. Repeated stillbirths in a woman are likely to be related to chromosomal abnormality during intrauterine life (IUL) and the abnormality will be:
A. Mosaicism

B. Isochromosome
C. Inversion
D. Deletion only
E. All of the above

52. In a genetically determined disease, one of the parents is genetically normal and the other is abnormal, then the condition is equally distributed among offsprings of either sex, however 50% will have a chance of getting manifest disease. This trait is called as:
A. Autosomal dominant trait
B. Autosomal recessive trait
C. X-linked dominant
D. Y-linked
E. X-linked recessive trait

53. Consider the following Statemente(s):
I. If mutation is confined to a single gene it is called "point" mutation
II. An individual with an autosomal dominant trait will produce two kind of gametes with respect to the mutant gene—half with mutant gene and half with normal allele
III. Abnormalities caused by recessive genes occur when both the parents are heterozygotes

Choose the true answer as per code given below:
A. I only
B. II only
C. I and II only
D. I, II and III All

54. Following are recognised examples of X-linked dominant traits, *save* for one:
A. Familial hypophosphatemia
B. Hydrocephalous
C. Blood group Xg
D. Vit. D resistant rickets

55. Which is NOT inherited as X-linked recessive trait?
A. Mega colon (Hirschprung's disease)
B. Agammaglobulinaemia (bruten type)
C. Retinitis pigmentosa
D. G_6 PD deficiency

56. Following are inherited as autosomal dominant trait, *save* for one:
A. ABO blood group system
B. Polycystic kidney
C. Familial polyposis coli
D. Huntington's chorea
E. Duchenne type of muscular dystrophy

57. All are inherited as autosomal recessive traits, *but* one of the following:
A. Albinism
B. Brachydactyly
C. Cystic fibrosis
D. Haemoglobinopathies
E. Tay-Sachs disease

58. At present, how many blood groups are discovered in human?
A. Three
B. Five
C. Seven
D. Twelve
E. Fourteen

59. In the ABO system, the most common blood group observed in Indian population is:
A. Group B
B. Group AB
C. Group 'O'
D. Group A only

60. In the ABO system the rarest blood group seen in Indian people is:
A. Group 'B'
B. Group 'O'
C. Group 'A'
D. Group 'AB' only

61. The Rh system have been demonstrated in a:
A. 3 months old foetus
B. 38 days old foetus
C. 60 days old foetus
D. Foetus at term

62. What % of Indian population is Rh positive?
A. 75%
B. 85%
C. 93%
D. 97%
E. 50%

63. Following diseases are seen in blood group 'A' individuals, *save* for one:
A. Gastric ulcer
B. Gastric C_A
C. C_A uterine C_X
D. Pernicious anaemia
E. Thrombosis

64. A classic example of disease caused by a point mutation in DNA is:
A. Thalassemias
B. Sickle cell anemia
C. PKU
D. Hemophilia
E. Cystic fibrosis

65. Sickle cell anemia usually manifests during:
A. 1st year of life
B. 2nd year of life
C. IUL only
D. 5th year of life
E. Adolescence

66. A 10-year-old boy had hemophilia. The disease will not occur in:
A. His sister
B. His daughter
C. His sons
D. All of the above

67. Following diseases are associated with multifactorial aetiology, *except* for one:
A. Essential hypertension
B. Duodenal ulcer
C. Schizophrenia
D. None of these

68. Gene therapy may be used in the following ways:
A. To correct a genetic mutation (in cystic fibrosis)
B. To kill a cell (cancer)
C. To modify susceptibility (CAD)
D. Both A and B above
E. All of these

69. "The relative frequency of each gene allele tends to remain constant from generation to generation. This law was enunciated by:
A. Hardy
B. Hardy-Wienberg law
C. Campbell law
D. Dalton's law
E. Galton's law

70. Following factors influence the human gene pool, *except:*
A. Mutation and natural selection
B. Breeding structure
C. Struggle for existence
D. Population movement
E. Public health measure

71. The science which aims to improve the genetic "endowment of human population is known as:
A. Eugenics
B. Anthropology
C. Euthenics
D. Genetic counselling

72. "EUGENICS" is credited to whom?
A. Hitler
B. Galton
C. Rambler
D. Dalton
E. Gibbon

73. All the following methods are suggested under retrospective genetic counselling, *except* for:
A. Contraception
B. Pregnancy termination
C. Consanguineous marriage
D. Sterilization

74. **Prospective genetic counselling has got its application in the:**
A. Sickle cell anemia
B. Thalassemia
C. Both
D. Neither

75. **If the incidence of Down's syndrome in mother at age 20 is only 1 : 3000, then at the age of 40 its incidence would be:**
A. 1 : 3000
B. 1 : 2000
C. 1 : 200
D. 1 : 80
E. 1 : 40

76. **Carriers can be detected in the following, *but* one:**
A. Haemophilia
B. PKU
C. Galactosaemia
D. Alkaptonuria

77. **"Amniocentesis" is indicated for all, *save* for one:**
A. Screening for neural tube defects
B. IUGR
C. Advanced maternal age
D. Previous child with chromosome defects

78. **"Guthrie card test" is done for:**
A. Congenital adrenal hyperplasia
B. PKU
C. Cystic fibrosis
D. Congenital hypothyroidism

79. **Neonatal screening for cystic fibrosis (CF) is based on measurement of immuno-reactive trypsin in:**
A. Sweat test
B. Sweat NaCl test
C. Guthrie blood spots
D. Both A and B above
E. All of the above

80. **Biochemical screening of newborn infants was first used for PKU in which year?**
A. 1946
B. 1952
C. 1986
D. 1966
E. 1996

81. **Consanguineous marriages more likely to produce the following outcomes:**
A. Albinism
B. Alkaptonuria
C. PKU
D. Increased risk of premature death
E. All of the above

82. **Hardy-Weinberg law related to:**
A. Population genetics
B. Health economics
C. Social medicine
D. None of these

83. **Holandric inheritance is transmitted as:**
A. X-linked
B. Y-linked
C. AR
D. AD

84. **The genotype of cri du chat syndrome is:**
A. $13q^-$
B. Trisomy 18
C. $5p^-$
D. None of the above

85. **Robertsonian translocation is:**
A. 8:14t
B. 5:11t
C. 10/21t
D. 14/21 translocation

86. **An example of intermediate inheritance is:**
A. Sickle cell anemia
B. PKU
C. Haemophilia
D. Xq blood group

87. **Robertsonian translocation is a transloation between:**
A. Two submetacentric chromosomes

B. Two acrocentric chromosomes
C. Two metacentric chromosomes
D. An submetacentric and metacentric chromosomes

88. An example of co-dominant inheritance is:
A. Albinism
B. Haemophilia
C. AB blood group
D. Testicular feminization syndrome

89. The type of chromosomes *not* seen in human is:
A. Acrocentric
B. Telocentric
C. Metacentric
D. Submetacentric

90. Chromosomal constitution of primary oocyte is:
A. 23XX
B. 46XY
C. 23X
D. 46XX

91. The mode of inheritance of testicular feminisation syndrome is:
A. X-linked recessive
B. AD
C. X-linked dominant
D. AR

92. Edward's syndrome is due to:
A. Trisomy 13
B. Trisomy 18
C. Trisomy 21
D. Trisomy 9

93. Patau's syndrome is due to:
A. Trisomy 13
B. Trisomy 9
C. Trisomy 21
D. Trisomy 18

94. The disease transmitted as X-linked dominant is:
A. Wilson's disease
B. Total colour blindness
C. Vitamin D resistant rickets
D. Albinism

95. The mode of inheritance of testicular feminization syndrome is:
A. X-linked dominant
B. X-linked recessive
C. AD
D. AR

96. All are transmitted as AD mode of inheritance, *but* one:
A. Achondroplasia
B. Brachydactyly
C. Yellow-blue colour blindness
D. Duchenne muscular dystrophy

97. All are transmitted as AR mode of inheritance, *but* one:
A. Total colour blindness
B. Tuberous sclerosis
C. Hepatolenticular degeneration
D. Ataxia-telangiectasia

98. All are inherited as X-linked recessive manner, *except* for:
A. Cervico-oculo acoustic syndrome
B. Fabry's disease
C. Lesch-Nyhan syndrome
D. Reifenstein's syndrome

99. Hyperammonemia is inherited as:
A. AD
B. AR
C. XLD
D. XLR

Answers

1 E	2 D	3 B	4 D	5 C	6 E	7 A	8 C	9 B	10 D
11 A	12 B	13 E	14 A	15 C	16 C	17 E	18 A	19 D	20 E
21 C	22 A	23 B	24 D	25 A	26 E	27 B	28 A	29 B	30 E
31 A	32 C	33 D	34 C	35 B	36 E	37 B	38 A	39 C	40 B
41 C	42 A	43 B	44 E	45 C	46 B	47 C	48 C	49 B	50 C
51 D	52 A	53 D	54 B	55 A	56 E	57 B	58 E	59 C	60 D
61 B	62 C	63 A	64 B	65 A	66 C	67 E	68 E	69 B	70 C
71 A	72 B	73 C	74 C	75 E	76 D	77 A	78 B	79 C	80 D
81 E	82 A	83 B	84 C	85 D	86 A	87 B	88 C	89 B	90 D
91 A	92 B	93 A	94 C	95 B	96 D	97 B	98 A	99 C	

C•H•A•P•T•E•R **ELEVEN**

Mental Health

DIRECTION: Following MCQ's are provided with a few suggestive answers/completions. Only one answer is correct. You have to identify the *BEST* one in each case.

1. The mental illness morbidity rate in India is not less than ....

A. 10 per 1000
B. 15 per 1000
C. 18 to 20 per 1000
D. 25 per 1000
E. 30 per 1000 of total population

2. The number of mental hospital beds in the country, as per a 1991 survey is:

A. 5000
B. 10,000
C. 18,000
D. 21,147
E. 48,500

3. The "warning signals of poor mental health" has been devised by whom?

A. William C. Menninger
B. Sigmund Freud
C. C. Jung
D. David Morley
E. None of the above

4. Following are major psychiatric illnesses called psychoses:

I. Schizophrenia
II. Manic depressive psychosis
III. Paronia
IV. Neurosis only

Select the true response from the code given below:

A. I and II only
B. II and III only
C. I, II and III
D. I, II, III and IV

5. Following peculiar symptoms has been exhibited by psychoneurotics, *except* for one:

A. Morbid fears only
B. Split personality only
C. Compulsions only
D. Obsessions only

6. Following are recognized characteristics of a mentally healthy person, *save* for one:

A. Neither underestimates nor overestimates his own ability
B. Feels rights towards others
C. Able to like and trust others
D. Does not accept his shortcomings
E. Shoulders his daily responsibilities

7. **Following are major mental illnesses, *but* one:**
   A. Paronia only
   B. Schizophrenia
   C. Psychoneurosis only
   D. Manic depressive psychosis
   E. None of these

8. **Following mineral deficiencies are related to mental ill health:**
   I. Iodine only
   II. Iron only
   III. Calcium only
   IV. Zinc only
   Select the true response from the code given below:
   A. I only
   B. I and II only
   C. II and III only
   D. I, II and III
   E. I, II, III and IV

9. **Psychic and physical state resulting from interaction between a living organism and a drug is called:**
   A. Drug abuse
   B. Drug dependence
   C. Drug intoxication
   D. Adverse drug effect
   E. None of these

10. **Statement (S): Personality and character disorders are of major psychiatric illnesses.**
    Reason (R): Because most of these individuals show split personality.
    A. Both (S) and (R) are true and related to cause and effect
    B. Both (S) and (R) are true but unrelated to cause and effect
    C. (S) is true but (R) is false
    D. Both (S) and (R) are false

11. **In which of the following psychiatric illness symptoms varies from heights of excitement to depths of depression?**
    A. Schizophrenia only
    B. Psychoneurosis only
    C. Manic-depressive psychosis
    D. Paronia only

12. **Which psychiatric illness is associated with undue and extreme suspicion and a progressive tendency to regard the whole world in a framework of delusions?**
    A. Personality and character disorders
    B. Psychoneurosis
    C. Schizophrenia
    D. Manic-depressive-psychosis
    E. Paronia

13. **Statement (S): In schizophrenia, the patient lives in a dream world of his own.**
    Reason (R): Because he possesses a split personality.
    A. Both (S) and (R) are true and related to cause and effect
    B. Both (S) and (R) are true but unrelated to cause and effect
    C. (S) is true but (R) is false
    D. Both (S) and (R) are false

14. **Following chronic diseases produce mental illness:**
    I. Tuberculosis
    II. Leprosy
    III. Epilepsy
    Select the true answer from the code given below:
    A. I and II only
    B. I and III only
    C. I, II and III
    D. II and III only

15. **The child of 2 schizophrenic parents is .... more likely to develop schizophrenia than is the child of healthy parents.**
    A. 10 times
    B. 20 times
    C. 30 times
    D. 40 times
    E. 50 times

16. Mental illnesses may have their origin in organic conditions like:

I. Cerebral arteriosclerosis
II. Metabolic diseases
III. Neurological diseases
IV. Neoplasms
V. Endocrine diseases

Select the true response from the code given below:

A. I, II, III, IV and V All
B. I, II and III
C. I, II, III and IV
D. II, III, IV and V

17. Following toxic substances are related to abnormal human behaviour, *except* for one:

A. Mercury
B. Barbiturates
C. Carbondisulphide only
D. Manganese and tin only
E. Lead compounds

18. Following psychotropic drugs produce abnormal human behaviour, *save* for one:

A. Alcohol only
B. Barbiturates
C. Chlorpromazine
D. Griseofulvin only
E. None of these

19. Which of the following vitamin deficiency causes mental ill health?

A. Ascorbic acid
B. Thiamine
C. Pyridoxine only
D. Both B and C above
E. All of the above

20. Following infectious disease during the prenatal, perinatal and postnatal periods causes mental illness:

A. Measles only
B. Rubella only
C. Chickenpox
D. All of the above
E. Both A and B

21. Statement (S): Nervous system is most sensitive to radiation during the period of neural development.

Reason (R): Because involvement of nervous system during organogenesis causes mental ill health.

A. Both (S) and (R) are true and related to cause and effect
B. Both (S) and (R) are true but not related to each other
C. (S) is true but (R) is false
D. Both (S) and (R) are false

22. The basic needs of the adolescents are:

A. The need to be needed by others
B. The need for increasing independence
C. The need to achieve adequate adjustment to the opposite sex
D. The need to rethink the cherished beliefs of one's elders
E. All of the above

23. The causes of mental illness in the aged are organic conditions of the brain, economic insecurity, lack of a home, poor status and insecurity.

A. True
B. False

24. The mental health services comprise the following:

I. Early diagnosis and treatment
II. Rehabilitation
III. Group and individual psychotherapy
IV. Mental health education
V. Use of modern psychoactive drugs
VI. After care services

Select the true response from the code given below:

A. I and II only
B. I, II and IV only
C. I, IV, V and VI only
D. I, II, III, IV and V only
E. I, II, III, IV, V and VI All

25. The philosophy of community Mental Health Programme consists of the following essential elements:
I. Inpatient services
II. Out-patient services
III. Partial hospitalization
IV. Emergency services
V. Diagnostic services
VI. Pre-care and aftercare services including foster home placement and home visiting
VII. Education services
VIII. Training
IX. Research and evaluation

Select the true answer from the code given below:
A. I, III, V and VII
B. II, IV, VI and VIII
C. III, IV, V, VI and IX
D. I, III, IV, V, VI, VIII and IX
E. I, II, III, IV, V, VI, VIII, IX All true

26. WHO has defined drug as "any substasnce that, when taken into the living organism, may modify one or more of its functions".
A. True
B. False

27. How may people smoke marijuana in the U.S.A.?
A. 5 million
B. 7 million
C. 8 to 10 million
D. 12 to 20 million

28. What percentage of all high school students has made marijuana an accepted part of life?
A. 10 to 12%
B. 30 to 50%
C. 20 to 30%
D. 50 to 60%

29. How many drugs are in use now-a-days?
A. Only one
B. Three
C. Five
D. Six only
E. Eight

30. Amphetamines are synthetic drugs, structurally resembles which of the following drugs?
A. Alcohol
B. Barbiturates
C. Cannabis only
D. LSD only
E. Adrenaline only

31. Amphetamines are used in medical practice to treat the following:
I. Obesity
II. Mild depression
III. Narcolepsy
IV. Certain behaviour disorders in children

Select the correct response from the code given below:
A. I, II and III only
B. I, II, III and IV All
C. I and III only
D. I, III and IV

32. Statement (S): Amphetamines are called "Superman" drugs.
Reason (R): Because they give a tremendous boost to self-confidence and energy.
A. Both (S) and (R) are true and correctly explain to each other
B. Both (S) and (R) are true but not related to each other
C. (S) is true but (R) is false
D. Both (S) and (R) are true

33. Following statements are true regarding amphetamines:
A. These drug act on the CNS
B. They produce mood elevation, elation and a feeling of well-being
C. They increased alertness and a sense of heightened awareness
D. All of above
E. Both B and C but not A above

34. Statement (S): Psychic dependence with amphetamines is dose dependent.

Reason (R): Because with large doses, such dependence, is often rapid and strong.

A. Both (S) and (R) are true but not related to each other
B. Both (S) and (R) are true and related to each other
C. (S) is true, (R) is false
D. Both (S) and (R) are false

35. Following are true statements regarding barbiturates, *except* for one:

A. They are the major ingredient in sleeping pills
B. The drug-users generally prefer long acting barbiturates than short acting barbiturates
C. The addiction to barbiturates is one of the worst forms of suffering
D. It leads to craving, or both physical and psychic dependence

36. The chewing of coca leaves is a very common practice in Bolivia and Peru in South America.

A. True
B. False

37. Perhaps, the most widely used drug today is:

A. Amphetamines
B. Barbiturates only
C. Cannabis only
D. LSD only
E. Alcohol only

38. In U.S.A. the term MARIJUANA is used to refer to any part of the Cannabis plant which induces somatic and psychic changes in man.

A. True
B. False

39. Perhaps, the most widely used drug today is:

A. Alcohol
B. Barbiturates
C. Cannabis
D. LSD
E. Heroin

40. Cannabis is a very ancient drug obtained from the hemp plants:

A. Cannabis sativa
B. C. indica
C. Cannabis americana
D. All of the above
E. Both B and C but not A above

41. Regarding cannabis, following statements are true:

A. The resinous exudate from the flowering tops of the female plant contains most of the active ingredients called hashish or charas
B. The dried leaves and flowering shoots are called bhang
C. The resinous mass from the small leaves and brackets of inflorescence is called ganja
D. Both A and C above
E. All the above

42. Following are narcotic analgesic, *save* for one:

A. Alcohol
B. Heroine
C. Morphine
D. Methadone only

43. LSD was synthesized in 1938 by whom?

A. Aldermann (Glaxo)
B. Hoffmann (Sandoz lab)
C. Carletti (Ciba-Geigy)
D. Daveshon (Hochest)

44. "Physical dependence" does not develop with:

A. Alcohol
B. Barbiturates

C. LSD
D. All of the above
E. Both A and B above

45. **"Alcohol" is incriminated in the causation of following cancers in human, *save* for one:**
A. C_A mouth
B. C_A pharynx
C. C_A larynx and oesophagus
D. C_A colon and rectum
E. None of these

46. **Statement (S): Addiction to heroin is perhaps the worst type of addiction.**
Reason (R): Because it produces craving.
A. Both (S) and (R) are true and (R) is the true explanation of (S)
B. Both (S) and (R) are true but (R) is not the true explanation of (S)
C. (S) is true but (R) is false
D. Both (S) and (R) are false

47. **Statement (S): There is no addiction liability with LSD.**
Reason (R): Aecause physical dependence does not develop with LSD.
A. Both (S) and (R) are true but (R) is not the true explanation of (S)
B. Both (S) and (R) are true and (R) is the true explanation of (S)
C. (S) is true but (R) is false
D. Both (S) and (R) are false

48. **"Psychic dependence" is seen with following drugs:**
A. Amphetamine
B. Barbiturates
C. Cannabis
D. Heroin only
E. All of the above

49. **Mental retardation is defined if I.Q. is below how much?**
A. < 50
B. < 60
C. < 70
D. < 90

50. **The approximate number of mentally retarded persons in India is around:**
A. 4 to 8 millions
B. 10 to 15 millions
C. 15 to 20 millions
D. 20 to 25 millions

51. **Globally about .... people are suffering from mental retardation.**
A. 83 millions
B. 93 millions
C. 103 millions
D. 203 millions

52. **The most commonly abused drug causing addiction among Indians is:**
A. Amphetamine
B. Barbiturates
C. Cannabis
D. LSD
E. Crack

53. **The incidence of mental illness is the maximum if the causal factors affect a particular period of life:**
A. Perinatal period
B. 1st 5 years of life
C. School age
D. Adolescence

Answers

1 C	2 D	3 A	4 C	5 B	6 D	7 C	8 A	9 B	10 D
11 C	12 E	13 A	14 C	15 D	16 A	17 B	18 C	19 D	20 E
21 A	22 E	23 A	24 E	25 E	26 A	27 D	28 B	29 D	30 E
31 B	32 A	33 D	34 B	35 B	36 A	37 C	38 A	39 C	40 D
41 E	42 A	43 B	44 C	45 D	46 A	47 B	48 C	49 C	50 D
51 A	52 C	53 B							

C•H•A•P•T•E•R **TWELVE**

Health Care of the Community

DIRECTION: Following MCQ's are provided with a few suggestive answers/completions. Only one answer is correct. You have to identify the *BEST* one in each case.

1. **The current criticism against health care services includes all, *but* one:**
   A. Faced only by developing nations not by developed one
   B. Predominantly urban oriented
   C. Mostly curative in nature
   D. Accessible mainly to a small part of the population
   E. None of these

2. **Statement (S): The current social policy throughout the world is to build up health systems based on primary health care.**
   Reason (R): Because policy objectivce of Health for All by 2000 AD has only been achieved through primary health care.
   Select the true answer as per code given below:
   A. Both (S) and (R) are ture, but are unrelated to cause and effect
   B. Both (S) and (R) are true and are related to cause and effect
   C. (S) is true, (R) is false
   D. (R) is true, (S) is false
   E. Both (S) and (R) are false

3. **In India, which of the following serve as the 1st referral level hospital?**
   A. Subcentres
   B. PHCs
   C. Community health centres
   D. District hospital
   E. Both C and D

4. **The AIIMS at New Delhi is serving as a:**
   A. Primary care level hospital
   B. Secondary care level hospital
   C. Tertiary care level hospital
   D. None of the above

5. **The term "comprehensive health care" was 1st used by whom?**
   A. Kartar Singh Committee
   B. Bhore Committee
   C. Srivastava Committee
   D. Jungalwala Committee
   E. Chadah Committee

6. **The term "basic health services" was used by:**
   A. Indian Red Cross
   B. UNICEF
   C. WHO

D. Both B and C above
E. All of these

7. The term "Primary health care" has come into existence at Alma-Ata in:
A. 1946
B. 1965
C. 1978
D. 1981
E. 1983

8. The 1st key principle in the primary health care strategy is:
A. Equitable distribution of health services
B. Social injustice
C. Irrespective of ability to pay
D. Failure to reach the majority

9. In which country of the world "bare foot doctors" are found?
A. Australia
B. Bangladesh
C. China
D. Denmark
E. Equador

10. An essential feature of primary health care in India is:
A. Health guides
B. Trained dais
C. Both of these
D. None of these

11. "Health for All by 2000 AD" was decided in the World Health Assembly in:
A. 1977
B. 1978
C. 1981
D. 1982
E. 1983

12. "Attainment of a level of health that will enable every individual to lead a socially and economically productive life". This is the definition of:
A. Primary health care
B. Health for all
C. Comprehensive care
D. Basic health care
E. None of the above

13. A global strategy for HFA was evolved by WHO in which year?
A. 1978
B. 1980
C. 1981
D. 1997
E. 2000 AD

14. The WHO has established how many global indicators as the basic point of reference for assessing the progress towards HFA?
A. Three
B. Five
C. Seven
D. Ten
E. Twelve

15. In the context of the national health policy and WHO call for HFA and Alma Ata declaration, the following goals has to be achieved by 2000 AD *save* for one:
A. Reduction of IMR from the level of 125 (1978) to 60
B. To raise the expectation of life at birth from 52 years to 64 years
C. To reduce CBR from 33/1000 population to 21
D. To reduce CDR from 14/1000 population to 9
E. To provide potable water to entire rural population

16. An assessment of the health status and health problems is:
A. Social pathology
B. Social medicare
C. Community diagnosis
D. Health care delivery
E. Epidemiology

17. In 1947, the annual incidence of malaria was:
A. 15 million
B. 30 million

C. 45 million
D. 60 million
E. 75 million

18. By which year, the incidence of malaria was drastically reduced to about 0.1 million with no deaths?
A. 1953
B. 1958
C. 1960
D. 1965
E. 1970

19. In which year, the resurgence of malaria has been noted in India?
A. 1953 B. 1958
C. 1976 D. 1962
E. 1965

20. A modified action plan against malaria control was put into operation in the year:
A. 1977
B. 1958
C. 1966
D. 1979
E. 1980

21. In recent years, malaria due to which species of plasmodium are gradually increasing in India?
A. Plasmodium vivax
B. Plasmodium falciparum
C. P. ovale only
D. P. malariae
E. Almost all are equally vulnerable

22. The % of tuberculin positive cases in india out of total population is:
A. 15.2%
B. 25.2%
C. 30%
D. 40.3%
E. 50% only

23. What % of Indians are radiologically active T.B. Lung disease?
A. 0.4%
B. 0.9%
C. 1.0%
D. 1.5% only
E. 5.6% only

24. What % of Indians are sputum positive case of tuberculosis?
A. 0.1 %
B. 0.2%
C. 0.5%
D. 0.3%
E. 0.4% only

25. India has nearly 12.7 million cases of pulmonary T.B. of which about .... are sputum positive.
A. 1.2 million
B. 3.4 million
C. 4.3 million
D. 2.1 million

26. Diarrhoeal diseases constitute one of the major causes of morbidity and mortality in the following age groups:
A. < 1 month
B. < 1 year
C. < 2 years
D. < 3 years
E. < 5 years

27. It is estimated that about 13.6% hospital admissions and .... inpatient deaths in paediatric wards are due to ARI.
A. 6.5%
B. 13.0%
C. 16.0%
D. 18.2%
E. 20.0% only

28. In India, the number of leprosy case is:
A. 0.61 million
B. 0.71 million
C. 0.81 million
D. 0.91 million

29. What % of total new cases of leprosy in India are multibacillary?
A. 1 to 5%
B. 5 to 10%

C. 10 to 15%
D. 35 to 39%
E. 20 to 25%

30. The prevalence rate of leprosy in India is about .... per 10,000 population.
A. 1.6
B. 2.3
C. 6.7
D. 4.8
E. 8.9 per 1000 population

31. Consider the following statements about leprosy.
I. About 15% of the cases are children below the age of 15 years
II. The proportion of infectious cases varies between 6 to 8%
III. The 1.8% cases suffer from deformities
IV. India accounts for 60% of leprosy cases in world

Select the correct answer as per code given below:
A. I and II
B. II, III and IV
C. I, II and III
D. I, II and IV
E. I, II, III and IV All

32. About what % of people in India are at risk to filariasis?
A. 420 million
B. 25 million
C. 19 million
D. 100 million

33. It is estimated that .... manifest filariasis in India.
A. 5 million
B. 19 million
C. 12 million
D. 25 million
E. 15 million

34. What proportion of Indians shows filarial parasites in their blood?
A. 15 million
B. 19 million
C. 25 million
D. 50 million
E. 100 million

35. What proportion of cases are seropositive for HIV in India?
A. 10,000
B. 20,000
C. 33,000
D. 5.1 million
E. 1.2 lakhs

36. In India, AIDS was 1st detected in which year?
A. 1986
B. 1988
C. 1990
D. 1991
E. 1981

37. The period .... was designated as the "International water supply and sanitation decade".
A. 1961-1970
B. 1971-1980
C. 1951-1960
D. 1991-2000
E. 1981-1990

38. At present what % of rural population in India has been getting safe water?
A. 30%
B. 45%
C. 55%
D. 85%
E. 65%

39. Consider the following statements about PEM:
I. "Food gap" appears to be the chief cause of PEM
II. Nearly 80% of PEM cases are mild and moderate
III. The incidence of severe cases is 1 to 2% in pre school age children
IV. The Marasmus is more frequent than Kwashiorkor

Choose the correct answer as per code given below:

A. I, II, III, IV All
B. I, II and III only
C. I and II only
D. I and III only
E. I and IV only

40. The specific nutritional problem in India includes:

I. Protein energy malnutrition (PEM)
II. Nutritional anaemia
III. Xerophthalmia
IV. Low birth weight
V. Iodine deficiency disorders

Select the true answer as per code given below:

A. I and II only
B. I, II and III only
C. I, II and IV only
D. I, II, III, IV and V All
E. I, III and V

41. In world, probably the highest prevalance of nutritional anaemia in women and children are seen in:

A. South Africa
B. India
C. Bangladesh
D. Indonesia
E. Srilanka

42. The most frequent cause of nutritional anaemia in India is:

A. Folate deficiency
B. B_{12} deficiency
C. Iron deficiency
D. All of the above
E. Both A and C above

43. What % of babies born in India are of low birth weight?

A. 5%
B. 10%
C. 20%
D. 30%
E. 40%

44. Consider the following statements about nutritional blindness:

I. About 0.04% of total blindness in India is attributed to Vitamin A deficiency
II. Keratomalacia has been the major cause of nutritional blindness in children usually between 1 to 3 years of age
III. Subclinical deficiency of Vitamin A is also widespread and is associated with increased morbidity and mortality from respiratory and GIT infections

Choose the false answer as per code given below:

A. I only
B. II only
C. I and II both
D. I, II and III All
E. None of the above

45. The maximum prevalance rate for I.D.D. has been found in:

A. Sirmor (HP)
B. Mandi (HP)
C. Champaran (Bihar)
D. Darjeeling (WB)

46. The most difficult problem to tackle in India is:

A. AIDS
B. PEM
C. Communicable diseases
D. Environmental sanitation

47. What proportions of modern medicare facilities are available in urban area?

A. 80%
B. 60%
C. 50%
D. 62%
E. 69% only

48. Currently, India's growth rate is:

A. 1.93%
B. 2.1%

C. 2.5%
D. 3.1%
E. Just 1%

49. India is producing per year how many allopathic doctors?
A. 7,000
B. 10,000
C. 12,000
D. 15,000
E. 20,000

50. The suggested norms for doctor to population is:
A. 1 per 3,000
B. 1 per 3,500
C. 1 per 4,000
D. 1 per 5,000

51. The suggested norm for nurses to population is:
A. 1 per 3,000
B. 1 per 35,000
C. 1 per 4,000
D. 1 per 5,000
E. 1 per 10,000

52. The suggested norm for health assistant (male and female) in tribal and hilly areas is ......population.
A. 1 per 5,000
B. 1 per 10,000
C. 1 per 20,000
D. 1 per 30,000
E. 1 per 50,000

53. In India, there are how many community health centres by 1996?
A. 5,000
B. 10,000
C. 7,000
D. 2,424
E. 3,000 only

54. To achieve HFA, WHO has set as a goal the expenditure of what % of each country's GNP on health care?
A. 1%
B. 2%
C. 3%
D. 4%
E. 5%

55. At present India is spending about .... of GNP on health and family welfare development.
A. 1%
B. 2%
C. 3% only
D. 4%
E. 5%

56. The Government of India launched a Rural Health Scheme, based on the principle of "placing people's health in people's hands" in:
A. 1977
B. 1978
C. 1981
D. 1983
E. 1986

57. The village health guides scheme was introduced on 2nd October:
A. 1952
B. 1967
C. 1977
D. 1981
E. 1968

58. The village health guide scheme is NOT applicable in following Indian states, *but* one:
A. Arunachal Pradesh
B. Bihar only
C. Kerala and Karnataka
D. Tamil Nadu
E. Jammu and Kashmir only

59. The guidelines for selection of village health guides include all the following, but one:
A. A parttime Government functionary
B. Educated upto 6th class
C. Acceptable to all sections of community
D. Preferably female
E. Able to spare atleast 1 to 3 hours every day for community health work

60. Currently, in India how many village health guides are functioning?
A. 2.2 lakhs

B. 3.23 lakhs
C. 6.2 lakhs
D. 10.2 lakhs

61. **The training period of each local dais is:**
A. 15 days
B. 21 days
C. 30 days
D. 60 days
E. 90 days

62. **After successful training each dai is entitled to receive an amount of Rs......... per delivery provided the case is registered with subcentre/PHC:**
A. 10 only
B. 25
C. 50
D. 75
E. 100

63. **To each infant registered by local dais, she will receive Rs. ....**
A. One
B. Two
C. Three
D. Four
E. Five only

64. **During per training each dai is required to conduct atleast how many deliveries under the guidance and supervision of the HW, ANM or HA?**
A. One
B. Two
C. Three
D. Four
E. Five

65. **In each ICDS blocks, how many Aanganwadi workers?**
A. Only one
B. Hundred
C. Twenty-five
D. Fifty
E. Thousands

66. **How many ICDS blocks are functioning in India to date?**
A. 1000
B. 2000
C. 3050
D. 4035
E. 5320

67. **The peripheral outpost of the existing health delivery system in rural areas in India is:**
A. Additional PHC
B. PHC
C. Subcentres
D. Community health centre

68. **At present, the functions of subcentre are limited to all, *except:***
A. MCH
B. Family planning
C. Immunization
D. IUCD insertions

69. **In India, the total requirement of subcentre is estimated to be:**
A. 1 lakh
B. 1.38 lakh
C. 1.5 lakh
D. 1.75 lakh
E. 2.2 lakh

70. **In India, the total requirement of PHC is about:**
A. 5,000
B. 10,000
C. 15,000
D. 20,000
E. 23,000

71. **In community health centres, the following specialists (doctor) posts has been sanctioned to function, *but* one:**
A. Surgery
B. Pathology
C. Medicine
D. Obs and Gynae
E. Paediatrics

72. **The specialist at the community health centre may refer a patient directly to:**
A. State level hospital/Medical college

B. Subdivisional hospital
C. District hospital
D. All of these
E. Both B and C above

73. The ESI Act covers employees drawing wages not exceeding Rs....... per month.
A. 3,500
B. 5,500
C. 6,500
D. 7,500
E. 8,300

74. The CGHS scheme for Central Government employees was 1st introduced in:
A. Bombay 1950
B. Baroda 1952
C. Calcutta 1953
D. New Delhi 1954

75. The existing doctor-population ratio for the country as a whole is:
A. 1 : 5000
B. 1 : 3500
C. 1 : 3000
D. 1 : 2100
E. 1 : 1500

76. The National Institute of Ayurveda is established at:
A. Jaipur
B. Bombay
C. Calicut
D. Bhopal
E. Bhubaneshwar

77. The National Institute of Homeopathy is situated at:
A. Delhi
B. Mumbai
C. Kolkata
D. Chennai
E. Ernaculum

78. A Central Council of Indian Medicine was established in which year to prescribe minimum standards of education in Indian Medicine?
A. 1951
B. 1971
C. 1961
D. 1981
E. 1991

79. Recognised activities of Indian Red Cross includes:
A. Relief work, milk and medical supplies
B. Armed forces and MCH care
C. Family planning, blood bank and first aid
D. All of the above

80. The recognised function of central social welfare board includes:

I. Surveying the needs and requirements of voluntary welfare organisations

II. Promoting and setting up of social welfare organisations on voluntary basis

III. Financial aid to deserving existing organisations and institutions

Select the true answer as per following code:
A. I and II only
B. I and III
C. I, II and III All
D. II and III
E. None of these

81. In which year Millennium Development Summit (MDS), in which 189 nations of the world participated, ensued?
A. March 2001
B. September 2000
C. December 2002
D. October 2003

82. MDS took place in which city of the world under United Nations Millennium declaration?
A. New York
B. Geneva
C. New Delhi
D. London

83. Government have set what date by which they would meet "Millennium development goals" (MDGs) like eradicate extreme poverty and hunger, achieve universal primary education, promote gender equality, improve maternal health, combat HIV/AIDS, malaria and other communicable diseases, ensures environmental sustainability, and develop a global partnership for development?
A. 2005
B. 2010
C. 2015
D. 2007

84. Hind Kusht Nivaran Sangh was founded in 1950, but prior to 1950 its precursor was known as:
A. ICCW
B. BELRA
C. Bharat Sevak Samaj (BSS)
D. The Kasturba Memorial Fund

85. A quarterly published journal named "Leprosy in India" is published by:
A. JIMA
B. JAMA
C. Hind Kusht Nivaran Sangh
D. BMJ

86. The Family Planning Association of India was formed in 1949 with its headquarters at:
A. Mumbai
B. Bangalore
C. Kolkata
D. New Delhi

87. Health for All by the WHO was announced at:
A. U.S.A.
B. Geneva
C. U.S.S.R.
D. Denmark

88. Following is not a voluntary health agency:
A. Family Planning Association of India
B. Ford/Rockfeller Foundation
C. National Institute of Nutrition
D. Indian Council for Child Welfare

89. An Anganwadi worker is trained for:
A. 3 months
B. 4 months
C. 6 months
D. 9 months

90. All are peripheral level health workers, *but* one:
A. Gram sevak
B. VHNS
C. Anganwadi workers
D. Trained dais

91. Principles of PHC (Primary health care) include all, *except:*
A. Community involvement
B. Resource allocation
C. Political commitment to HFA
D. Disability prevalence

92. All are grass roots workers, *except:*
A. Health assistant
B. Traditional birth attendants
C. Village health guide
D. Anganwadi workers

93. Village health guide scheme is *not* seen in:
A. Karnataka
B. J and K
C. Tamil Nadu
D. All of the above

94. In an hospital ideal bed space should be:
A. 5 feet
B. 7 feet
C. 8 feet
D. 12 feet

95. Not a duty of raditional birth attendants is:
A. Aseptic delivery
B. Injection of TT
C. Birth registration
D. Health education

96. **According to the World Health Report 2000, India's health expenditure is:**
A. 4.8% of GDP
B. 5.2% of GDP
C. 6.8% of GDP
D. 7% of GDP

97. **Indian (economic) real GDP growth for the year 2003 is:**
A. 6.0
B. 6.5 to 6.8
C. 7.8
D. 10.5

98. **According to a joint study "Healthcare in India" the road ahead is done by CII and Mekinsey and Company in 2002. India's executing bed population rate is:**
A. 2 : 1000
B. 1.5 : 1000
C. 2.5 : 1000
D. 9 : 1000

Answers

1 A	2 B	3 C	4 C	5 B	6 D	7 C	8 A	9 C	10 C
11 A	12 B	13 C	14 E	15 A	16 C	17 E	18 D	19 C	20 A
21 B	22 C	23 D	24 E	25 B	26 E	27 B	28 A	29 D	30 B
31 E	32 A	33 B	34 C	35 D	36 A	37 E	38 D	39 A	40 D
41 B	42 C	43 D	44 E	45 C	46 D	47 A	48 A	49 C	50 B
51 D	52 C	53 D	54 E	55 C	56 A	57 C	58 B	59 A	60 B
61 C	62 A	63 C	64 B	65 B	66 E	67 C	68 D	69 B	70 E
71 B	72 A	73 D	74 D	75 D	76 A	77 C	78 B	79 D	80 C
81 B	82 A	83 C	84 B	85 C	86 A	87 B	88 C	89 B	90 A
91 D	92 A	93 D	94 D	95 B	96 B	97 B	98 C		

C•H•A•P•T•E•R **THIRTEEN**

International Health

DIRECTION: Following MCQ's are provided with a few suggestive answers/completions. Only one answer is correct. You have to identify the *BEST* one in each case.

1. Who said, "Nothing on earth is more international than disease"?
A. Paul Russel
B. Rene Sand
C. James Lind
D. Linga Tu
E. Lamuhar Kalakki

2. In which century, a procedure known as "quarantine" was introduced in Europe to protect against the importation of plague?
A. 13th century
B. 14th century
C. 15th century
D. 16th century
E. 17th century

3. The 1st international sanitary conference was held in 1851 in which country (city)?
A. Great Britain (London)
B. Italy (Rome)
C. France (Paris)
D. U.S.A. (Washington DC)

4. "OIHP" stands for:
A. On Indian hospital programme
B. On international health programme
C. Our Indian horticulture programme
D. Office International D' Hygiene Publique

5. Statement (S): The existence of OIHP is only upto 1950.

Reason (R): Because after that its responsibilities has been taken over by the WHO.
A. Both (S) and (R) are true and (R) is the true explanation of (S)
B. Both (S) and (R) are true and (R) is not the true explanation of (S)
C. (R) is false and (S) is true
D. Both (S) and (R) are false

6. Which of the following statements is/are true?
A. The United Nations Relief and Rehabilitation Administration (UNRRA) was set up in 1943
B. UNRRA did outstanding work of preventing the spread of typhus and other diseases
C. UNRRA terminated its official existence in 1946
D. All of the above
E. Both A and C but not B above

7. The WHO has its origin in April:
A. 1945
B. 1946
C. 1947
D. 1948
E. None of these

8. The WHO health day is celebrated every year on:
A. 7th Jan
B. 7th April
C. 7th July
D. 7th October
E. None of the above

9. The current objective of WHO is:
A. HFA by 2000 AD
B. To help in medical research
C. To supervise national health programmes in the countries
D. To help international cooperation in the field of health

10. The headquarter of WHO is situated at:
A. Rome
B. Paris
C. Geneva
D. New York

11. The WHO is unique among the UN specialized agencies because:
A. It has its own constitution
B. Own governing bodies
C. Own membership
D. Own budget
E. All of the above

12. In 1948, the WHO had how many members?
A. 48
B. 56
C. 84
D. 65
E. None of these

13. By 1996 WHO had how many members?
A. 56 **B.** 87
C. 104 **D.** 140
E. 190 only

14. The following diseases are target of the WHO special programmes for research and training in tropical nations, *except* for one:
A. Tuberculosis and AIDS
B. Malaria and Filaria
C. Leprosy and Leishmaniasis
D. Schistosomiasis and Trypanosomiasis

15. The 30th world health assembly adopted a resolution aimed at ensuring immunization of all children by:
A. 1985
B. 1990
C. 1995
D. 2000
E. None of the above

16. Regarding the role of WHO in family health:
I. Maternal and child health
II. Nutrition
III. Human reproduction
IV. Health education

Select the true answer from the following code given:
A. I only
B. I and II only
C. I, II and IV only
D. I, II, III and IV All

17. The WHO is committed to attain the target adopted to have "Water for All" by:
A. 1987 **B.** 1995
C. 1990 **D.** 1997
E. 2000

18. The only fully computerised indexing system covering the whole of medicine on an international basis is:
A. Stedman's index
B. Medlar's index
C. Dorland's index
D. All of the above
E. Both B and C above

19. The WHO consists of the following:
- **A.** World health assembly
- **B.** The executive board
- **C.** The secretariat
- **D.** All of the above
- **E.** Both B and C but not A above

20. In which year the 14th World Health Assembly met in New Delhi?
- **A.** 1961
- **B.** 1965
- **C.** 1971
- **D.** 1981
- **E.** 1991

21. The main functions of the Health Assembly includes:
- **I. To determine international health policy and programmes**
- **II. To review the work of the past year**
- **III. To approve the budget needed for the following year**
- **IV. To elect member states to designate a person to serve for three years on the executive board and to replace the retiring members**

Select the correct answer from the following code:
- **A.** I and IV
- **B.** II and III
- **C.** I, II, III and IV All
- **D.** I, II and III
- **E.** I, III and IV

22. The executive board had originally 18 members, what is the number of existing members?
- **A.** 18
- **B.** 24
- **C.** 26
- **D.** 30
- **E.** None of these

23. The South-East Asian regional headquarter of WHO is situated at:
- **A.** Tokyo
- **B.** New Delhi
- **C.** Kolkata
- **D.** Mumbai

24. Which of the following South-East Asian region country is *not* a member of WHO?
- **A.** India
- **B.** Bhutan
- **C.** Maldive Islands
- **D.** Sri Lanka
- **E.** Pakistan only

25. The executive board has power to take action in emergency like:
- **A.** Epidemics
- **B.** Earthquake
- **C.** Floods only
- **D.** All of the above
- **E.** Both A and B only

26. The following South-East Asian region became WHO member in 1948, *except* for one:
- **A.** Bangladesh
- **B.** Burma
- **C.** India
- **D.** Sri Lanka

27. UNICEF (United Nations International Children's Emergency Fund) was established in which year?
- **A.** 1986
- **B.** 1976
- **C.** 1966
- **D.** 1956
- **E.** 1946

28. Following statements or facts are true about UNICEF *except* for one:
- **A.** It was established by the United Nations General Assembly to deal with rehabilitation of children in war ravaged nations
- **B.** In 1953, its name has been changed to: U.N. Children's Fund, but retained the initials UNICEF
- **C.** It is governed by 50 member (nations) executive board
- **D.** The headquarters of the UNICEF is at United Nations, New York
- **E.** None of these

29. The UNICEF's South Central Asian Region, regional office is located at which place?
A. New Delhi
B. Sri Lanka
C. Dubai
D. Maldive Islands

30. UNICEF works in close collaboration with:
A. WHO
B. UNDP
C. FAO
D. UNESCO
E. All of the above

31. UNICEF provides aid in:
A. Child health
B. Child nutrition
C. Education
D. Family and child welfare
E. All of the above

32. Following statements are true about child health in India under UNICEF, *except* for:
A. Supported India's BCG vaccination programme
B. Has not assisted in environmental sanitation
C. Assisted in the erection of penicillin plant near Pune
D. Donated a DDT plant
E. Donated two plants for the manufacture of triple vaccine and iodized salt

33. GOBI campaign of UNICEF includes the following:
I. Growth charts
II. Oral rehydration
III. Breast feeding
IV. Immunization
V. Iodine supplementation
Select the true answer from the code given below:
A. I, II, III and V
B. I and II
C. I, II, III and IV
D. I, II and III

34. Following is recognised association of UNICEF in India:
I. Education
II. Health
III. Nutrition
IV. Water supply
V. Social welfare
Select the true answer from the code given below:
A. I, II, III, IV and V All
B. I, II and III
C. I, II, III and IV
D. I, II, III and V

35. UNICEF has been participating in Urban Basic Services (UBS) since:
A. 1986
B. 1956
C. 1966
D. 1976
E. 1952

36. The United Nations Development Programme (UNDP) was established in which year?
A. 1956
B. 1966
C. 1976
D. 1986
E. None of these

37. The United Nations Fund for Population Activities (UNFPA) has been providing assistance to India since:
A. 1954
B. 1964
C. 1974
D. 1984
E. 1994

38. How many districts of Bihar state has been taken into consideration under UNFPA?
A. Three
B. Four
C. Nine
D. Eleven
E. Twelve

39. Besides Bihar UNFPA has also been implemented in which Indian States?
A. Andhra Pradesh
B. West Bengal
C. Rajasthan only
D. Madhya Pradesh
E. Any of the above

40. In which year the Food and Agriculture Organization (FAO) was formed?
A. 1945
B. 1948
C. 1956
D. 1962
E. None of these

41. The headquarter of FAO is in:
A. Geneva
B. Rome
C. New York
D. London

42. Which of the following is acknowledged as the first United Nations Organization specialized agency created?
A. UNICEF
B. UNDP
C. FAO
D. ILO
E. WHO

43. The chief aims of FAO is:
A. To help nations raise living standard
B. To improve nutrition of the people of all countries
C. To increase the efficiency of farming, forestry and fisheries
D. To better the condition of rural people
E. All of the above

44. The FAO has organised a world "Freedom from hunger campaign" (FFHC) in which year?
A. 1950
B. 1960
C. 1970
D. 1980
E. 1990

45. The joint WHO/FAO expert committees have provided the basis for many co-operative activities like:
A. Nutritional surveys
B. Training courses
C. Seminars and the coordination of research programmes on brucellosis and other zoonoses
D. All of the above
E. Both A and C but not B above

46. In which year International Labour Organization (ILO) was established?
A. 1919
B. 1945
C. 1948
D. 1952
E. 1962

47. Following are the purposes of ILO:
I. To contribute to the establishment of lasting peace by promoting social justice
II. To improve, through international action, labour conditions, and living standards
III. To promote economic and social stability

Select the true answer from the code given below:
A. I only
B. I and III
C. I, II and III
D. II and III
E. I and II

48. The headquarter of ILO is in:
A. London, England
B. Geneva, Switzerland
C. Washington DC, USA
D. Copenhagen, Denmark

49. Cooperative programmes that exist between WHO and the World Bank includes the following *save* for one:
A. Projects for water supply

B. World Food Programme
C. Population control
D. The control of onchocer ciasis programme in West Africa
E. None of these

50. The US Government presently extends aid to India through three agencies:
I. World Bank
II. USAID
III. The Public Law 480 (Food for Peace) Programme
IV. The US Export-Import Bank

Select the true answer from the code given below:
A. I and II only
B. II and III only
C. II, III and IV
D. I, II, III and IV All

51. In which year United States Agency for International Development (USAID) was created?
A. 1951
B. 1961
C. 1971
D. 1981
E. 1991

52. Under the Colombo Plan how many regional developing countries are members?
A. 5 only
B. 12
C. 20
D. 26
E. None of these

53. How many non-regional members are included under the Colombo Plan?
A. 6
B. 12
C. 18
D. 24
E. 30 only

54. The bulk of Colombo Plan assistance goes to:
A. Industrial development
B. Health promotion
C. Agricultural development
D. All of the above
E. Both A and C but not B above

55. The AIIMS at New Delhi was established with financial assistance from:
A. Australia
B. Newzealand
C. Russia
D. USA
E. United Kingdom

56. The cobalt therapy units to medical institutions in India is contributed by .... under Colombo Plan.
A. USA
B. UK
C. Canada
D. West Germany

57. The Rockefeller Foundation is a:
A. Political organization
B. Philanthropic organization
C. Both of the above
D. None of the above

58. Who was the founder of Rockefeller organization?
A. John D Rockefeller
B. Sir Ronald Jackson
C. Ian Rockefeller
D. Henry Dunant

59. The work of the Rockefeller Foundation in India began in 1920 with a scheme for:
A. The control of amoebiasis
B. The control of hookworm
C. The control of tuberculosis
D. The control of leprosy

60. The National Institute of Virology at Pune was established in close cooperation with:
A. WHO
B. UNICEF
C. Rockefeller Foundation

D. CARE

61. "NIHAE" (National Institute of Health Administration and Education at Delhi) has been set up with the help of:

A. WHO
B. UNICEF
C. CARE
D. Ford Foundation

62. "CARE" stands for:

A. Cooperative for Americans Relief Everywhere
B. Cooperative for Australian Relief Everywhere
C. Cooperative for Arabian Relief Everywhere
D. Cooperative for Asian Relief Everywhere

63. "CARE" has been helping India in:

A. Family welfare
B. Mid-day meal scheme
C. Sanitation programme
D. All of these
E. Both A and C above

64. "CARE" was created in which year?

A. 1946
B. 1956
C. 1966
D. 1976
E. 1986

65. The International Red Cross was founded by:

A. Mr JD Rockefeller
B. Henry Dunant
C. Alfred Noble
D. Annie Besant

66. Who wrote the book "Un Souvenir de Solferine"?

A. Annie Besant
B. Martin Luther King
C. Henry Dunant
D. Alfred Noble

67. In which year the league of the Red Cross Society was created?

A. 1859
B. 1864
C. 1901
D. 1919
E. 1948

68. The headquarter of Red Cross Society is in:

A. Geneva
B. Copenhagen
C. Toronto
D. Washington DC
E. Bonn

69. The Indian Red Cross Society was established in:

A. 1919
B. 1920
C. 1948
D. 1958
E. 1962

70. Recognised objectives of Indian Red Cross includes:

A. Improvement of health
B. Prevention of disease
C. Mitigation of suffering
D. All of the above

71. The world health day theme for the year 2001 focuses on:

A. Mental health
B. Safe blood transfusion
C. Reproductive and child health
D. Disaster management

Answers

1 A	2 B	3 C	4 D	5 A	6 D	7 A	8 B	9 A	10 C
11 E	12 B	13 E	14 A	15 B	16 D	17 C	18 B	19 D	20 A
21 C	22 D	23 B	24 E	25 D	26 A	27 E	28 C	29 A	30 E
31 E	32 B	33 C	34 A	35 D	36 B	37 C	38 D	39 C	40 A
41 B	42 C	43 E	44 B	45 D	46 A	47 C	48 B	49 E	50 C
51 B	52 C	53 A	54 E	55 B	56 C	57 B	58 A	59 B	60 C
61 D	62 A	63 B	64 A	65 B	66 C	67 D	68 A	69 B	70 D
71 A									

C·H·A·P·T·E·R **FOURTEEN**

Health Information and Basic Medical Statistics

DIRECTION: Following MCQ's are provided with a few suggestive answers/completions. Only one answer is correct. You have to identify the *BEST* one in each case.

1. In which year, the World Health Assembly stressed the need for complete reconstruction of the health information systems?
A. 1973
B. 1953
C. 1963
D. 1983
E. 1993

2. Consider the following statements:
I. Data consists of discrete observations of attributes or events that carry little meaning when considered alone
II. Data as collected from operating health care systems or institutions are inadequate for planning
III. Data need to be transformed into information by reducing them, summarising them and adjusting them for variations
Choose the correct answer as per following code:
A. I only
B. I and II only
C. I, II and III All
D. I and III only
E. II and III only

3. Following requirements to be satisfied by health information systems:
I. The system should be population based
II. The system should be problem oriented
III. The system should avoid the unnecessary agglomeration of data
IV. The system should make provision for the feedback of data
Choose the correct answer as per code given below:
A. I, II and III
B. I, II, III and IV All
C. I, III and IV only
D. I and IV only
E. II, III and IV only

4. Recognised components of health information system includes:
I. Demography and vital events
II. Health status and health resources
III. Indices of outcome of medical care
IV. Environmental health statistics

Choose the correct answer as per code given below:
A. I, II and III only
B. I and II only
C. I and IV only
D. I, II, III and IV All
E. II, III and IV only

5. **Following are uses of health information:**
   I. **To measure the health status of the people**
   II. **For local, national international comparisons of health status**
   III. **For planning administration and effective management of health services and programmes**
   IV. **For research into particular problems of health and disease**

   Select the false answer as per code given below:
   A. I only
   B. I, II and III only
   C. I and II only
   D. I, II, III and IV only
   E. None of these

6. **Regarding CENSUS, all statements are true, *save* for one:**
   A. The census in India was taken first in 1881
   B. The census is not an important source of health information
   C. The last census was held in India in 2001 at the interval of 10 years
   D. The legal basis of census is provided by the Census Act of 1948

7. **The Government of India had passed the births, death and marriage, registration Act on voluntary basis in which year?**
   A. 1873
   B. 1893
   C. 1973
   D. 1923
   E. 1943

8. **According to central births and deaths registration Act, 1969, the time limit for registering the events of births is 14 days and that of deaths is 7 days. In case of default a fine upto how much in rupee can be imposed?**
   A. Rs. 10
   B. Rs. 50
   C. Rs. 100
   D. Rs. 250
   E. Rs. 500 only

9. **The sample registration system (SRS) was initiated in which year?**
   A. Mid 50's
   B. Mid 90's
   C. Mid 60's
   D. Mid 70's
   E. Mid 80's

10. **Regarding sample registration system (SRS) all are true, *but* one:**
    A. Provides reliable estimates of birth and death rate at the national and state levels
    B. It is an half yearly survey
    C. It is a dual record system
    D. It is a major source of health information
    E. It does not cover the entire country

11. **In sample registration system, survey is done every .... :**
    A. 3 months
    B. 6 months
    C. 9 months
    D. 12 months
    E. 15 months

12. **Following diseases are notifiable to WHO in Geneva under the International Health Regulations (IHR), *save* for one:**
    A. Polio
    B. Cholera
    C. Plague
    D. Yellow fever
    E. None of these

13. Statements (S) : Hospital records are not good source of health information.

Reason (R): Because the hospital statistics provide only the numerator.

Select the true answer as per code given below:

A. Both (S) and (R) are true but unrelated to each other
B. Both (S) and (R) are true, but related to cause and effect
C. (S) is true, (R) is false
D. (R) is false, (S) is false

14. A continuous account of the frequency of disease in the community is provided by:

A. Hospital records
B. Record linkage
C. Notification of diseases
D. Disease registers
E. All of the above

15. In practice record linkage has been applied to:

A. Twin studies
B. Measurement of morbidity
C. Family and genetic studies
D. Chronic disease epidemiology
E. All of the above

16. Health surveys on a permanent basis are in operation in the following countries, *save* for one:

A. India
B. Japan
C. USA
D. UK
E. None of these

17. The cheapest method of collecting data is:

A. Health manpower statistics
B. Health records survey
C. Record linkage
D. Epidemiology surveillance
E. All of these

18. Health records survey has several disadvantages:

A. The estimates obtained from the records are not population-based
B. Reliability of data is open to question
C. Lack of uniform procedures and standardization in the recording of data
D. All of the above
E. Both B and C above

19. Consider the following statements:

I. The health information system concentrated mainly on statistical data to the population

II. The collection of data about the health and sickness of a population is primary data

IV. Primary data gives the precise information wanted which the secondary data may not give

Choose the true answer as per code given below:

A. I, II and III
B. I, II and IV
C. I, II, III and IV All
D. I and III
E. I and IV only

20. Most satisfactory method of collecting data is:

A. Oral questionnaires
B. First hand reports
C. Results of experiments
D. All of these
E. Both B and C above

21. Biostatistics is the cornerstone of epidemiology who was the father of statistics?

A. Henry Dunant
B. John Gruant
C. John Snow
D. Galton

22. The 1st step before the data is used for analysis or interpretation is:

A. Special curves

B. Graphs
C. Tables
D. Charts
E. Diagrams

23. Statement (S): Most people find a vertical arrangement better than a horizontal one in a tabulation.
Reasons (R): Because, it is easier to scan the data from top to bottom than from left to right.
Select the true answer from the code given below:
A. Both (S) and (R) are true but are related to cause and effect
B. Both (S) and (R) are true but are not related to cause and effect
C. (S) is true, (R) is false
D. (R) is true, (S) is false
E. Both (S) and (R) are false

24. In a frequency distribution table, the data is first split up into:
A. Class intervals
B. Frequency
C. Both of these
D. Neither A nor B above

25. A popular media of expressing statistical data, especially in newspapers and magazines is:
A. Table
B. Charts
C. Diagrams
D. Both B and C above
E. All of these

26. Statement (S) : Bar charts are a popular media of presenting statistical data.
Reasons (R) : Because they are easy to prepare, and enable values to be compared visually.
Select the true answer from the code given below:
A. Both (S) and (R) are true but are unrelated to cause and effect
B. Both (S) and (R) are true and are related to cause and effect
C. (S) is true, (R) is false
D. (R) is true, (S) is false
E. Both (S) and (R) are false

27. Quantitative data can be represented in:
A. Pie diagram
B. Pictogram
C. Bar diagram
D. Line diagram

28. A pictorial diagram of frequency distribution is denoted by:
A. Histogram
B. Pictogram
C. Pie charts
D. Bar diagram
E. All of the above

29. "Line diagrams" are used to show:
A. Frequency distribution
B. Trend of events with passage of time
C. Frequency polygon
D. Relationship between two variables

30. To denote the percentages in a segment which is used?
A. Pictogram
B. Bar charts
C. Pie chart
D. Histogram
E. All of the above

31. "Man in the Street" referred to:
A. Line diagram
B. Histogram
C. Diagram
D. Pictogram

32. Following graphical method of presentation of data are suitable for a quantitative continuous data:
I. Histogram
II. Bar diagram
III. Frequency curve
IV. Pie chart

Select the true answer from the following code:
A. I and III only
B. I and II only
C. I, II and III only
D. I, II, III and IV only
E. I and IV only

33. **"Median" is preferred to arithmatic mean because:**
A. Skew deviation is seen in reading
B. Population is very large
C. Uniform distribution of variable
D. Low variance is seen

34. **Graph showing relationship between two variables is:**
A. Scatter diagram
B. Frequency polygon
C. Pie charts
D. Histogram

35. **A suitable chart to depict clearly the decadal total census will be:**
A. Histogram
B. Simple bar chart
C. Line diagram
D. Frequency polygon

36. **Median is almost equivalent to .... the percentile:**
A. 25th
B. 40th
C. 50th
D. 75th
E. 95th

37. **Middle value of a series arranged in ascending or descending order of magnitude is termed as:**
A. Median
B. Average
C. Mode
D. Mean
E. Range

38. **In a statistical analysis, average mean is mentioned to describe the dispersion of data, best is:**
A. Mode
B. Range
C. Geometric mean
D. Standard error of means

39. **Standard deviation means:**
A. Sumtotal of the means
B. Middle value
C. Root mean square
D. All of the above

40. **All are measures of central tendency of given observations, *except* for:**
A. Median
B. Mode
C. Range
D. Arithmatic mean
E. None of these

41. **The most frequently occurring value in a data is:**
A. Median
B. Mode
C. Mean
D. Standard deviation

42. **Following is maximally used as measure of dispersion:**
A. Median
B. Mode
C. Mean
D. Standard deviation

43. **Which is denoted by Greek letter "σ" (sigma)?**
A. Mean
B. Mode
C. Median
D. Standard deviation
E. Standard error

44. **"Spread" of the dispersion of (numerical) is:**
A. Standard deviation
B. Mean
C. Mode
D. Median

45. If the mean cholesterol value of a group of normal subjects is 230 mg% with a standard error of 10. The 95% confidence limit for the population is:
A. 210 and 240
B. 210 and 250
C. 220 and 240
D. 200 and 260

46. In a normal distribution with mean '55' and standard deviation '10', the areas to the right of the 55 is:
A. 0.4
B. 0.6
C. 0.8
D. 0.9
E. None of these

47. In a normal distribution curve, the area between one standard deviation on either side of the mean is:
A. 68%
B. 95%
C. 99%
D. 80%
E. 100%

48. Regarding standard normal curve all are true, *but* one:
A. The mean, median and mode all coincide
B. Its mean is zero
C. The total area of the curve is one
D. Its S.D. is one
E. Its standard normal variate is denoted by 'x'

49. In a normal distribution curve, the area between "three" standard deviation on either side of the mean is:
A. 68%
B. 90%
C. 95%
D. 99.7%
E. 100%

50. "Standard error" is the measure of:
A. Sampling error
B. Observer error
C. Conceptual error
D. Instrumental error

51. Systemic random sample:
A. Is done by assigning a number to each of the units in the sampling form
B. Is done by picking every 5th or 10th units at regular intervals
C. Is a haphazard collection of certain numbers
D. Is deliberately drawn in a systematic way

52. Which of the following is a dependent variable?
A. Association
B. Relative proportion
C. Cause
D. Effect

53. $\sqrt{\frac{pq}{n}}$ indicates what?
A. Standard error of mean
B. Standard deviation from the mean
C. Standard error of proportion
D. Difference between proportion

54. The statistical analysis of two unrelated big data (N = 200) is by:
A. Paired 't'
B. Z test
C. uni 't'
D. X^2 test only
E. All of the above

55. Following is unrelated to the chisquare test of statistical significance:
A. Life table
B. Qualitative data
C. Significance level
D. Degree of freedom

56. A 2" × 2" contingency table construction is applicable in the calculation of the following, *except* for one:
A. Relative risk
B. Odds ratio
C. Validity of a screening test
D. Regression coefficient
E. None of these

57. The test of significance used while investigating discrete variables is:
A. 'Z' test
B. Standard error of difference between two means
C. Chi-square test
D. 't' test
E. All of these

58. When the variables are nonmeasurable, which of the following is used to be represented?
A. Variation
B. Ratio
C. Nominal
D. Ordinal

59. Student 't' test:
A. Is used to calculate attributable risk
B. To find out degree of significance
C. Is used to calculate relative risk
D. To calculate disease generation time

60. In a 4" × 4" table, number of degree of freedom is:
A. 4
B. 8
C. 9
D. 16
E. None of these

61. Between weight and height, there is:
A. Association
B. Index
C. Causation
D. Correlation

62. If there is no participation by 40% of study group, it is:
A. Response bias
B. Selection bias
C. Berkesonian bias
D. Interviewer's bias

63. "Weight measurement" is what type of variation?
A. Normal
B. Discrete
C. Continuous
D. Unpredictable

64. In a 2" × 2" contingency table, the degree of freedom will be:
A. Only one
B. Two
C. Three
D. Four
E. Five

65. Variation in two variables with different units of measurement can be compared by:
A. Standard deviation
B. Coefficient of variation
C. Variance
D. X^2 test

66. Correlation coefficient (r) quantifies the relationship between:
A. Two qualitative variables
B. Two quantitative variables
C. Both of the above
D. None of the above

67. In three comparable groups of 100 patients each, an antianaemic drug was given and Hb levels were measured after 6 months. Mean Hb levels of each group were calculated. Which test of significance would you apply to test the null hypothesis?
A. Analysis of variance
B. X^2 test
C. Correlation coefficient
D. Standard error of difference between means

68. Correlation between two quantitative variables is to be estimated. Only one of these variables shows normal distribution. With which test would you quantify the correlation?
A. Analysis of variance
B. Spearman's ranking test
C. Correlation coefficient
D. Both A and C above
E. All of these

69. For X^2 test in which there are three rows and two columns the degree of freedom will be:
A. One
B. Two
C. Three
D. Four
E. Five

70. In students 't' test the calculated t value is less than 't' value in the table of probability. Then the null hypothesis will be:
A. Accepted
B. Rejected
C. Further analysed
D. All of these

71. The degree of reedom for chisquare test (x^2) is:
A. n – 1
B. (R – 1) (C – 1)
C. (n + 1)
D. $(n_1 + n_2 - 2)$

72. The degree of freedom for unpaired 't' test is:
A. (R – 1) (C – 1)
B. n–1
C. $n_1 + n_2 - 2$
D. n – 1

73. The degree of freedom for paired 't' test is:
A. n + 1
B. (R – 1) (C – 1)
C. $n_1 + n_2 - 2$
D. n – 1

74. When the sample size is less than 30 and the study group serves as its own control group the statistical test which should be applied is:
A. Paired 't'
B. Unpaired 't'
C. X^2 with yates correction
D. All of the above

75. $x^2 = \sum \frac{(O - E \pm 0.5)^2}{E}$ is used when:
A. Expected frequency in any cell is <5
B. The DF is >1
C. Expected frequency in all cells is >5
D. Both A and B above
E. All of the above

76. Mean and standard deviation can be worked out only if data is on:
A. Interval/ratio scale
B. Dichotomous scale
C. Nominal scale
D. Ordinal scale

77. For a negatively skewed data mean will be:
A. Less than medium
B. More than median
C. Equal to median
D. One

78. The national level system that provides annual national as well as state level reliable estimates of fertility and mortality is:
A. Ad hoc survey
B. Sample registration system
C. Census
D. Civil registration system

79. National family health survey has successfully completed:
A. One round
B. Two rounds
C. Three rounds
D. Four rounds

80. The age and sex structure of a population may be described by a:
A. Life table
B. Bar chart
C. Population pyramid
D. Correlation coefficient

81. The rate adjusted to allow for the age distribution of the population is:
A. Age standardized mortality rate

B. Fertility rate
C. Crude mortality rate
D. Perinatal mortality rate

82. After applying a statistical test, an investigator gets the 'P value' as 0.01. It means that:
A. The probability of finding a significant difference is 1%
B. The probability of declaring a significant difference, when there is truly no difference, is 1%
C. The difference is not significant 1% times and significant 99% times
D. The power of the test used is 99%

83. A bacterium can divide every 20 mts. Beginning with a single individual, how many bacteria will be there in the population if there is exponential growth for 3 hours:
A. 18
B. 440
C. 512
D. 1024

84. The carrying capacity of any given population is determined by its:
A. Population growth rate
B. Birth rate
C. Limiting resource
D. Death rate

85. The standard normal distribution:
A. Is skewed to the left
B. Has mean = 1.0
C. Has standard deviation = 0.0
D. Has variance = 1.0

86. The PEFR of a group of 11-year-old girls follow a normal distribution with mean 300 L/min and standard deviation 20 L/min:
A. About 95% of the girls have PEFR between 260 and 340 L/min
B. The girls have healthy lungs
C. About 5% of girls have FEFR below 260 L/min
D. All the PEFR must be less than 340 L/min

87. The event A and B are mutually exclusive, so,
A. Prob (A or B) = Prob (A) + Prob (B)
B. Prob (A and B) = Prob (A) × Prob (B)
C. Prob (A) = Prob (B)
D. Prob (A) + Prob (B) = 1

88. Total cholesterol level = a + b (calorie intake) + c (physical activity) + d (body mass index); is an example of:
A. Simple linear regression
B. Simple curvilinear regression
C. Multiple linear regression
D. Multiple logistic regression

89. In a village having population of 1000, we found, patients with certain disease. The results of a new diagnostic test on that disease are as follows:

	Disease	
Test result	*Present*	*Absent*
+	180	400
–	20	400

What is the percent prevalence of disease?
A. 0.20
B. 2
C. 18
D. 20

90. The Hb level in healthy women has mean 13.5 gm/dL and standard deviation 1.5 gm/dL. What is the Z score for a woman with Hb level 15.0 gm/dL?
A. 9.0
B. 10.0
C. 2.0
D. 1.0

91. The table below shows the screening test results of disease Z in relation to the true

disease status of the population being tested:

Screening test results	*Disease (z)*		*Total*
Positive	400	200	600
Negative	100	600	700
Total	500	800	1300

A. 70%
B. 75%
C. 79%
D. 86%

92. If prevalence of diabetes is 10%, the probability that three people selected at random from the population will have diabetes is:
A. 0.01
B. 0.03
C. 0.001
D. 0.003

93. If each value of a given group of observation is multiplied by 10 the standard deviation of the resulting observations is:
A. Original standard deviation × 10
B. Original standard deviation/10
C. Original standard deviation – 10
D. Original standard deviation itself

94. If the systolic B.P. in a population has a mean of 130 mm Hg and a median of 140 mm Hg, the distribution is said to be:
A. Symmetrical
B. Positively skewed
C. Negatively skewed
D. Either positively or negatively skewed depending on standard deviation

95. A measure of location which divides the distribution in the ratio of 3:1 is:
A. Median
B. First quartile
C. Third quartile
D. Mode

96. The 'P' value of a randomized controlled trial comparing operation A (new procedure) and operation B (Gold standard is 0.04). From this, we conclude that:
A. Type II error is small and we can accept the findings of the study
B. The probability of false negative conclusion that operation A is better than operation B, when in truth it is not, is 4%
C. The power of study to detect a difference between operation A and B is 96%
D. The probability of a false positive conclusion that operation A is better than operation B, when in truth it is not, is 4%

97. Chi-square test is used to measure the degree of:
A. Agreement between two variables
B. Association between two variables
C. Correlation between two variables
D. Causal relationship between exposure and effect

98. For a 60 kg Indian male, the minimum daily protein requirement has been calculated to be 40 gm (mean) and standard deviation is 10. The recommended daily allowance of protein would be:
A. 40 gm/day
B. 50 gm/day
C. 60 gm/day
D. 70 gm/day

99. A population study showed a mean glucose of 86 mg/dL. In a sample of 100 showing normal curve distribution, what % of people have glucose above 86%?
A. 50%
B. 60%
C. 65%
D. 75%

100. The best method to show the association between height and weight of children in a class is by:
A. Bar chart

B. Line diagram
C. Scatter diagram
D. Histogram

101. The correlation between variables A and B in a study was found to be 1.1. This indicates:
A. Very strong correlation
B. Moderately strong correlation
C. Weak correlation
D. Computational mistake in calculating correlation

102. In a study, variation in cholesterol was seen before and after giving a drug. The test which would give its significance is:
A. Unpaired 't' test
B. Paired 't' test
C. Chi-square test
D. Fisher test

103. Sampling error is classified as:
A. Alpha error
B. Beta error
C. Gamma error
D. Delta error

104. The most common channel of communi-cation is:
A. Printed media
B. Radio
C. Interpersonal or face to face
D. T.V.

105. Following folk media has been regarded as a channel of communications in respective states in India, *except:*
A. Bhojpuri—Bihar
B. Nautanki—U.P.
C. Burrakatha—A.P.
D. Harikatha—Western India (Gujarat and Maharashtra)

106. The recognised examples of point-to-point systems closer to interpersonal commu-nication is:
A. TV
B. Telephone
C. Radio
D. Internet

107. Which has become the most popular of all media?
A. Radio
B. Newspaper
C. TV
D. Printed materials

108. In which year the Government of India established a Central Health Education Bureau (CHEB) in the Ministry of Health, New Delhi, to promote and coordinate health education work in the country?
A. 1947
B. 1950
C. 1956
D. 1966

109. The headquarter for International Union for Health Education is in:
A. Geneva
B. New York
C. London
D. Paris

110. The South-East Asia Regional Bureau (SEARB) of the International Union for Health Education was established in 1983 with headquater at:
A. Mumbai
B. Islamabad
C. Bangalore
D. Dhaka

111. Confidence limits can be calculated using:
A. Mean and range
B. Mean and standard error
C. Median and range
D. Median and standard error

112. Limits of confidence of a hypothesis is determined by:
A. Level of significance

B. Power factor
C. 1-Power factor
D. 1-level of significance

113. A non-symmetrical frequency distribution is known as:
A. Normal distribution
B. Skewed distribution
C. Cumulative frequency distribution
D. None of the above

114. A total of 3500 patients with thyroid C_A are identified and surveyed by patient interviews with reference to past exposure to radiation. The study design most appropriately illustrates:
A. Clinical trial
B. Case control study groups
C. Case series report
D. Case report

115. Which is a pre-requisite for the chi-square test to compare?
A. Both samples should be mutually exclusive
B. Both sample need not be mutually exclusive
C. Normal distribution
D. All of the above

116. Regression co-efficient is between:
A. 0–1
B. –1 to + 1
C. 0 to + 1
D. + 1 to + 2

117. When the height and weight is perfectly correlated, coefficient of correlation is:
A. + 1
B. – 1
C. Zero (0)
D. > 1

118. Continuous quantitative variables are expressed by:
A. Bar chart
B. Histogram and frequency polygon
C. Ogive
D. Pie chart

119. Ten readings of BP taken before and after treatment is studied by:
A. Paired 't' test
B. Student's 't' test
C. 'Z' test
D. Correlation test

120. If we reject Null hypothesis, when actually it is true it is known as:
A. Power
B. Specificity
C. Type I error
D. Type II error

121. In the WHO recommended EPI cluster sampling for assessing primary immunization coverage, the age group of children to be surveyed is:
A. 0–12 months
B. 6 to 12 months
C. 9 to 12 months
D. 12 to 23 months

Answers

1 A	2 C	3 B	4 D	5 E	6 B	7 A	8 B	9 C	10 E
11 B	12 A	13 B	14 D	15 E	16 A	17 B	18 D	19 C	20 A
21 B	22 C	23 A	24 C	25 D	26 B	27 C	28 A	29 B	30 C
31 D	32 C	33 B	34 A	35 B	36 C	37 A	38 B	39 C	40 A
41 B	42 B	43 D	44 A	45 B	46 C	47 A	48 E	49 D	50 A
51 B	52 D	53 C	54 B	55 A	56 C	57 D	58 A	59 B	60 C
61 D	62 A	63 B	64 A	65 B	66 B	67 A	68 B	69 B	70 A
71 B	72 C	73 D	74 A	75 D	76 A	77 A	78 B	79 B	80 C
81 A	82 B	83 C	84 C	85 D	86 A	87 A	88 C	89 D	90 D
91 B	92 C	93 A	94 C	95 C	96 D	97 B	98 C	99 A	100 C
101 D	102 B	103 A	104 C	105 A	106 B	107 C	108 C	109 D	110 C
111 B	112 A	113 B	114 C	115 A	116 B	117 A	118 B	119 A	120 C
121 D									

C•H•A•P•T•E•R **FIFTEEN**

Principles of Epidemiology and Epidemiologic Methods

DIRECTION: Following MCQ's are provided with a few suggestive answers/completions. Only one answer is correct. You have to identify the *BEST* one in each case.

1. **"The study of the distribution and determinants of health-related states or events in specified populations, and the application of this study to the control of health problems." This is the most recent definition of epidemiology given by whom in which year?**
   A. Parkin (1973)
   B. Frost (1997)
   C. Mac Mahon (1990)
   D. John M Last (1988)
2. **The foundations of epidemiology was laid in which century?**
   A. 17th
   B. 18th
   C. 19th
   D. 20th
   E. Hippocratic era
3. **W.H. Frost (1927) became the 1st professor of epidemiology is USA, who defined epidemiology as:**
   A. That branch of medical science which treats the epidemics
   B. The science of the mass phenomena of infectious diseases
   C. The study of disease, any disease, as a mass phenomenon
   D. The study of the distribution and determinants of disease frequency in man
4. **Who became the 1st professor of epidemiology and medical statistics in the University of London?**
   A. Major Greenwood
   B. Parkin
   C. Mac Mahon
   D. Frost
   E. John M. Last
5. **According to the International Epidemiological Association (IEA) epidemiology has following main aims:**
   I. To describe the distribution and magnitude of health and disease problems in human population
   II. To identify aetiological factors (risk factors) in the pathogenesis of disease
   III. To provide the data essential to the planning, implementation and evolution of services for the prevention, control and treatment of disease and to the setting up of priorities among those services
   IV. To eliminate or reduce the health problem or its consequences

V. To promote the health and well-being of society as a whole

Select the true answer as per code given below:

A. I, III and V
B. I, II and III
C. III, IV and V
D. II, III and IV
E. II, IV and IV

6. Descriptive epidemiology of disease is concerned with:

A. Description of natural history
B. Description of underlying cause
C. Description of distribution
D. Description of clinical spectrum

7. Analytical epidemiology of disease is concerned with the following:

A. Analysis of underlying cause
B. Analysis of clinical spectrum
C. Analysis of natural history
D. Analysis of distribution

8. Epidemiology is concerned with the following:

I. Health
II. Communicable disease
III. Non-communicable disease

Select the true answer as per code given below:

A. I only
B. I and II only
C. I, II and III All
D. I and III only
E. II and III only

9. In what respect epidemiology differs from clinical medicine?

A. Defined population
B. Case
C. Sick and healthy
D. Conceptual

10. What is true about "making comparison" in epidemiological approach?

A. Like can be compared with like
B. Randomization or random allocation
C. In case control and cohort studies random allocation is not possible
D. All of the above
E. Both A and B above

11. Recognised example of discrete variables are all the following, *save* for one:

A. C_A lung
B. Broken leg
C. Rash in measles
D. Leucocyte count
E. None of the above

12. Which is NOT regarded as a continuous variables?

A. Weight
B. Height
C. Blood pressure
D. Serum cholesterol

13. The basic tools of measurement in epidemiology includes:

I. Rate
II. Ratios
III. Proportions
IV. Frequency distribution

Choose the correct answer as per code given below:

A. I and II only
B. I, II and III
C. II and IV only
D. I, II, III and IV All
E. II, III and IV only

14. The numerator is not a component of the denominator in:

A. Proportion
B. Rate
C. Ratio
D. Frequency distribution

15. The numerator is a component of the denominator while calculating the:

A. Ratio
B. Rate
C. Proportion
D. Frequency distribution

16. **Numerator refers to:**
A. Sickness only
B. Birth only
C. Deaths only
D. Episodes of sickness
E. All of the above

17. **What is true about "proportion"?**
A. A proportion is a ratio which indicates the relation in magnitude of a part of the whole
B. A proportion is usually expressed as a percentage
C. The numerator is always included in the denominator
D. Both A and B above
E. All of the above

18. **The simplest measure of mortality is:**
A. Crude death rate
B. Age specific death rate
C. Case fatality rate
D. Proportional mortality rate
E. Survival rate

19. **Following, *but* one, are true regarding "case fatality rate":**
A. The killing power of a disease
B. The time interval is always specified
C. Typically used in acute infectious disease
D. It is closely related to virulence

20. **Statement (S): The case fatality rate for some diseases may vary in different epidemics.**
Reason (R): Because of changes in the agent, host and environmental factors.
Choose the correct response as per code given below:
A. Both (S) and (R) are true, and are related to cause and effect
B. Both (S) and (R) are true, but are not related to cause and effect
C. (S) is true, (R) is false
D. (R) is true, (S) is false
E. Both (S) and (R) are false

21. **Regarding proportional mortality rate, which is false?**
A. Computed usually for a broad disease group and for a specific disease of major public health importance
B. Used when population data are not available
C. Of great value in making comparison between population groups or different time periods
D. Proportional mortality rate does not indicate the risk of members of the population contracting or dying from the disease

22. **Which can be used as a yardstick for the assessment of standards of therapy?**
A. Crude death rate
B. Specific death rate
C. Case fatality rate
D. Survival rate
E. Proportional mortality rate

23. **Calculate the standardized death rate for city x where the standard population of different age groups is 93,000 and expected deaths is 609.94:**
A. 3.0
B. 3.1
C. 4.4
D. 5.3
E. 6.56

24. **Calculate the standardized mortality rate (SMR) for coal workers, where the observed death is 9 and expected death is 7.0:**
A. 16
B. 32
C. 64
D. 129
E. 96

25. **The simplest and most useful form of indirect standardization is:**
A. Standardized mortality ratio
B. Life table

C. Regression techniques
D. Multivariate analysis
E. None of the above

26. In England, the basis for the allocation of Government money to the health regions of the country is:
A. Index death rate
B. Standardized mortality rates
C. Life table
D. Regression techniques
E. Multivariate analysis

27. Consider the following statements:
I. Three aspects of morbidity are commonly measured by morbidity rates or ratios
II. Disease frequency is measured by incidence and prevalence rate
III. Morbidity means any departure, subjective or objective, from a state of physiological well being
IV. Incidence rate is defined as the number of new case occurring in a defined population during a specified period of time

Select the true answer as per code given below:
A. I, II only
B. I, II and III
C. I, II, III and IV All
D. II and IV
E. II, III and IV only

28. There had been 500 new cases of an illness in a population of 30,000 in a year. The incidence rate would be:
A. 9.0
B. 7.1
C. 10.2
D. 60.7
E. 19.2 per 1000 per year

29. Regarding attack rate, which is false?
A. It is an incidence rate
B. It relates to the number of cases in the population at risk
C. It reflects the extent of the epidemic
D. All of these
E. None of these

30. The relationship between incidence and prevalence can be expressed as:
A. $P = I \times D$
B. $P = \frac{I}{D}$
C. $P \times I = D$
D. $P \times D = I$
E. $D = \frac{I}{P}$

31. In a village with 1000 population have 10 cases per year of leprosy. The mean duration of disease is 5 years. Prevalence would be:
A. 10
B. 20
C. 30
D. 40
E. 50 per 1000 population

32. Following statements are true about prevalence, *save* for one:
A. It is not the ideal measure for studying disease aetiology or causation
B. Two factors determine prevalence namely incidence and duration
C. It has got no limitations
D. Prevalence helps to estimate the magnitude of health/disease problems in the community
E. Prevalence rates are especially useful for administrative and planning purposes (hospital beds, manpower needs, rehabilitation)

33. "Burkitt's lymphoma" a type of cancer seen in Africa caused by Epstein Barr Virus (EBV). The name "Burkitt" has come after:
A. Its inventer or observer
B. The patient on whom it was 1st recognised
C. The place in Africa where it was 1st seen
D. Malaria infection

34. The concept of "defined population" (or population at risk) is crucial in epidemiological studies because:
A. It provides the denominator for calculating rates
B. To measure the frequency of disease
C. Study its distribution and determinants
D. All of the above
E. Both A and C but not B above

35. The best known short term fluctuation in the occurrence of a disease in an:
A. Endemic
B. Epidemic
C. Emporiatrics
D. Exotic

36. Which is NOT true regarding common source, single exposure epidemics?
A. These are also called as "Point source" epidemics
B. Median incubation period
C. The curve has usually only one peak
D. It is the time required for 100% of the cases to occur following exposure

37. The main feature of "Point source" epidemic includes the following:
I. The epidemic curve rises and falls rapidly, with no secondary waves
II. The epidemic tends to be explosive, there is clustering of cases within a narrow interval of time
III. All the cases develop within one incubation period of disease
Choose the correct answer as per code given below:
A. I and II only
B. II and III only
C. I and III only
D. III only
E. I, II and III All

38. "Minamata disease" in Japan resulting from consumption of fish containing high concentration of "material mercury" is an example of:
A. Point source epidemic
B. Propagated epidemic
C. Slow epidemic
D. Continuous epidemic
E. None of the above

39. Recognised examples of common source, continuous or repeated exposure includes:
I. Prostitute having gonorrhoea infection
II. A well of contaminated water
III. A nationally distributed brand of Polio vaccine
IV. A contaminated food
Select the wrong answer from the code given below:
A. I and II
B. I, III and IV
C. I, II, III and IV All
D. None of the above

40. The outbreak of respiratory illness, the Legionnaire's disease, in the summer of 1976 in Philadelphia (USA) was a recognised example of:
A. Point source epidemics
B. Common source, continuous or repeated exposure
C. Propagated epidemics
D. Slow modern epidemics

41. In propagated epidemics the speed of spread depends upon:
A. Herd immunity
B. Opportunities for contact
C. Secondary attack rate
D. Both B and C above
E. All of the above

42. An epidemics of "hepatitis A" and "Polio" is:
A. Point source epidemics
B. Multiple exposure epidemics
C. Propagated epidemics
D. Repeated exposure

43. Statement (S): GIT infections are prominent in summer months.

Reason (R): Because of warm weather and rapid multiplication of flies.

Select the true answer from following code:

A. Both (S) and (R) are true and are related to cause and effect
B. Both (S) and (R) are true are not related to cause and effect
C. (S) is true, (R) is false
D. (R) is true, (S) is false
E. Both (S) and (R) are false

44. "Seasonal variation" is well known characteristic of the following:

I. Varicella
II. Measles
III. Cerebro-spinal meningitis
IV. Malaria

Select the true answer as per the following code:

A. II and IV
B. I and II
C. I, II and III
D. I, II, III and IV All
E. I, II and IV only

45. Statement (S): Influenza pandemics are known to occur at intervals of 7 to 10 years.

Reasons (R): Because of antigenic variations.

Select the true answer from the following code:

A. Both (S) and (R) are true, but are not related to each other
B. Both (S) and (R) are true and are related to each other
C. (S) is true, (R) false
D. (R) true, (S) false
E. Both (S) and (R) are false

46. Automobile accidents in USA are more frequents on which day?

A. Sunday
B. Monday
C. Saturday
D. Wednesday
E. Friday

47. Secular trend has NOT been shown by the following:

A. Tuberculosis
B. Measles
C. Lung cancer
D. Diabetes mellitus

48. The prevalence of breast cancer is lowest in:

A. Japan
B. USA
C. India
D. Australia
E. Israel

49. The classic examples of place-related diseases include all, *but* one:

A. Yellow fever
B. Schistosomiasis
C. Sleeping sickness
D. Endemic goiter
E. None of the above

50. Bimodality is seen in following disease conditions, *except* for:

A. Measles
B. Females breast C_A
C. Leukaemia
D. Hodgkin's disease

51. Following diseases are more common in women than men, *save* for:

A. Obesity
B. Coronary artery disease
C. Hyperthyroidism
D. Diabetes

52. Following diseases are more common in males than women:

A. Lung C_A
B. CAD
C. Duodenal ulcer

D. All of these
E. Both A and B above

53. C_A C_X is rare among:
A. American Indians
B. Indians
C. Nuns
D. Devdasis
E. All of the above

54. Following diseases are seen in upper social class peoples, *but* one:
A. Scabies
B. CAD
C. Hypertension
D. Diabetes mellitus
E. None of the above

55. Following behavioural factors which have attracted greatest attention is:
A. Cigarette smoking
B. Sedentary life
C. Over-eating
D. Drug abuse
E. All of the above

56. Regarding cross-sectional studies which is not true?
A. It is the simplest form of an observational study
B. It is also known as incidence study
C. It is more useful for chronic than short-lived diseases
D. It is useful for finding out incidence rate

57. Following are not true about longitudinal studies:
A. It is useful to study the natural history of disease and its future outcome
B. It is useful for identifying risk factors of disease
C. Longitudinal studies are easy to organise and less time taking
D. It is useful for finding out incidence rate

58. Case control studies have been used effectively for studying following:
A. Various cancers
B. Cirrhosis of liver
C. Lupus erythematosus
D. Congestive heart failure
E. All of these

59. There are 4 basic steps in conducting a case control study:
I. Selection of cases and controls
II. Matching
III. Measurement of exposure
IV. Analysis and interpretation
The correct sequence of study as per code is:
A. I, II, III and IV
B. I, III, IV and II
C. I, IV, III and II
D. II, I, III and IV

60. A "confounding factor" is defined as one which is associated with both exposure and disease and is distributed unequally in study and control groups. In the study of the role of alcohol in the aetiology of Oesophageal C_A, SMOKING is a confounding factor because:
A. It is associated with the consumption of alcohol
B. It is an independent risk factor for Oesophageal C_A
C. Both of these
D. None of the above

61. Statement (S): A typical case control study does not provide incidence rates from which relative risk can be calculated directly.
Reason (R): Because there is no appropriate denominator or population at risk to calculate these rates.
Select the true answer as per code given below:
A. Both (S) and (R) are true but are unrelated to cause and effect
B. Both (S) and (R) are true and are related to cause and effect
C. (S) true, (R) false

D. (R) true, (S) false
E. Both (S) and (R) are false

62. A key parameter in the analysis of case control studies is:
A. Relative risk
B. 'P' value
C. Odds ratio
D. All of these
E. Both A and B above

63. A confounding variable may relate closely in time to the onset of disease that:
A. Cannot be alleviated through disease prevention programmes
B. Is one of several causal agents
C. Exacerbates rather than cause it
D. Is not necessary for its occurrence
E. Any of these

64. Confounding variable is:
A. Not a cause of disease
B. By removing it, disease can be prevented
C. Help in assessing causal relationship
D. All of these

65. The bias arises because of the different rates of admission to hospitals for people with different diseases is called as:
A. Confounding bias
B. Memory or recall bias
C. Berkesonian bias
D. Selection bias
E. Interviewer's bias

66. Recognised advantages of case control studies includes all, *but* one:
A. Relatively easy to carry out
B. Problem of bias
C. No risk to subjects
D. Rapid and inexpensive
E. Risk factors can be identified

67. Recognised examples of case control studies includes:
A. Maternal smoking and congenital malformations
B. Radiation and leukaemia
C. Oral contraceptive use and hepatocellular adenoma
D. All of the above
E. Both A and C above

68. THALIDOMIDE was 1st marketed as safe, non-barbiturate hypnotic in Britain in 1958. In which year its teratogenic effects has been noticed and attention drawn by gynecologists?
A. 1961
B. 1962
C. 1963
D. 1964
E. 1965

69. Cohort study is also known by the following:
A. Prospective study
B. Longitudinal study
C. Incidence study
D. Forward-looking study
E. All of these

70. Recognised indications of cohort studies include all, *save* for:
A. When there is a good evidence of an association between exposure and disease
B. When exposure is rare, but the incidence of diseases high among exposed
C. When attrition of study population can be minimised
D. When ample funds are not available
E. None of these

71. Court-Brown and Doll (1957) applied combination of retrospective and prospective cohort studies in the:
A. C_A lung
B. Effects of radiation
C. Effects of alcohol
D. All of the above

72. In epidemiological studies, important criterion for control group is that it should be:
A. Age and socio-economic status matched
B. Equal in number

C. That the factor to be studied should be absent
D. That the factor to be studied should be present

73. Which of the following is NOT true of cohort study?
A. Expensive
B. Always prospective
C. Incidence can be calculated
D. Used to study chronic diseases
E. All of the above

74. All, *but* one, are true about case control study:
A. Sequence of events not known
B. Many aetiological factors can be studied
C. Presence of bias
D. Several possible outcomes can be studied

75. Following are true about Randomized controlled trial, *save* for one:
A. In a single blind trial the doctor does not know of group allocation
B. Bias may arise during evaluation
C. Both study and control group should be comparable
D. The groups should be representative of the population

76. The likelihood of a causal relationship is increased by:
A. Temporal association
B. Biological plausibility
C. Strength of association
D. All of the above
E. Both A and C above

77. Which is NOT a likely explanation for cyclic trend of disease?
A. Antigenic variation
B. Build up susceptible
C. Environmental conditions
D. Herd immunity variations
E. None of these

78. Seasonal variation of a disease can be assessed by:
A. Comparing prevalence of disease
B. Comparing incidence of disease
C. Using mortality rates
D. Using survival rates
E. All of these

79. Relative risk can show an association between:
A. Smoking and lung cancer
B. Efficacy of two drugs
C. OCP and pregnancy
D. Altitude and endemic goiter
E. All of the above

80. Sampling in a village of 200 houses and 1000 population to screen 100 persons is best taken:
A. Selecting one person per house
B. Selecting every 5th person
C. Selecting every 10th person
D. Selecting randomly any 100 patients from a random chart

81. In a population prevalence of a disease can be rapidly determined by:
A. Surveillance
B. Cross sectional study
C. Case control study
D. Double blind study
E. Any of the above

82. Which of the following is an odd ratio?
A. PMR
B. Attributable risk
C. Association of risk of outcome
D. Relative risk
E. All of the above

83. Randomization is:
A. Mixing control with cases
B. Selecting case for study
C. Mixing different types of controls
D. Selecting characteristics of case group
E. All of the above

84. Cohort is:
A. People of same community
B. People with different communities forming a group for study

C. People with same experience
D. People of a geographical area
E. All of the above

85. Relative risk can be obtained from:
A. Case study
B. Experimental study
C. Cohort study
D. Case cohort study
E. None of these

86. Epidemic occurring every three years is called:
A. Pandemic
B. Secular trend
C. Cyclical trend
D. None of these

87. Following are true about cohort study, *save* for one:
A. Both groups must be disease free
B. Similar except the factor under study
C. Both should be equally susceptible to disease
D. The disease criteria can be defined later as the study progresses

88. Growth, development and morbidity of two hundred babies born on 1st January 1970 were studied for five years. You could call such a study:
A. Secular
B. Prospective
C. Cross-sectional
D. Retrospective

89. Method of choice to know success of immunization programme is:
A. Random sampling
B. Systematic sampling
C. Cluster testing
D. Stratified random sampling
E. All of these

90. Secular trend refers to:
A. Gradual change in particular direction
B. Increase in prevalence
C. Change of pattern over a long period of time
D. Decrease in prevalence of disease

91. Longitudinal studies:
A. Efficient
B. Single outcome
C. Economical
D. Give incidence

92. Case control study has all the following features, *but* one:
A. Provides attributable risk
B. Reliable
C. Cost-effective
D. Quick result

93. Cross over study is characterised by all, *save* for one:
A. Case is also control
B. Suitable for disease with rapidly changing features
C. All persons involved receive treatment
D. Smaller group required for study

94. If a new drug is invented which prevent mortality from a disease but does not affect a cure then:
A. Incidence will increase
B. Prevalence will decrease
C. Prevalence will increase
D. Incidence will decrease

95. Double blind study means:
A. Interpreters and analysers blind about the study
B. Observer is blind about the study
C. Person or group being observed are blind about the study
D. Both observer and group are blind about the study

96. Randomization is useful to eliminate:
A. Patient bias
B. Sampling bias
C. Confounding bias
D. Observer bias

97. Which one of the following is the principal problem in cohort?
A. Lack of follow up
B. Difficult coming back to original study
C. Selection bias
D. All of these
E. Both B and C above

98. Which is NOT true about cohort study?
A. Prospective study
B. Cheap and quick
C. Yields incidence rate
D. Reserved for formulated hypothesis
E. None of these

99. Cyclical occurrence:
A. All of susceptible
B. Seasonal change
C. Occurring in cycles
D. Changes in occurrence over decades

100. Amount of disease which can be decreased by intervention strategy:
A. Attributable risk
B. Relative risk
C. Odds ratio
D. Population attributable risk
E. All of these

101. Random sampling:
A. Stratified random sampling is used when no particular characteristic is used
B. Is systematic random type, every 5th or 10th case is used
C. A table of random numbers is used to determine which units to be used
D. Simple random type provides maximum number of possible samples

102. Attrition in Randomized controlled trials means:
A. Inevitable confounding due to non-binding
B. Inevitable losses during follow up
C. Single binding that goes wrong inevitably
D. Inevitable cross-over type of study in blinding techniques

103. In Randomization, "blinding" can be done in how many ways?
A. One
B. Two
C. Three
D. Four
E. Five ways

104. Of the following methodology of "blinding" the most frequently used method when a blind trial is conducted is:
A. Single blind trial
B. Double blind trial
C. Triple blind trial
D. All of these
E. None of these

105. Ideally which of the following blinding should be used?
A. Single blind trial
B. Double blind trial
C. Triple blind trial
D. All of these
E. None of these

106. The major risk factors of coronary heart disease includes:
A. Elevated blood cholesterol
B. Smoking
C. Hypertension
D. Sedentary habits
E. All of these

107. The most frequently occurring type of preventive trials include:
A. Trials of vaccines
B. Trials of chemo-prophylactic drugs
C. Smoking trials
D. Both A and B above
E. All of these

108. Retrolental fibroplasia was originally observed and reported by:
A. T.L. Terry (1944)
B. Parson's (1938)
C. Duke (1040)
D. Elder (1944)

109. John Snow's discovery that cholera is a water-borne disease was the outcome of:

A. An uncontrolled trials
B. Natural experiments
C. Before and after comparison studies
D. All of the above
E. Both A and C above

110. The classic examples of "before and after comparison studies" includes the following:

A. Prevention of scurvy among sailors by James Lind (1750) by providing fresh fruit
B. Studies on the transmission of cholera by John Snow (1954)
C. Prevention of Polio by Salk and Sabin vaccines
D. Both A and B above
E. All of the above

111. Consider the following statement about correlation:

I. Correlation indicates degree of association between two characteristics
II. The correlation coefficients range from –1.0 to +1.0
III. A correlation coefficient of 1.0 means that the two variables exhibit a perfect linear relationship
IV. Causation implies correlation but correlation does not imply causation
V. Correlation does not measure risk

Select the true answer as per code given below:

A. I, II and III
B. I, II, III and IV
C. I, II, III, IV and V All
D. I, III and V
E. I, II and IV only

112. Following can be obtained from prospective study, *except* for:

A. Attributable risk
B. Prevalence rate
C. Relative risk
D. Incidence rate

113. The likelihood of a causal relationship is increased by the presence of the following criteria:

I. Temporal association
II. Strength of association
III. Biological plausibility
IV. Specificity of the association
V. Consistency of the association
VI. Coherence of the association

Select the true answer as per code given below:

A. I, II and III
B. I, II, III and IV
C. I, II, III, IV and V
D. I, II, III, IV, V and VI All

114. Subclinical or inapparent infection is seen in:

A. Polio
B. Staph aureus
C. Herpes simplex
D. All of the above
E. Both B and C above

115. Following are examples of contagious disease, *except* for:

A. Scabies
B. Bornholm disease
C. Trachoma
D. STD
E. Leprosy

116. "Malaria" is an example of:

A. Epidemic
B. Hyperendemic
C. Holoendemic
D. All of the above

117. An endemic disease when conditions are favourable may burst into an epidemic is:

A. Hepatitis 'A'
B. Typhoid fever
C. Malaria
D. Both A and B above
E. All of the above

118. When cases occur irregularly, haphazardly from time to time, and generally infrequently are called as:
A. Sporadic
B. Pandemic
C. Zoonosis
D. Exotic
E. Epornithic

119. Recognised examples of Pandemic occurring and recorded includes:
A. Influenza
B. Cholera el tor
C. Acute hemorrhagic conjunctivitis
D. All of the above

120. Infections maintained in both man and lower vertebrate animals that may be transmitted in either direction is called:
A. Anthropozoonoses
B. Zooanthroponoses
C. Amphixenoses
D. Zoonosis

121. "New zoonosis" is the name given to following disease, *but* one:
A. KFD
B. Bovine TB
C. Monkeypox
D. Lassa fever
E. None of these

122. An endemic occurring in animals include the following, *save* for one:
A. Anthrax
B. Brucellosis
C. Japanese encephalitis
D. Bovine T.B.

123. Disease which are imported into a country in which they does not otherwise exists/occur is called as:
A. Epizootic
B. Sporadic
C. Epornithic
D. Enzootic
E. Exotic

124. An infection acquired in health care facility/hospital places are called:
A. Nosocomial
B. Opportunistic
C. Exotic
D. Sporadic

125. Recongnised examples of nosocomial infection includes all, *but* one:
A. Infection of surgical wounds
B. Hepatitis 'B'
C. UTI
D. None of these

126. Iatrogenic disease includes:
A. Physician induced
B. The professionals activity of the health professionals
C. Physician's professional activity
D. Both B and C above
E. All of the above

127. Eradication is:
A. An absolute process
B. An "all or phenomenon
C. Restricted to termination of an infection from the entire world
D. All of these
E. Both A and C above

128. Diseases which are amenable to eradication includes all, *except*:
A. Smallpox
B. Measles
C. Polio
D. Diphtheria
E. Guineaworm

129. The subclinical cases are also referred to as:
A. Inapparent
B. Covert
C. Missed or abortive cases
D. All of the above

130. The chain of infection (endemicity) in the community is maintained by:
A. Clinical cases
B. Subclinical infection

C. Latent infection
D. All of the above

131. A great deal of covert infection is seen in all, *but* one:
A. Measles
B. Rubella
C. Mumps
D. Polio
E. Influenza

132. "Latent infection" occur in the following, *save* for one:
A. Herpes simplex
B. Brill-Zinsser disease
C. Japanese encephalitis
D. Ankylostomiasis
E. Slow viral infections

133. In which of the following infection incubatory, convalescent and healthy carriers are seen?
A. Mumps
B. Polio
C. Cholera
D. Diphtheria only
E. Whooping cough

134. Following are called as Temporary carriers:
A. Incubatory
B. Convalescent
C. Healthy
D. Both B and C above
E. All of the above

135. In Diphtheria, carrier state is associated with:
A. Infected tonsils
B. Infected gallbladder
C. Myocarditis
D. All of the above

136. "Histoplasmosis" is carried all over the world by:
A. Animals
B. Birds
C. Cows
D. Dogs
E. Alligator

137. Soil may harbour agents that may cause all *but* one:
A. Tetanus
B. Anthrax
C. Influenza
D. Coccidioidomycosis
E. Mycetoma

138. Vertical transmission is NOT seen in:
A. Varicella
B. HBV
C. Coxsachie 'B'
D. Polio
E. Rubella

139. "Meningococcal meningitis" is transmitted through:
A. Droplet infection
B. Direct contact
C. Contact with soil
D. Inoculation

140. Diseases transmitted by water and food include:
A. Malaria
B. Polio
C. Chagas disease
D. CMV infection

141. Which infection is NOT transmitted by blood?
A. Hepatitis 'B'
B. Brucellosis
C. Typhoid fever
D. Syphilis
E. Trypanosomes

142. Kidney transplantation is more likely to result in the introduction of which disease agent?
A. AIDS
B. HBV
C. CMV
D. Dengue
E. None of these

143. Transmission of the disease agent from one stage of the life cycle to another:
A. Trans-stadial
B. Propagative
C. Cyclo-propagative
D. Cyclo-developmental

144. "Malarial parasites" in mosquito is an example of:
A. Transovarian transmission
B. Cyclo-propagative
C. Propagative
D. Cyclodevelopmental
E. Trans-stadial transmission

145. "Propagative" mode of transmission is seen in:
A. Nymph to adults
B. Microfilariae in mosquito
C. Plague bacilli in rat flea
D. Malarial parasite mosquito

146. Disease spread by droplet nuclei include all, *but* one:
A. Measles
B. T.B.
C. Varicella
D. Poliomyelitis
E. Fever

147. Diseases carried by infected dust includes all, *save* for one:
A. T.B.
B. Streptococcal staphylococcal infections
C. Coccidioidomycosis
D. Psittacosis
E. None of these

148. Diseases transmitted by FOMITES includes all, *except* for one:
A. Typhoid fever
B. Hepatitis 'B'
C. Bacillary dysentery only
D. Diphtheria
E. Eye and skin infections

149. Following organisms has more than one portal of entry, *but* one:
A. Hepatitis 'A'
B. Hepatitis 'B'
C. Brucellosis
D. Fever only

150. Which of the following is regarded as dead-end infection?
A. Rabies
B. Bubonic plague
C. Tetanus
D. Trichinosis
E. All of these

151. The time required for 50% of the cases to occur following exposure is:
A. Minimum IP
B. Median IP
C. Estimate of average IP
D. All of the above

152. Following infectious diseases are communicable during the later part of the incubation period, *save* for one:
A. Hepatitis 'A'
B. Measles
C. Varicella
D. Pertussis
E. None of these

153. Diseases having very short I.P. includes all, *but* one:
A. Measles
B. Influenza
C. Cholera
D. Bacillary dysentery

154. Infections with longer I.P. includes the following:
A. Rabies
B. Hepatitis A and B
C. Leprosy
D. Slow virus disease
E. All of the above

155. Which of the following non-infectious disease have I.P.?
A. Cancer
B. Heart disease
C. Mental illness

D. All of the above
E. Both A and B above

156. **"The period from disease initiation to disease detection" is called as:**
A. Latent period
B. I.P.
C. Serial interval
D. Generation time

157. **"The gap in time between the onset of the primary case and the secondary case is called" as:**
A. I.P.
B. Serial interval
C. Communicable period
D. Generation time

158. **"The interval of time between receipt of infection by a host maximal infectivity of that host" is known as:**
A. I.P.
B. Serial interval
C. Generation time
D. Communicable period

159. **An important measure of communicability is:**
A. Serial interval
B. Generation time
C. Communicable period
D. Secondary attack rate

160. **The denominator in secondary attack rate (SAR) consists of:**
A. All persons exposed to the case
B. No. of exposed persons developing the disease
C. Per thousand live population
D. None of these

161. **Following antigenic exposure, the antibody elicited first is of .... type.**
A. IgG
B. IgM
C. IgA
D. IgD
E. IgE

162. **Active immunity can be acquired by the following:**
A. Following clinical infection
B. Following subclinical or in apparent infection
C. Following immunisation with an antigen
D. All of these
E. Both A and C above

163. **The antigenic dose required for the induction of IgG is about .... that which is required to induce IgM antibody.**
A. 10 times
B. 20 times
C. 30 times
D. 40 times
E. 50 times

164. **Following are true about secondary (booster) response, *but* one:**
A. Large latent period
B. Production of antibody more rapid
C. More abundant antibody
D. Antibody response maintained at higher levels for a longer period of time

165. **A child born with a defect in humoral immunity (antibody production) may survive for as long as .... without replacement therapy.**
A. 1 year
B. 2 years
C. 3 years
D. 6 years
E. 12 years

166. **A child born with a severe defect in CMI will result in death within the first:**
A. 1 month of life
B. 6 months of life
C. 6 years of life
D. 12 years of life

167. **In which disease, herd immunity does not protect the individuals?**
A. Tetanus
B. Polio
C. Small pox

D. Diphtheria
E. All of the above

168. Following are live attenuated bacterial vaccines, *but* one:
A. Typhoid oral
B. BCG
C. Cholera
D. Plague
E. None of the above

169. Hepatitis 'B' vaccine was developed in which year?
A. 1956
B. 1966
C. 1986
D. 1976
E. 1996

170. The 1st bacterial vaccine prepared was of:
A. Small pox
B. Rabies
C. Cholera
D. Diphtheria
E. BCG

171. Live attenuated vaccine is prepared for which rickettsial infections?
A. Epidemic typhus
B. RMSF
C. Q fever
D. Endemic typhus
E. All of the above

172. Killed viral vaccine includes all, *except* for one:
A. KFD
B. Yellow fever
C. Salk polio
D. Rabies
E. Japanese encephalitis

173. Which is a polypeptide vaccine?
A. Meningococcal
B. BCG
C. Hepatitis 'B'
D. Pneumococcal vaccine

174. Which is a polyvalent vaccine?
A. Polio
B. Influenza
C. DPT
D. Both A and B above
E. All of the above

175. Adjuvants are substances that are added to vaccines with the intent of potentiating the:
A. Potency
B. Immune response
C. Both of the above
D. None of the above

176. More stable vaccine preparation is:
A. Freeze dried
B. Liquid vaccine
C. Both of the above
D. None of the above

177. Following are freeze-dried vaccines, *except* for:
A. BCG
B. Yellow fever
C. Salk polio
D. Measles only

178. The normal human Ig preparation should contain atleast how much percent of intact IgG?
A. 25%
B. 50%
C. 75%
D. 90%
E. 100%

179. Antitoxins are prepared from the following:
A. Monkeys
B. Man
C. Horses
D. Dogs
E. All of these

180. The most heat sensitive vaccine is:
A. Polio
B. BCG

C. Measles
D. DPT
E. All of the above

181. Vaccines which must be stored in the freeze compartment includes all, *except:*
A. Polio
B. Measles
C. BCG
D. DPT
E. None of these

182. At the health centre, most vaccines can be stored upto 5 weeks if the refrigerator temperature is strictly kept between:
A. 0 to 5°C
B. –01 to –20°C
C. 4 to 8°C
D. 10 to 12°C

183. Opened multi-dose vials which have not been fully used should be discarded within ...., if no preservative is used.
A. One hour
B. Two hours
C. Three hours
D. 6 hours
E. 12 hours

184. All vaccines at PHC level are stored in the:
A. Deep freeze
B. Ice lined refrigerators
C. Cold chain
D. WIC

185. Ice packs contain:
A. Water only
B. Salt
C. Water and salt both
D. Neither

186. "Guillain-Barre syndrome" is associated with:
A. Antirabies vaccine
B. Small pox vaccine
C. Swine influenza vaccine
D. All of the above

187. Under IHR following diseases are notified by the national health authority to WHO:
A. Cholera
B. Plague
C. Yellow fever
D. All of these
E. Both B and C above

188. Isolation has failed in the control of following disease, *except* for:
A. T.B.
B. Hansen's disease
C. STD
D. Diphtheria
E. None of these

189. Periods of isolation recommended in Hepatitis 'A' infection is:
A. One week
B. Two weeks
C. Three weeks
D. Four weeks
E. Six weeks

190. Duration of "period of quarantine" is:
A. Period of infectivity
B. Longest I.P.
C. Shortest I.P.
D. None of the above

191. The WHO officially launched a global immunization programme called as EPI (Expanded programme on immunization) to protect all children of the world against six vaccine preventable diseases in which year?
A. 1974
B. 1978
C. 1984
D. 1985
E. 1996

192. Hepatitis 'B' vaccine and Hepatitis 'B' Ig. Should be given simultaneously.
A. True
B. False

193. Following disease need combined passive and active immunization:
A. Tetanus
B. Diphtheria
C. Rabies
D. All of these
E. None of these

194. Recognised chemoprophylaxis for household contacts for cholera is:
A. Tetracycline
B. Furazolidine
C. Erythromycin
D. All of the above
E. Both A and B above

195. How many dose of hepatitis "B' vaccine constitute the complete course?
A. Only one
B. Two
C. Three
D. Four
E. Six

196. "Autoclaving" is the most effective method for sterilization of all, *except:*
A. Gloves
B. Sharp instruments
C. Culture media
D. Dressings
E. Syringes

197. The most effective skin antiseptics are alcoholic solutions of chlorhexidine and iodine.
A. True
B. False

198. The cheapest of all disinfectant is:
A. Sunlight
B. Burning
C. Lime
D. Phenol
E. Alcohols

199. Formaldehyde gas is most commonly used for disinfection of rooms.
A. True
B. False

200. For disinfecting one litre of faeces and urine the amount of bleaching power needed is 50 gm of what percentage concentration?
A. 1%
B. 2%
C. 3%
D. 4%
E. 5%

201. The 1st step in an epidemic investigation is:
A. Obtaining a map of the area
B. Counting the population
C. Confirming of the existence of an epidemic
D. Verification of diagnosis

202. The objectives of an epidemic investigation includes:
A. To define the magnitude of the epidemic outbreak or involvement in terms of time, place and person
B. To determine the particular conditions and factors responsible for the occurrence of the epidemic
C. To identify the cause, source of infection and modes of transmission to determine measures necessary to control the epidemic
D. To make recommendations to prevent recurrence
E. All of the above

203. Following steps should be taken in investigation of an epidemic *save* for one:
A. Confirmation of diagnosis
B. Isolation of cases
C. Study of ecological factors
D. Confirm that the epidemic exists

204. Ecological factors which have made the epidemic possible includes:
A. Sanitary status of eating establishments
B. Water and milk supply
C. Breakdown in water supply system
D. Movements of human population
E. All of the above

205. Who observed, that an epidemiological investigation is more than the collection of established facts?
A. William Budd
B. Frost
C. Collins
D. Davenport

206. Following statement about pre-post clinical trial is most appropriate:
A. They cannot be randomized
B. They are useful in studies involving mortality
C. They use the patient as his or her own control
D. They are usually easier to interpret than the comparable parallel clinical trial

207. Following is true about prevalence and incidence:
A. Both are rates
B. Prevalence is a rate but incidence is not
C. Incidence is a rate but prevalence is not
D. Both are not rates

208. Following is characteristic of a single exposure common vehicle outbreak:
A. Frequent secondary cases
B. Explosive
C. Cases occur continuously beyond the longest I.P.
D. Severity increases with increasing age

209. Following statement is true about BCG vaccination:
A. Distilled water is used as diluent for BCG vaccine
B. WHO recommends Danish 1331 strain for vaccine production
C. The site of infection should be cleaned thoroughly with spirit
D. Mantoux test becomes positive after 48 hours of vaccination

210. The most important function of sentinel surveillance is:
A. To find the total amount of disease in a population
B. To plan effective control measures
C. To determine the trend of disease in a population
D. To notify disease

211. Following are advantages of case control studies, *except:*
A. Useful in rare disease
B. Relative risk can be calculated
C. Odds ratio can be calculated
D. Cost-effective and inexpensive

212. The association between coronary artery disease (CAD) and smoking was found to be as follows:

	CAD	NO CAD
Smokers	30	20
Non-smokers	20	30

The odds ratio can be estimated as:
A. 0.65
B. 0.8
C. 1.3
D. 2.25

213. Modern epidemiology refers to:
A. Study of health services
B. Incidence study
C. Prevalence study
D. Morbidity study

214. Incidence is best measured by:
A. Cross sectional study
B. Cohort study
C. Case control study
D. Double blind study

215. Attributable risk means:
A. Strength of association
B. Temporal relation
C. Potential for prevention
D. Causal relation

216. Recognised features of point source epidemic includes all, *except:*
A. Rapid rise
B. No secondary waves
C. Rapid fall
D. Gradual fall

217. Epidemiological studies is carried for a period of:
A. Twice the IP
B. IP
C. Half the IP
D. 4 times the IP

218. Non-bias study is:
A. Case control study
B. Randomized controlled trials
C. Cohort study
D. Unrandomized trials

219. No-subclinical infection exists in:
A. Polio
B. HAV
C. Varicella
D. Mumps

220. Isolation is not carried out in:
A. Plague
B. Varicella
C. Cholera
D. HIV (AIDS)

221. The rate adjusted to allow for the age distribution of the population is:
A. Age standardized mortality rate
B. Fertility rate
C. Curde mortality rate
D. Perinatal mortality rate

222. Iceberg phenomena is *not* seen in:
A. AIDS
B. Measles
C. Polio
D. Rubella

223. Test of association between two variables is done by:
A. X^2
B. Regression
C. Correlation
D. All of the above

224. Following is the best indicator of severity of a short duration acute disease:
A. Cause specific death rate
B. Case fatality rate
C. 5-year survival
D. Standardized mortality ratio

225. If a new effective treatment is initiated and all other factors remain the same, which of the following is most likely to happen?
A. Incidence will not change
B. Prevalence will not change
C. Both incidence and prevalence will change
D. Neither incidence nor prevalence will change

226. In the context of epidermiology, the following are important criteria for making casual inferences, *except:*
A. Strength of association
B. Predictive value
C. Coherence of association
D. Consistency of association

227. The purpose of double-blind study is to:
A. Reduce the effects of sampling variation
B. Avoid observer and subject bias
C. Avoid observer bias and sampling variation
D. Avoid subject bias and sampling variation

228. A case control study is not characterized by:
A. Cases with the disease are compared to controls without the disease
B. Assessment of past exposure may be biased
C. Definition of cases may be difficult
D. Incidence rates may be computed directly

229. The major purpose of randomization in a clinical trial is to:
A. Ensure the groups are comparable on baseline characteristics
B. Reduce selection bias in allocation to treatment
C. Facilitate double blinding
D. Help ensure the study subjects are representative of general population

230. The purpose of double blinding in clinical trials is to:

A. Avoid observer bias
B. Avoid observer and subject bias
C. Avoid subject bias
D. Achieve comparability between study and control group

231. Following are true in a RCT, *except:*

A. Baseline characteristics of intervention and control groups should be similar
B. Investigator's bias is minimized by double blinding
C. The dropouts from the trial should be excluded from the analysis
D. The sample size required depends on the hypothesis

Answers

1 D	2 C	3 B	4 A	5 B	6 C	7 A	8 C	9 B	10 D
11 E	12 A	13 B	14 C	15 B	16 E	17 E	18 A	19 B	20 A
21 C	22 D	23 E	24 D	25 A	26 B	27 C	28 D	29 E	30 A
31 E	32 C	33 A	34 D	35 B	36 D	37 E	38 A	39 D	40 B
41 E	42 C	43 A	44 D	45 B	46 C	47 B	48 A	49 E	50 A
51 B	52 D	53 C	54 A	55 E	56 B	57 C	58 E	59 A	60 C
61 B	62 C	63 D	64 A	65 C	66 B	67 D	68 A	69 E	70 D

71 B	72 C	73 A	74 D	75 A	76 D	77 C	78 B	79 A	80 C
81 B	82 A	83 B	84 C	85 D	86 C	87 D	88 A	89 B	90 C
91 D	92 A	93 B	94 C	95 D	96 B	97 A	98 B	99 C	100 D
101 A	102 B	103 C	104 B	105 C	106 E	107 D	108 A	109 B	110 E
111 C	112 B	113 D	114 A	115 B	116 C	117 D	118 A	119 D	120 C
121 B	122 C	123 E	124 A	125 D	126 E	127 D	128 A	129 D	130 B
131 A	132 C	133 D	134 E	135 A	136 B	137 C	138 D	139 A	140 B
141 C	142 C	143 A	144 B	145 C	146 D	147 E	148 B	149 A	150 E
151 B	152 E	153 A	154 E	155 D	156 A	157 B	158 C	159 D	160 A
161 B	162 D	163 E	164 A	165 D	166 B	167 A	168 C	169 D	170 C
171 A	172 B	173 C	174 D	175 B	176 A	177 C	178 D	179 C	180 A
181 D	182 C	183 A	184 B	185 A	186 C	187 D	188 D	189 C	190 B
191 A	192 A	193 D	194 E	195 C	196 B	197 A	198 C	199 A	200 E
201 D	202 E	203 B	204 E	205 B	206 C	207 C	208 B	209 B	210 A
211 B	212 D	213 A	214 B	215 C	216 D	217 A	218 B	219 C	220 D
221 A	222 B	223 C	224 B	225 A	226 B	227 C	228 D	229 A	230 B
231 C									

C•H•A•P•T•E•R **SIXTEEN**

Screening for Disease

DIRECTION: Following MCQ's are provided with a few suggestive answers/completions. Only one answer is correct. You have to identify the *BEST* one in each case.

1. Following submerged portion of the iceberg represents the hidden mass of disease, *save* for one:
   A. Clinical case
   B. Subclinical cases
   C. Carriers
   D. Undiagnosed cases
   E. None of these

2. "Floating tip of an iceberg "represents what?
   A. Undiagnosed cases
   B. The physician sees in his practice
   C. Subclinical cases
   D. Carriers only
   E. All of these

3. Active search for recognized disease among apparently healthy people is:
   A. Notification
   B. Surveillance
   C. Case finding
   D. Screening

4. The screening differs from periodic health examination in the following respect:
   I. Physician is required to administer the test
   II. Capable of wide application
   III. Relatively inexpensive, recognized apparently
   IV. Requires little physician time
   Select the true answer from the code given below:
   A. I and II only
   B. II and III only
   C. II, III and IV
   D. I, II and III
   E. I, III, II and IV

5. "Screening" has been defined as:
   A. "The search for unrecognized disease or defect by means of rapidly applied tests, examinations or other procedures in apparently healthy individuals"
   B. The annual health examinations which are meant for the early detection of "occult" disease among diseased
   C. The search for unrecognized disease or defect by means of rapidly applied tests, examination or other procedures in apparently unhealthy individuals
   D. All of the above
   E. Both B and C but not A above

6. **Following are recognized features of screening tests, *save* for one:**
   A. Done on apparently healthy
   B. More expensive
   C. Tests results are arbitrary and final
   D. Based on one criterion or cut-off point
   E. Less accurate

7. **Following are *not* a feature of diagnostic tests:**
   A. The initiative comes from a patient with a complaint
   B. More accurate
   C. Applied to groups
   D. More expensive
   E. Used as a basis for treatment

8. **"Screening" means separation of:**
   A. Healthy from diseased
   B. Apparently diseased from healthy
   C. Apparently diseased from apparently healthy
   D. Definitely diseased from apparently individuals

9. **Following tests are used both for screening and diagnosis:**
   I. Test for anemia
   II. Test for tolerance
   III. Test for cancer
   IV. Test for glaucoma

   Select the true answer from the code given below:
   A. I and II only
   B. I and III only
   C. I and IV only
   D. I, II and III
   E. I, II, III and IV

10. **The time interval between diagnosis by early detection and diagnosis by other means is:**
    A. Serial interval
    B. Incubation period
    C. Lead time
    D. Latent period
    E. None of the above

11. **Following are the main uses of screening, *except* for:**
    A. Case detection
    B. Control of disease
    C. Research purpose
    D. Educational opportunities
    E. None of the above

12. **"Prospective screening" is done for:**
    A. Case detection
    B. Prevention of disease
    C. Research purpose
    D. Control of disease

13. **"Prescriptive screening" is done for what?**
    A. Case detection
    B. Control of disease
    C. Research purpose
    D. None of these

14. **The time interval between first possible detection and usual time of detection of a case is termed as:**
    A. Latent period
    B. Lead time
    C. Lag time
    D. Serial interval
    E. None of these

15. **Application of screening test to entire population of an area is termed as:**
    A. Multiphasic screening
    B. Multiple screening
    C. Multicentric screening
    D. Mass screening

16. **In a community, identification of high risk individuals of risk factors is:**
    A. Mass screening
    B. Surveillance
    C. Selective screening
    D. Multiphasic screening

17. **A good screening test should be:**
    A. Valid
    B. Acceptable
    C. Repeatable

D. All of the above
E. Both A and B but not C above

18. The best and the most economical method of screening for a disease is:
A. Mass screening
B. High risk screening
C. Multiphasic screening
D. Retrospective screening

19. Selective screening refers to screening test applied to the following:
I. High risk groups only
II. Groups of volunteers
III. Group selected by random sampling
Select the true answer from the code given below:
A. I only
B. I and II only
C. I and III only
D. I, II and III

20. Application of two or more screening tests in combination to a large number of people at one time is called as:
A. Mass screening
B. Multiple screening
C. Multicentric screening
D. Multiphasic screening

21. Statement (S): High risk or selective screening has got important role in detecting coronany heart disease.
Reason (R): Because elevated serum cholesterol is associated with a high risk of developing such.
A. Both (S) and (R) are true and (R) correctly explains (S)
B. Both (S) and (R) are true and (R) does not correctly explains (S)
C. (S) is true but (R) is false
D. (R) is true but (S) is false
E. Both (S) and (R) are false

22. Testing for presence of infection/disease in those who seek health care for other reason is termed as:
A. Selective screening
B. Powerful screening
C. Case finding
D. Acceptability

23. Which screening test is applied to selected population with high prevalence?
A. Multiphasic screening
B. High risk screening
C. Multiple screening
D. Purposeful screening

24. The disease to be screened should fulfill the following criteria:
I. Prevalence should be high
II. There is an effective treatment
III. Facilities should be available for confirmation of the diagnosis
IV. There should not be a recognizable latent or early asymptomatic stage
Select the true answer from the code given below:
A. I only
B. I and II only
C. I, II and IV only
D. I, II and III
E. I, II, III and IV

25. The repeatability of the test depends upon three major factors:
I. Observe variation
II. Biological variation
III. Errors relating to technical methods
IV. Subject variation
Select the true answer from the code given below:
A. I, II and III only
B. I only
C. II and IV only
D. I, III and IV
E. I, II, III and IV

26. The variation in measurement readings checked by repeated measurements at one and the same time is:
A. Sample variation

B. Biological variation
C. Observer variation
D. Instrumental variation
E. Environmental variation

27. Intra-observer variation may often be minimised by taking the average of several replicate measurements at the same time.
A. True
B. False

28. "Observational errors" are common in the following:
I. Interpretation of X-rays
II. ECG tracings
III. Readings of blood pressure
IV. Studies of histopathological specimens
Select the correct answer from the code given below:
A. I only
B. II only
C. III only
D. I, II and III
E. I, II, III and IV All

29. "Observer errors" can be minimised by:
A. Standardization of procedures for obtaining measurements and classifications
B. Intense training of all the observers
C. Making use of two or more observers for independent assessment
D. All of the above
E. Both A and B but not C above

30. Sensitivity and specificity, together with "predictive accuracy" are inherent properties of a screening test.
A. True
B. False

31. Ability of a test to detect correctly all those who have the disease that is, true positives is called:
A. Specificity
B. Sensitivity
C. Negativity
D. Productivity
E. Any of the above

32. Ability of a test to detect correctly all those who do not have the disease, that is, true negatives is termed as:
A. Productivity
B. Sensitivity
C. Specificity
D. Negativity
E. Positivity

33. The ratio "true negatives divided by false negatives" is termed as:
A. Predictive power of a negative test
B. Productivity
C. Productivity power of a true test
D. Relative specificity

34. The ratio, "true positives divided by false positives" is termed as:
A. Predictivity
B. Predictive power of a positive test
C. Predictive power of a negative test
D. Relative sensitivity

35. The ratio "true negatives divided by false negatives" is termed as:
A. Relative specificity
B. Predictive power of a positive test
C. Productivity
D. Predictive power of a negative test

36. A test which gives minimum false negatives is termed:
A. Sensitive
B. Specific
C. Confirmatory
D. Association test
E. Any of the above

37. A test which gives minimum false positive is termed:
A. Sensitive
B. Specific
C. Predictive
D. Association test
E. Correlation test

38. The variation in measurement readings checked by repeated measurements at one and the same time is:
A. Sample variation
B. Biological variation
C. Observer variation
D. Instrumental variation

39. In India the screening for $C_A C_X$ is desirable more than the screening for phenylketonuria (PKU) because the former is:
A. More common
B. Less serious than the latter
C. Less common
D. More serious

40. The usual course of action for persons "apparently abnormal" after screening is:
A. Surveillance
B. Periodic screening
C. Monitoring
D. Treatment presumptive

41. MMR (mass miniature radiography) for diagnosis of tuberculosis has following limitation:
A. High cost
B. Less variability
C. Less sensitivity
D. Radiation hazard

42. The usual course of action for persons apparently abnormal after screening includes:
I. Periodic screening
II. Monitoring
III. Surveillance
IV. Treatment
Select the true answer from the code given below:
A. I and II only
B. II and III only
C. I, II and III
D. I, III and IV

43. Difference in two measurements by the same observer on the same subject is:
A. Intra-observer variation
B. Inter observer variation
C. Observer variation
D. Inevitable observer variation

44. Urinary glucose testing as screening has following "most important advantage":
A. Acceptability
B. Rapidity
C. Less subjective
D. Less variation

45. The term "sensitivity" was introduced by whom?
A. Virchow
B. CEA Winslow
C. Yerushalmy
D. Davenport
E. None of the above

46. Diagnostic power of the test is reflected by:
A. Population attributable risk
B. Sensitivity
C. Specificity
D. Predictive value

47. The predictive accuracy depends upon the following:
I. Sensitivity
II. Specificity
III. Disease prevalence
Select the true response from the code given below:
A. I, II and III All
B. I only
C. II only
D. I and II

48. An ideal screening test should have all, *except:*
A. High specificity
B. Low specificity
C. High yield
D. High sensitivity
E. None of the above

49. Prevalence of a disease affects:
A. Sensitivity

B. Specificity
C. Predictive value
D. Relative risk
E. None of the above

50. Which of the following statements is/are true?
A. The CT scan test is more sensitive and more specific than EEG in the diagnosis of brain tumor
B. The predictive value of a positive result falls as disease prevalence declines
C. The lower the sensitivity the larger will be the number of false negatives
D. All of the above
E. Both A and B above

51. Yield depends upon many factors:
A. Sensitivity and specificity of a test
B. Prevalence of the disease
C. Participation of individual in the detection programme
D. Both A and B above
E. All of the above

52. Statement (S): All syphilis screens are first evaluated by an RPR test.
Reason (R): Because RPR test is the most specific test for syphilis cases.
Select the correct answer as per following code:
A. Both (S) and (R) are true and are related to cause and effect
B. Both (S) and (R) are true but are not related to cause and effect
C. (S) is true, (R) is false
D. (R) is true, (S) false
E. Both (S) and (R) are false

53. Consider the following statements:
I. High specificity is necessary when false-positive errors must be avoided
II. The predictive value of a positive test measures the percentage of positive results that are true positives
III. Garfield has stressed the need to meet demands for medical care by separating screenees into well asymptomatic risk and sick groups
Choose the false answer as per code given below:
A. I only
B. II only
C. I and II both
D. I, II and III All
E. None of these

54. During pregnancy, to rule out syphilis, following screening tests is usually recommended:
A. VDRL only
B. RPR test
C. FTA-ABS
D. WR test

55. Screening tests are done in pregnancy, *except* for:
A. Anemia
B. Hypertension
C. PKU
D. Diabetes mellitus
E. Neural tube defects

56. Screening tests are usually recommended to be done in middle aged men and women for following:
I. Hypertension
II. Cancer
III. Diabetes mellitus
IV. Serum cholesterol
V. Obesity only
Select the true answer as per code given below:
A. I, II and III
B. I, II, III, IV and V All
C. II, III and V only
D. I, II, III and IV only
E. I, II, III and V only

57. If the prevalence is very low as compared to the incidence for a disease, it implies:
A. Disease is very fatal and/or easily curable
B. Disease is non fatal

C. Calculation of incidence or prevalence is wrong
D. Nothing can be said, as they are independent

58. The diagnostic power of a test to correctly exclude the disease is reflected by:
A. Sensitivity
B. Specificity
C. Positive predictivity
D. Negative predictivity

59. Denominator whilc calculating the secondary attack rate includes:
A. All the people living in next fifty houses
B. All the close contacts
C. All susceptible amongst close contact
D. All susceptible in the whole village

60. Study this formula carefully.

$$\frac{\textbf{True positives}}{\textbf{True +ves + False –ves}} \times 100.$$

This denotes:
A. Sensitivity
B. Specificity
C. Positive predictive value
D. Negative predictive value

61. For the calculation of positive predictive value of a screening test, the demominator is comprised:
A. True positive + false negatives
B. True positive + false positive
C. False positive + true negatives
D. True positives + true negatives

62. The parameters of sensitivity and specificity are used for assessing:
A. Content validity
B. Construct validity
C. Criterion validity
D. Discriminant validity

63. The response which is graded by an observer on an agree or disagree continuum is based on:
A. Adjective scale
B. Guttman scale
C. Visual analog scale
D. Likert scale

64. The time interval between diagnosis by early detection and diagnosis by other means is:
A. Lead time
B. IP
C. Serial interval
D. Latent period

65. It is found that the risks of C_AC_X is 5 times increased in females with multiple sex partners than with monogamy. Calculate the attributable risk:
A. 5%
B. 80%
C. 10%
D. 20%

66. Calculated positive predictive value of ELISA test for HIV with sensitivity 99%, specificity 99%, prevalence of HIV in population 5/1000 is:
A. 10
B. 70
C. 33
D. 99

Answers

1 A	2 B	3 D	4 C	5 A	6 B	7 C	8 B	9 A	10 C
11 E	12 D	13 A	14 B	15 D	16 C	17 D	18 B	19 A	20 D
21 A	22 C	23 B	24 D	25 E	26 C	27 A	28 E	29 D	30 A
31 B	32 C	33 A	34 B	35 D	36 A	37 B	38 C	39 A	40 B
41 C	42 D	43 A	44 B	45 C	46 D	47 A	48 B	49 C	50 D
51 E	52 C	53 E	54 A	55 C	56 B	57 A	58 D	59 C	60 A
61 B	62 C	63 D	64 A	65 B	66 C				

C·H·A·P·T·E·R **SEVENTEEN**

Demography and Family Planning

DIRECTION: Following MCQ's are provided with a few suggestive answers/completions. Only one answer is correct. You have to identify the *BEST* one in each case.

1. **Demography refers to:**
   A. Population statistics
   B. Medical statistics
   C. Health statistics
   D. Vital statistics
   E. Any of the above
2. **Statement (S): Community medicine is vitally concerned with population.**

   Reason (R): Because group health depends upon the dynamic relationship between the numbers of people, the space which they occupy and the skill that they have acquired in providing for their needs.

   Select the true statement from the code given below:
   A. Both (S) and (R) are true but are not related to cause and effect
   B. Both (S) and (R) are true, and are related to cause and effect
   C. (S) is true, (R) is false
   D. (R) is true, (S) is false
   E. Both (S) and (R) are false
3. **The main sources of demographic statistics in India includes:**

   I. Population census
   II. National sample surveys
   III. Registration of vital events
   IV. Ad hoc demographic studies

   Select the true answer as per code given below:
   A. I and IV only
   B. I, II and III only
   C. I, II, III and IV All
   D. I and II only
   E. I and III only
4. **Till 1920, India was surviving under which phase of demographic cycle?**
   A. Low stationary
   B. Declining phase
   C. Late expanding
   D. High stationary
   E. Early expanding
5. **In Demographic cycle, which state is characterised by high birth rate and high death rate?**
   A. Early expanding
   B. Late expanding
   C. Low stationary
   D. Phase of decline
   E. High stationary

6. "Zero" population growth has been recorded in which country?
A. Austria
B. Belgium
C. Sweden
D. Denmark
E. Germany

7. Currently Germany and Hungary are surviving under which phase of demographic cycle?
A. High stationary
B. Phase of decline
C. Late expanding
D. Low stationary
E. Early expanding

8. Nearly half of the world population live in:
A. China and India
B. India, USA and Russian Federations
C. Both of the above
D. None of the above

9. At present approximately what % of the world's population is living in the developing nations of Asia, Africa and Latin America?
A. 50% B. 60%
C. 70% D. 80%
E. 86.66

10. Which of the following is the LEAST populous nation of the world?
A. Switzerland
B. Italy
C. Germany
D. Srilanka
E. Myanmar only

11. The world's birth rate fell below 30 for the 1st time around:
A. 1921
B. 1947
C. 1975
D. 1980
E. 1985

12. The world population growth rate was at, or near its peak around:
A. 1960
B. 1970
C. 1978
D. 1977
E. 1980

13. A population growing at 0.5% per year will double in about:
A. 50 years
B. 75 years
C. 100 years
D. 125 years
E. 140 years

14. Currently what % of world's population is under 15 years of age?
A. 15%
B. 25%
C. 30%
D. 33.33%
E. 44.44%

15. The UNFPA estimates that world population is most likely to nearly double to 10 billion people in or around:
A. 2025
B. 2030
C. 2050
D. 2040
E. 2060

16. World's population is currently growing at the following rate:
I. 176 people per minute
II. 10,564 people per hour
III. 253,542 people per day
IV. 92,543,000 people per year
Select the true answer as per following code:
A. I and II only
B. I, II, III and IV All
C. I, II and III
D. I and IV
E. I, III and IV

17. **Facts about India includes the following, *but* one:**
A. India has 7.2% of the total world's land area
B. Population 944.5 million (1996)
C. Supporting 16% of world's population
D. India is 7th nation in world in land area

18. **Statement (S): The year 1921 is called the "big-divide".**
Reason (R): Because the absolute number of people added to the population during each decade has been on increase since 1921.
Select the true answer as per code given below:
A. Both (S) and (R) are true but are unrelated to cause and effect
B. Both (S) and (R) are true and are related to cause and effect
C. (S) is true, (R) is false
D. (R) is true, (S) is false
E. Both (S) and (R) are false

19. **India's population is currently increasing at the rate of .... per year.**
A. 12 million
B. 16 million
C. 20 million
D. 24 million
E. 26 million

20. **The average annual exponential growth rate (%) of population of India in 1996 is:**
A. 2.1%
B. 1.96%
C. 2.20%
D. 2.22%
E. 2.11%

21. **According to 1991 census, which of the following Indian states has been accorded as fifth stage in respect of population size?**
A. West Bengal
B. Karnataka
C. Tamil Nadu
D. Andhra Pradesh

22. **Ranking of following states as per population size (1991 census) are as follows:**
I. U.P.
II. Bihar
III. Madhya Pradesh
IV. Maharashtra
V. West Bengal
The correct sequence of 1st four states is:
A. I, II, III and IV
B. I, III, II and IV
C. I, II, IV and V
D. I, II, III and V
E. I, III, IV and V

23. **Approximate magnitude of completed family size can be obtained from:**
A. Total fertility rate
B. Pregnancy rate
C. Gross reproduction rate
D. All of the above

24. **In India, the percentage of urbanization in 1993 is:**
A. 19%
B. 22%
C. 17%
D. 26%
E. 34%

25. **Upto 1993, the % of urbanisation of the entire world is:**
A. 22%
B. 34%
C. 44%
D. 58%
E. 76%

26. **Consider the following statements:**
I. For the purpose of census, a person is deemed as literate if he or she can read and write with understanding in any language

II. **A person who can merely read but cannot write is not considered literate**

III. **In the last few census children below 7 years of age were treated as illetrates**

IV. **In the last census (1991) children above 7 years are considered for literacy**

V. **In 1995 the total number of literate person in India is about 52%**

Select the true answer as per following code:

A. I, II and III
B. I, II, III, IV and V All
C. III, IV and V
D. II, III and V
E. I, III and V only

27. **One of the best indicators of a country's level of development and of the overall health status of its population is:**
A. Infant mortality rate
B. MMR
C. Life expectancy
D. Birth rate

28. **For both males and females, which is the leading nations of the world in respect of life expectancy?**
A. Japan
B. U.S.A.
C. U.K.
D. Denmark
E. Germany

29. **Among the following Asian nations, which has got the best life expectancy?**
A. Nepal
B. Bangladesh
C. Myanmar
D. India
E. Srilanka

30. **If the life expectancy at birth in India during Independence (1947) was 32, then the current life expectancy is:**
A. 57
B. 58
C. 61
D. 62
E. 64

31. **In which year, the Sarada Act was enacted forbidding the practice of child marriage?**
A. 1947
B. 1952
C. 1962
D. 1929
E. 1901

32. **Child Marriage Restraint Act (1978) raises the legal age at marriage:**
A. From 15 to 18 years for girls
B. From 18 to 21 years for boys
C. From 15 to 21 years for girls
D. From 18 to 24 years for boys
E. Both A and B above

33. **Following bear an inverse relationship with fertility, *save* for one:**
A. Age at marriage
B. Caste and religion
C. Educational status
D. Economic status

34. **Fertility rate can be increased by following methods, *save* for one:**
A. Female literacy
B. Spacing of pregnancies
C. Change of MTP Act
D. Late marriages
E. None of these

35. **Statements (S): General fertility rate is a better measure of fertility than the crude birth rate.**
Reason (R): Because the denominator is restricted to the number of women in the child-bearing age, rather than the whole population.
Select the true answer as per code given below:
A. Both (S) and (R) are true and are related to cause and effect

B. Both (S) and (R) true but are not related to cause and effect
C. (S) is true, (R) is false
D. (R) is true, (S) is false
E. Both (S) and (R) are false

36. Which is a more precise measure of fertility that throw light on the fertility pattern and regarded as sensitive indicators of family planning achievements?
A. Total fertility rate
B. Age specific fertility rate
C. Gross reproduction rate
D. General marital fertility rate
E. General fertility rate

37. The simplest indicator of fertility is:
A. Net reproduction rate
B. General fertility rate
C. Birth rate
D. Total fertility rate
E. Age-specific marital fertility rate

38. Which fertility measure gives the approximate magnitude of "completed family size"?
A. General fertility rate
B. Total fertility rate
C. Net reproduction rate
D. General marital fertility rate

39. Which of the following is regarded as a demographic indicator?
A. Marriage rate
B. Abortion rate
C. Child-women ratio only
D. Net reproduction rate
E. Pregnancy rate only

40. According to revised National Health Policy NRR of 1 is to be achieved by:
A. 2006
B. 2002
C. 1996
D. 2008
E. 2000

41. Statement (S): The goal of NRR of 1 can only be achieved if at least 60% of the eligible couples are effectively practising family planning.

Reason (R): Because NRR of 1 is equivalent to attaining approximately the two child norm.
A. Both (S) and (R) are true and are related to cause and effect
B. Both (S) and (R) are true but are not related to cause and effect
C. (S) true, (R) false
D. (R) true, (S) false
E. Both (S) and (R) are false

42. Statement (S): The general marriage rate is more sensitive and accurate when computed for women than for men.

Reason (R): Because more men than women marry at the older ages.
A. (S) is true, (R) is false
B. (R) is true, (S) is false
C. Both (S) and (R) are false
D. Both (S) and (R) are true and are related to cause and effect
E. Both (S) and (R) are true but are not related to cause and effect

43. The gross reproduction rate (rural + urban) in India (1991) is:
A. 1.3
B. 1.7
C. 1.8
D. 1.9
E. None of the above

44. Statement (S): Marriage rate is considered as a very unsatisfactory rate.

Reasons (R): Because the denominator is comprised primarily of population that is not eligible to marry.

Select the correct statement as per code given below:
A. Both (S) and (R) are true and are related to cause and effect
B. Both (S) and (R) are true but are not related to cause and effect

C. (S) is true, (R) is false
D. (R) is true, (S) is false
E. Both (S) and (R) are false

45. If the birth rate in India (1993) is 28.5, then what is its death rate?
A. 9.7
B. 9.8
C. 10.1
D. 9.2
E. 11.1

46. In India, eligible couples per 1000 population is:
A. 30 to 50
B. 50 to 80
C. 80 to 120
D. 120 to 150
E. 150 to 180

47. In India, upto 1990 number of eligible couples using contraception is:
A. 42%
B. 44.1%
C. 50.2%
D. 60.1%
E. 80.2%

48. High level of contraceptive acceptance is prevalent in the following Indian states, *save* for one:
A. Maharashtra
B. Punjab
C. M.P.
D. Haryana
E. None of the above

49. Recognised tools of couple protection rate includes:
I. Sterilization
II. IUCD
III. Condoms
IV. Oral pills
Select the true answer as per code given below:
A. I and II only
B. I and IV only
C. I, II and IV only
D. I, II and III only
E. I, II, III and IV All

50. In India, the couple protection rate in 1993 is:
A. 41.9
B. 43.3
C. 44.1
D. 43.5
E. 50.2

51. India framed its 1st "National Population Policy" in:
A. April 1976
B. May 1977
C. June 1978
D. July 1981

52. The goals set up for following indicators to be achieved by 2000 AD include the following, *except* for one:
A. CBR-21
B. CDR-7
C. Natural growth rate (NGR) 1.95%
D. IMR—<60
E. Couple protection rate—60

53. As per 1991 census, crude birth rate is:
A. 29.1
B. 21.0
C. 29.3
D. 33.9 per 1000 population

54. As per 1991 census crude death rate is:
A. 10.4
B. 9.0
C. 12.6
D. 9.8 per 1000 population

55. As per 1991 census natural growth rate is:
A. 1.87%
B. 1.95%
C. 1.2%
D. 2.13%
E. 3.2%

56. As per 1991 census, the infant mortality rate in India is:
A. 90
B. <60
C. 104
D. 75
E. 80 per 1000 live births

57. A dominant factor in the reduction of NRR is:
A. Couple protection rate
B. CBR
C. CDR
D. IMR
E. All of these

58. Targets to be achieved by the end of 8th five year plan includes all, *except:*
A. Effective CPR-56%
B. CBR-21
C. CDR-9
D. IMR-70
E. Immunization-Universal coverage

59. Recognised feature of revised national population policy (1986) includes:
I. Advancing age of girls (marriage) to 20 years and increasing female literacy
II. Promoting two child norm and spacing methods
III. Enhancing child survival through UIP and promoting ORT
IV. Securing maximum involvement of non-government agencies
Choose the true answer as per following code:
A. I and II only
B. I, II and III only
C. I, II, III and IV All
D. I and III only
E. I, III and IV

60. Statements (S): Contraceptive method which may be quite suitable for one group may be unsuitable for another.
Reason (R): Because of different cultural patterns, religious beliefs and socio-economic milieu.
Select the correct statement as per following code:
A. Both (S) and (R) are true and (R) is the correct explanation of 'S'
B. Both (S) and (R) are true but are not related to cause and effect
C. (S) is true, (R) is false
D. (R) is true, (S) is false
E. Both (S) and (R) are false

61. Recognised example of conventional contraceptive include all, *but* one:
A. Spermicidal jelly
B. IUD only
C. Condom
D. Diaphragm only

62. Which is NOT regarded as the barrier method of contraceptives?
A. Foams
B. Vaginal sponge
C. Condoms
D. Diaphragm
E. Lippes loop

63. Following contraceptive is marketed as a "TODAY" brand name.
A. Foam aerosols
B. Vaginal sponge
C. Condom
D. Diaphragm

64. Regarding condom, which is false?
A. It is the most widely used barrier device by males around the world
B. Easy to use donot require medical supervision
C. Light, compact and disposable without any side effects
D. Protects only men not women from STD
E. None of these

65. Regarding diaphragm, all are correct, *save* for one:
A. A vaginal barrier
B. Invented by English physician (1882)
C. Also called as "Dutch cap"
D. Side effects practically nil

66. The diaphragm is inserted before sexual intercourse and must remain in place for not less than .... after sexual intercourse.
A. Half an hour
B. One hour
C. Two hours
D. 4 hours
E. 6 hours

67. Diaphragm method of contraception combines with:
A. Spermicidal jelly
B. Condom
C. Vaginal sponge
D. Loop

68. The commonly used material in modern spermicides is:
A. Tartaric acid
B. Nonoxynol-9
C. Progesterone
D. Surface active agents
E. All of the above

69. In which year, the Government of India introduced the loop in its National Family Planning Programme?
A. 1952
B. 1959
C. 1965
D. 1974
E. 1977

70. The lippes loop exists in how many sizes?
A. Only one
B. Two
C. Three
D. Four
E. Five

71. Which is the largest of all lippes loop?
A. Size 'A'
B. Size 'D'
C. Size 'B'
D. Size 'C'
E. All are of equal size

72. Which of the following IUCD has become very popular in India?
A. Ota ring
B. Lippes loop
C. Copper devices
D. Progestagert

73. Concerning copper 'T', which of the following is/are false?
A. It is a 2nd generation IUCD's
B. Copper has a strong antifertility effect
C. It is smaller in size so that can be used in a nulliparous women
D. It is effective as post coital contraceptives, if inserted within 3 to 5 days of unprotected intercourse
E. None of these

74. Regarding progestasert, which of the following is/are incorrect?
A. A 3rd generation IUCD
B. The most widely used hormonal device
C. A 'U' shaped device filled with progesterone, the natural hormone
D. The hormone is released in the uterus at the rate of 65 mcg daily

75. Levonorgestral releasing IUD has following advantages over copper 'T', *except:*
A. Less expensive than copper devices
B. Revealed a low pregnancy rate
C. A 'T' shaped IUD releasing 20 mcg of levonorgestral (a potent synthetic steroid)
D. Lower menstrual blood loss
E. No ectopic pregnancy

76. Regarding mechanism of actions of IUCD, which is false?
A. Causes a foreign body reaction in the uterus

B. Causing cellular and biochemical changes in the endometrium
C. Affects the enzymes in the uterus
D. Copper ions may affect sperm motility, capacitation and survival
E. Hormone releasing device are unfavourable to fertilization than implantation

77. The Levonorgestrel releasing IUD has an effective life of:
A. 1 year
B. 3 years
C. 5 years
D. 7 years
E. 10 years

78. The overall effectiveness of IUD and oral contraceptives are about the .... in family planning programme.
A. Less
B. Same
C. 1/3rd
D. 2/3rd
E. None of these

79. The pregnancy rate for which IUD device is least?
A. Lippes loop 'D'
B. Progestasert
C. Nova T
D. Multiload 375

80. Absolute contraindications to IUD includes the following *but* one:
A. Purulent cervical discharge
B. Suspected pregnancy
C. PID
D. C_A C_X, C_A uterus adnexa
E. Ectopic gestation

81. Statement (S): IUD are not recommended for women who have not had children or who have multiple partners.
Reason (R): Because of the risk of PID and possible infertility.
Select the true answer as per code given below:
A. Both (S) and (R) are true but are not related to cause and effect
B. Both (S) and (R) are true and are related to cause and effect
C. (S) is true, (R) is false
D. (R) is true, (S) is false
E. Both (S) and (R) are false

82. Complications of IUD includes the following *save* for one:
A. Increased vaginal bleeding
B. Pain
C. Lactation suppression
D. Pelvic infection
E. Uterine perforation

83. IUD insertion is NOT recommended in all, *but* one:
A. Nulliparous women
B. Immediately after 2nd trimester abortion
C. Women having multiple partners
D. 6 to 8 weeks after delivery

84. The most favoured "Gonanes" is:
A. Levonorgestrol
B. Megestrol
C. Oestranes
D. Lynestrenol

85. Statement (S): The pregnane progestogens are now not recommended in oral contraceptives.
Reason (R): Because of doubts raised by the occurrence of breast tumors in beagle dogs.
Select the true answer as per code given below:
A. Both (S) and (R) are true but are not related to cause and effect
B. Both (S) and (R) are true and are related to cause and effect
C. (S) is true, (R) is false
D. (R) is true, (S) is false
E. Both (S) and (R) are false

86. **Recognised example of pregnane progestogens are all, *except:***
A. 19-nortestosterones
B. Megestrol
C. Chlormadinone only
D. Medroxy progesterone acetate
E. None of these

87. **Consider the following statements about oral pills:**
I. **Mala-N is supplied free of cost through all PHC's, urban family welfare centres**
II. **The commonly used progestogen in "Minipill" is norethisterone and levonorgestrel**
III. **POP could be given to old women for whom combined pill is contra-indicated because of cardiovascular risks**
IV. **POP may also be considered in young women with risk factors for neoplasia**

Select the true answer as per code given below:
A. I and II only
B. I and III only
C. I, II, III and IV All
D. I, II and III only
E. I and IV only

88. **The effectiveness of OCP may be affected by the following drugs, *except:***
A. Ampicillin
B. Phenobarbital
C. Rifampicin
D. None of these

89. **Oestrogen component of OCP may cause all, *save* for one:**
A. Myocardial infarction
B. Elevations of blood glucose
C. Venous thromboembolism
D. Decreased breast milk quantity

90. **Following, *but* one, are true about oral contraceptives:**
A. POP users have greater decline in milk volume
B. There is increased risk of C_A C_x with increased duration of use of OCP
C. Progestogen component causes decrease in HDL
D. Risk of ectopic pregnancy is more in POP pill only
E. Nonc of these

91. **Besides pregnancy the oral contraceptives protect against all, *save* for:**
A. Ovarian C_A
B. Fibroadenoma breast
C. Hepatocellular adenoma
D. PID only
E. Iron deficiency anemia

92. **Consider the following statements:**
I. **Pain and tenderness in breast are due to estrogen of OCP**
II. **Migraine may be aggravated or triggered by the OCP**
III. **Women using ergotamine should not take oral pills**
IV. **The single most significant benefit of the pill is its almost 100% effectiveness in preventing pregnancy**

Choose the correct answer from the following code:
A. I and II only
B. II and III only
C. I, II and III only
D. I, II, III and IV All

93. **Absolute contraindications to OCP includes all, *but* one:**
A. C_A breast and genitals
B. Undiagnosed abnormal uterine bleeding
C. Congenital hyperlipidaemia
D. Liver disease
E. Amenorrhoea

94. Statement (S): Beyond 40 years of age, the pill is not to be prescribed or continued.

Reason (R): Because of the sharp increase in the risk of cardiovascular complications.

Select the true answer as per code given below:

A. Both (S) and (R) are true and are related to cause and effect
B. Both (S) and (R) are true but are not related to cause and effect
C. (S) is true, (R) is false
D. (R) is true, (S) is false
E. Both (S) and (R) are false

95. Regarding DMPA or Depot provera (Depotmedroxyprogesterone acetate) all are true statements/facts, *save* for one:

A. The standard dose is an IM injection of 150 mg every 3 months
B. It has been in use since 1980s
C. It gives protection from pregnancy in 99% for at least 3 months
D. It exerts its contraceptive effect primarily by ovulation suppression
E. It does not affect lactation

96. It is true that the initial injection of both DMPA and NET-EN should be given:

A. During the first 5 days of the menstrual period
B By deep IM into the gluteus maximus
C. The site should never be massaged following injections
D. All of the above
E. Both A and B but not C above

97. The particular advantage of DMPA and NET-EN is that they are:

A. Highly effective
B. Long lasting
C. Reversible contraceptives
D. Both A and B above
E. All of the above

98. A one day census of inpatients in a mental hospital could:

A. Give good information about the patients in that hospital at that time
B. Give reliable estimates of seasonal factors in admissions
C. Enable us to draw conclusions about the mental hospitals of India
D. Enable us to estimate the distribution of different diagnosis in mental illness in the local area

99. As per 2001 census, total population of India is:

A. 843.0 million
B. 1027.0 million
C. 1090.0 million
D. 1072.0 million

100. As per 2001 census, which Indian states rank 1st, 2nd and 3rd in respect of population?

A. Uttar Pradesh, Maharashtra, Bihar
B. Uttar Pradesh, Bengal, Bihar
C. Uttar Pradesh, Tamilnadu, Madhya Pradesh
D. Uttar Pradesh, Madhya Pradesh, West Bengal

101. As per 2001 census, sex ratio in India is:

A. 927
B. 930
C. 933
D. 934

102. As per 2001 census, density of population in India is:

A. 267
B. 324
C. 216
D. 177

103. If the fertility rate in 2002 in Japan is 1.3, then what is the fertility rate in India in 2002?

A. 1.0
B. 1.3
C. 3.5
D. 3.1

104. As per 2001 census, the urban population in India is:
A. 200 million
B. 225 million
C. 250 million
D. 285 million

105. In India, all are included under mega-cities, *except:*
A. Hyderabad
B. Mumbai
C. Kolkata
D. Delhi

106. In 1950, which was the single "Megacity" in the world?
A. London
B. New York
C. Tokyo
D. Sanghai

107. As per 2001 census, Kerala tops the rank in respect of literacy then which state ranks at the bottom in terms of literacy?
A. Assam
B. Chhattisgarh
C. Bihar and Jharkhand
D. Orissa

108. If the birth rate in 2002 is 25.0 in India, then what is the death rate?
A. 9.0
B. 8.9
C. 8.7
D. 8.1

109. In India, under the NFWP, Cu T-200B is being used but from the year 2002 which type has been introduced?
A. Cu T-380A
B. Nova T
C. Cu-7
D. Levonorgestrel IUD

110. The most widely used hormonal IUCD is progestasert a T-shaped device that contains how much quantity of progesterone?
A. 25 mg
B. 38 mg
C. 50 mg
D. 65 mg

111. The most common complaint of women filled with IUD (inert or medicated) is:
A. ↑ed vaginal bleeding
B. Pain
C. PID
D. Fever

112. The United Nations defines "Mega-cities" as those with a population of .... or more.
A. One million
B. Three million
C. Seven million
D. Ten million

113. 100 women, followed up for 20 months, with OCPs, 5 became pregnant, calculate the Pearl Index?
A. 100
B. 200
C. 300
D. 400

114. Contraceptive efficacy (Pearl index) is expressed as:
A. 100 women years
B. 100 women months
C. 1000 women years
D. 10000 women months

115. People living in developing nations are:
A. 60%
B. 70%
C. 80%
D. 90%

116. The age and sex structure of a population may be best described by a:
A. Life table
B. Population pyramid
C. Bar chart
D. All of the above

117. NRR of 1 implies a couple protection rate is:
- **A.** 50%
- **B.** 60%
- **C.** 70%
- **D.** 80%

118. In census literacy rate is assessed by:
- **A.** Ability to read and write
- **B.** Ability to put a signature
- **C.** Ability to read a newspaper
- **D.** None of the above

119. DMPA is an injectable contraceptive given every:
- **A.** 3 weeks
- **B.** 2 months
- **C.** 3 months
- **D.** Three years

120. Population is said to be explosive when growth rate is more than:
- **A.** 1.5
- **B.** 2
- **C.** 2.5
- **D.** 3

Answers

I A	2 B	3 C	4 D	5 E	6 A	7 B	8 C	9 D	10 A
11 C	12 B	13 E	14 D	15 C	16 B	17 A	18 B	19 B	20 A
21 D	22 C	23 A	24 D	25 C	26 B	27 C	28 A	29 E	30 C
31 D	32 E	33 B	34 C	35 A	36 B	37 C	38 B	39 D	40 A
41 A	42 D	43 B	44 A	45 D	46 E	47 B	48 C	49 E	50 D
51 A	52 B	53 C	54 D	55 B	56 E	57 A	58 B	59 C	60 A
61 B	62 E	63 B	64 D	65 B	66 E	67 A	68 D	69 C	70 D
71 B	72 C	73 E	74 C	75 A	76 E	77 C	78 B	79 D	80 A
81 B	82 C	83 D	84 A	85 B	86 A	87 C	88 D	89 B	90 A
91 C	92 D	93 E	94 A	95 B	96 D	97 E	98 A	99 B	100 A
101 C	102 B	103 D	104 D	105 A	106 B	107 C	108 D	109 A	110 B
111 A	112 D	113 C	114 A	115 C	116 B	117 B	118 A	119 C	120 B

C•H•A•P•T•E•R **EIGHTEEN**

Health Programmes in India

DIRECTION: Following MCQ's are provided with a few suggestive answers/completions. Only one answer is correct. You have to identify the *BEST* one in each case.

1. **Which was the India's number one health problem in 1950's?**
   A. Malaria
   B. Filaria
   C. Leprosy
   D. Tuberculosis
   E. All of these

2. **The country faced a major resurgence of malaria in:**
   A. 1960's
   B. 1970's
   C. 1950's
   D. 1980's
   E. 1990's

3. **Following implementation of NMCP in 1953, the incidence of malaria from 75 million cases in 1952 was brought down to how much in 1958?**
   A. 50,000
   B. 1 million
   C. 2 million
   D. 5 million
   E. 7.5 million

4. **With the successful implementation of NMEP (1958), the annual incidence of malaria has further declined to an all-time low of 50,000 cases in which of the following year?**
   A. 1961 B. 1966
   C. 1968 D. 1971
   E. 1991

5. **A modified plan of operations, under the NMEP was evolved and put into operation with effect from 1st April, 1977 leading to reduction in malaria incidence from 6.4 million cases in 1976 to 1.7 million cases in which of the following year?**
   A. 1961
   B. 1978
   C. 1981
   D. 1986
   E. 1988

6. **Consider the following statement about malaria:**
   I. India's commitment to the goal of HFA by 2000 AD necessitated the integration of anti-malaria activities with primary health care
   II. PHCs are involved in the collection and examination of blood smears from fever cases through MPW's (multipurpose workers)

III. The drug distribution centres are manned by panchayat members, forest officials, village health guides and other community workers

IV. Fever treatment depots are manned by teachers forest and revenue officials

Choose the correct answer as per code given below:

A. I and II only
B. I and III only
C. II, III and IV only
D. I, II and III only
E. I, II, III and IV All

7. **Insecticide spraying operations in areas with API2 and above have been done under supervision of:**

A. Sanitary Inspector
B. District Malaria Officer
C. Health Commissioner
D. District Magistrate only
E. BDO/CO of that locality

8. **The malaria action plan (MAP) has come into existence following resurgence of malaria in which year?**

A. 1991
B. 1992
C. 1993
D. 1994
E. 1995

9. **The exercise of MAP-1994 has been completed in following states in India, *save* for one:**

A. Andhra Pradesh
B. Rajasthan
C. Gujarat only
D. Karnataka only
E. Maharashtra only

10. **Consider the following statement about National Filaria Control:**

I. According to recent estimate about 420 million people are exposed to the risk of filaria infection

II. In 1997 there are 206 filaria control units, 27 survey units and 195 filaria clinics functioning in the endemic areas

III. The population protected 47 million only out of 420 million at risk

IV. Training in filariology is being given at 3 regional filária training and research centre at Calicut (Kerala), Rajahamundry (A.P.) and Varanasi (U.P.) under National Institute of Communicable Disease, Delhi.

Select the true answer as per following code:

A. I, II and III only
B. I, II, III and IV All
C. II and IV only
D. I, II and IV only

11. **The operational component of the NFCP was merged with the urban malaria scheme for maximum utilization of available resources in which year?**

A. 1994
B. 1958
C. 1978
D. 1997
E. 1991

12. **Each leprosy control unit covering a population of:**

A. 1 lakhs
B. 2 lakhs
C. 3.5 lakhs
D. 4.5 lakhs
E. 5.6 lakhs

13. **SET centre have been established in areas with endemicity of less than .... per 1000 population.**

A. One
B. Two
C. Three
D. Four
E. Five

14. The main goal of leprosy control is:
- **A.** Interrupt transmission of infection
- **B.** Treatment and rehabilitation of patient
- **C.** Prevent the development of associated deformities
- **D.** All of the above
- **E.** Both A and B above

15. What % of leprosy patient were getting the benefit of MDT by March 1996:
- **A.** 33%
- **B.** 53%
- **C.** 92%
- **D.** 63%
- **E.** 72%

16. One urban leprosy centre is established for every .... thousand people.
- **A.** 5 to 10
- **B.** 10 to 20
- **C.** 20 to 30
- **D.** 30 to 40
- **E.** 50 to 1 lakh

17. The Central JALMA Institute of Leprosy is situated at:
- **A.** Agra
- **B.** Delhi
- **C.** Kolkata
- **D.** Chennai
- **E.** Mumbai

18. The Central Leprosy Training and Teaching Institute is located at:
- **A.** Bhopal
- **B.** Chingelput
- **C.** Orissa
- **D.** Raipur
- **E.** Gauripur

19. "Damien Foundation" helping India in the field of:
- **A.** Malaria control
- **B.** Filaria control
- **C.** Leprosy control
- **D.** T.B. control

20. The backbone of National Tuberculosis programme is:
- **A.** PHC
- **B.** UHC
- **C.** Developmental blocks
- **D.** District TB programme

21. The main strategy in NTCP (National T.B. control programme) is:
- **A.** To trace controls
- **B.** To give BCG vaccination to large population
- **C.** To provide free antikoch's drugs
- **D.** To detect and treat as many case of T.B. as possible
- **E.** All of these

22. Recognised principles of National Tuberculosis Control Programme includes all the following, *but* one:
- **A.** Isolation of TB case only
- **B.** BCG vaccination
- **C.** Early case detection
- **D.** Domicilliary chemotherapy
- **E.** None of these

23. At present out of 460 districts in the country, District T.B. centres have been established in how many districts?
- **A.** 460
- **B.** 466
- **C.** 346
- **D.** 246
- **E.** 459 districts

24. BCG vaccination was taken up under the National Immunization Programme with the goal of protecting all children by:
- **A.** 2000 AD
- **B.** 1997
- **C.** 1990
- **D.** 1998
- **E.** 1995

25. During the year 1995-96, the BCG coverage has gone upto how much?
- **A.** 75%
- **B.** 80%

C. 95%
D. 83.69%
E. Just 60.69%

26. Following International Agencies are providing the assistance to National Tuberculosis Programme (NTP), *except* for one:
A. WHO
B. SIDA
C. World Bank
D. DANIDA
E. None of these

27. Consider the following statements:
I. The Government of India had set up a BCG Vaccine Laboratory at Guindy, Madras (1948)
II. The BCG vaccine laboratory produces and supplies freeze-dried BCG vaccine and PPD tuberculin
III. Antikoch's drugs for free treatment are being supplied to the T.B. clinics run by state Government on a 50-50 sharing basis between the Centre and the states
IV. For Union Territory and Voluntary organisations the treatment assistance is 100%
V. 292 districts have been covered so far under short-term chemotherapy

Choose the true answer as per code given below:
A. I, II and III only
B. I, II, III, IV and V All
C. I, III and V only
D. I, II, III and IV only

28. The revised NTCP strategy has been introduced in the country as a pilot project since:
A. 1991
B. 1992
C. 1993
D. 1994
E. 1995

29. Consider the following statement:
I. Direct observed therapy short-term (DOTS) is a community based T.B. treatment
II. DOTS ensures high cure rates through its 3 components appropriate medical T/t, supervision and motivation by a health or non-health worker and monitoring of disease status by the health services
III. DOTS will be given by MPWs, teachers, anganwadi workers, Dais, expatients, social workers etc. known as DOT agent
IV. DOT agent will be paid incentive/ honorarium of Rs.150 per patient completing the treatment

Select the false answer as per code given below:
A. I only
B. I and II only
C. I, II and III
D. I, II, III and IV All
E. None of these

30. Under diarrhoeal disease control programme (DDCP), each village health guide is supplied packets of ORS per year:
A. 50
B. 100
C. 150
D. 200
E. 300 packets

31. Under CSSM programme, each kit contains how many ORS packets?
A. 50
B. 100
C. 150
D. 200
E. 500 packets

32. The aim of ARI control programme is to reduce mortality rate in children due to

acute respiratory infections by 20% by 1995 and how much % by the year 2000?

A. 20%
B. 25%
C. 30%
D. 35%
E. 40%

33. In CSSM districts, the treatment of Pneumonia is given by drug kit containing:

A. Cotrimoxazole
B. Ampicillin
C. Amoxycillin
D. Cephalosporin

34. The Government of India to launch the guineaworm eradication programme in 1983-84 during which five-year plan?

A. 3rd plan
B. 4th plan
C. 5th plan
D. 6th plan
E. 7th plan

35. Under guineaworm eradication, the concentration of Abate to be used to kill cyclops is:

A. 1 ppm
B. 2 ppm
C. 3 ppm
D. 4 ppm
E. 5 ppm

36. Consider the following statements:

I. Kala-azar is a serious public health problem in Bihar and West Bengal
II. Government of India provides the total costs of medicines and insecticides in Bihar
III. Since 1993, the total of 77101 cases with 1419 deaths in 1992, has been arrested

Select the true answer as per following code given below:

A. I only
B. II only
C. I and II only
D. I and III only
E. I, II and III All

37. The strategy for Kala-azar control broadly includes the following major activities, *save* for one:

A. Health education for community awareness
B. Prophylactic treatment of population
C. Reducing vector by doing indoor insecticidal spray twice annually
D. Early diagnosis and complete treatment of Kala-azar case
E. None of these

38. In the recent years majority of cases of Japanese encephalitis are reported from the following states, *save* for one:

A. Assam
B. Bihar
C. J and K
D. West Bengal
E. Karnataka

39. The strategies for control of Japanese encephalitis include:

I. Development of a safe and standard indigenous vaccine
II. Sentinel surveillance including clinical surveillance of suspected cases
III. Studies to identify the high risk groups by measuring the blood levels of antibodies
IV. Epidemiological monitoring of the disease for prevention and control

Select the true answer as per following code:

A. I and II only
B. II and III only
C. II and IV only
D. I, II, III and IV All
E. II, III and IV only

40. **In India, a goitre control programme has commenced in the year .... based on iodized salt.**
A. 1962
B. 1966
C. 1972
D. 1986
E. 1990

41. **In India, estimated number of people exposed to the risk of iodine deficiency disorder (IDD) is:**
A. 2.2 million
B. 6.6 million
C. 54 million
D. 167 million

42. **The aim of the national programme is to bring down the incidence of IDD to below how much % by the year 2000?**
A. 5 %
B. 10%
C. 12%
D. 15%
E. 20%

43. **In the following Indian states intensive IDD monitoring project has been finalised with the assistance of UNICEF, *except*:**
A. Assam
B. Bihar
C. U.P.
D. M.P.
E. Himachal Pradesh

44. **Under IDD programme the prevalence of goitre in 10 to 14 years age group is to be reduced below how much by 2000 AD?**
A. 1%
B. 3%
C. 5%
D. 10%
E. Zero%

45. **The ultimate goal of the national programme is to reduce blindness in the country from 1.4% to how much % by 2000 AD?**
A. 0.3%
B. 0.1%
C. Zero%
D. 1% only
E. 0.2% only

46. **In India, the approximate number of blind people is:**
A. 6 million
B. 9 million
C. 20 million
D. 12 million
E. 3 million

47. **In India, annual incidence of cataract induced blindness is:**
A. 1 million
B. 2 million
C. 3 million
D. 4 million
E. 5 million

48. **The rate of cataract operations being done each year in India is:**
A. 0.6 million
B. 1.0 million
C. 1.6 million
D. 2.0 million
E. 0.1 million

49. **Number of new cases of cancer in India per year is:**
A. 1.5 million
B. 0.1 million
C. 1.0 million
D. 0.6 million

50. **In which financial year Government of India has started the National Cancer Control Programme?**
A. 1971-72
B. 1972-73
C. 1973-74
D. 1974-75
E. 1975-76

51. Following activities are recommended under National Cancer Programme for district project, *but* one:
A. Setting up of cobalt therapy unit
B. Early detection of cancer
C. Pain relief measures
D. Preventive health education

52. Under National Cancer Control Programme, voluntary organisations would get financial assistance upto Rs. 5 lakhs, as per recommendations of State Government for health education and early detection. How many such organisations are functioning under such scheme?
A. 10 only
B. 15 only
C. 25 only
D. 50 only
E. 500 only

53. Child survival and safe motherhood (CSSM) is being implemented with financial assistance from:
A. WHO
B. UNICEF
C. World Bank
D. Both B and C above
E. All of the above

54. Following states have been taken up using to increased MMR under CSSM programme, *except* for one:
A. Assam and Bihar
B. M.P. and Orissa
C. Maharashtra and Gujarat
D. Rajasthan and U.P.

55. During the year 1995-96 (Upto Feb. 1996) the coverage level for following vaccines is maximum as well as minimum:
A. BCG, TT for pregnant mother
B. BCG, DPT
C. TT for pregnant, oral polio
D. Measles, TT for pregnant DPT, oral Polio

56. A "problem village" has been defined as one where:
A. No safe water is available within a distance of 1.6 km
B. Water is available at a depth of 15 metres
C. Water has excess salinity, iron, flourides, and other toxic elements
D. Water is exposed to the risk of cholera and guinea worm
E. All of these

57. Recognised components of MNP (minimum needs programme) includes all the following, *save* for one:
A. House for landless labourers
B. Rural industries
C. Rural health
D. Rural water supply
E. Rural electrification

58. According to latest assessment safe water is available to:
A. 25%
B. 45%
C. 65%
D. 85%
E. 100% of the total population

59. In the field of rural health, the objectives to be achieved by the end of the 8th five year plan, under the MNP includes:
A. One PHC for 30,000 in plains and 20,000 in tribal and hilly areas
B. One sub-centre for a population of 5,000 in plains and for 3,000 in tribal and hilly
C. One community health centre for a people of one lakh
D. One C.D. block by the year 2000
E. All of the above

60. Under MNP, in the field of nutrition, the objectives are to extend nutrition support to how many eligible persons?
A. 5 million
B. 11 million
C. 18 million
D. 36 million
E. 100 million

61. "Clean drinking water" has been incorporated under which 20-point programme?
A. Point 1
B. Point 5
C. Point 7
D. Point 8

62. Government of India has targeted to eliminate kala-azar by:
A. 2005
B. 2007
C. 2008
D. 2010

63. LEM (leprosy elimination monitoring) exercise was carried out with WHO assistance through the:
A. NIHFW (National Institute of Health and Family Welfare)
B. HKNS (Hind Kusht Nivaran Sangh)
C. NLCP
D. NLEP

64. The "Leprosy mission" is the World Bank supported .... NLEP.
A. 1st
B. 2nd
C. 3rd
D. 4th

65. The WHO has set a new target of elimination of leprosy by the year .... and has formed a global alliance for leprosy elimination.
A. 2005
B. 2006
C. 2007
D. 2010

66. Nearly 76% (about 851 million) of the Indian population in 26 states/UTs has been covered under RNTCP by:
A. January 2002
B. February 2001
C. March 2004
D. March 2005

67. India has become the .... largest nation in the world in terms of population coverage under DOTS.
A. 1st
B. 2nd
C. 3rd
D. 4th

68. Diagnostic facilities for RNTCP are available in .... labs. in India.
A. 780
B. 800
C. 8700
D. 7800

69. The death rate under RNTCP have been cut by how much fold?
A. Two fold
B. Five fold
C. Seven fold
D. Eleven fold

70. In India, out of estimated 4.58 million HIV +ve cases, around 1.6 million are estimated to be co-infected with HIV and TB. Action plan for TB/HIV coordination is being jointly implemented by:
A. DTP and NGO
B. RNTCP and NACO
C. RNTCP and NGO
D. RNTCP and DTO

71. In India, currently how many blood banks have been licensed?
A. 815
B. 950
C. 1055
D. 1233

72. From 1st June 2001 it is made mandatory to test blood for:
A. HIV
B. HCV
C. Babesia
D. Plasmodium

73. Voluntary counselling and testing (VCT) centre in AIDS is established by:
A. WHO
B. IMA
C. NACO
D. AIIMS

74. In India how many VCT centres have been formed by June 2004?
A. 62
B. 262
C. 907
D. 709

75. STD control programme has been in operation in India since:
A. 1946
B. 1956
C. 1966
D. 1976

76. The number of national AIDS telephone helpline is:
A. 1079
B. 1097
C. 9017
D. 7091

77. It is estimated that nearly 167 million persons are exposed to the risk of IDD of which how many are having goitre, cretins and mild neurological disorders?
A. 27 million
B. 47 million
C. 71 million
D. 67 million

78. Pulse Polio Immunization (PPI) programme was launched in which year in India?
A. 1995
B. 1996
C. 1997
D. 1998

79. A pilot project for the introduction of Hepatitis B vaccine in the national immunization programme was initiated in June 2002. Under this project Hepatitis B vaccine is being administered to infants along with the primary doses of DPT vaccine on:
A. 1st, 3rd and 6th week
B. 3rd, 6th and 9th week
C. 4th, 7th and 10th week
D. 6th, 10th and 14th week

80. Integrated Management of childhood Illness (IMCI) and its Indian version has been renamed as:
A. IMNCI
B. INMCI
C. ICMI
D. ICMNI

81. An empowered action group has been constituted in the Ministry of Health and Family Welfare with Union Minister for Health and Family Welfare as chairman on:
A. 20th March 2000
B. 20th March 2001
C. 20th January 2002
D. 20th January 2004

82. India has reported zero cases of guinea-worm since:
A. August 1996
B. September 1997
C. October 1998
D. November 1999

83. In which year the International Commission for the Certification of Dracunculiasis Eradication recommended that India be certified free of dracunculiasis transmission?
A. January 1999
B. February 2000
C. March 2001
D. April 2002

84. The number of Telcobalt-CS-137 units currently found in India is:
A. Nine
B. Twenty-nine
C. Thirty-nine
D. Forty-nine

85. Currently (31st March 2002) following Radiotherapy (RT) facilities are available in India, *but* one:
A. Total number of RT centres—500
B. No of Brachytherapy centres—113
C. No. of telecobalt units—243
D. Manual intracavitary units—76

86. The MNP was introduced during which year of 5th five-year plan (1974 to 78)?
A. 1st year
B. 2nd year
C. 3rd year
D. 5th year

87. Under 20-point programme, "Expansion of education" is incorporated under which point?
A. Point '1'
B. Point '8'
C. Point '10'
D. Point '14'

88. Under 20-point programme, point '17' is associated with:
A. Housing for the people
B. Health for all
C. Improvement of slums
D. Protection of the environment

89. Cancer control programme was launched in which year?
A. 1976
B. 1986
C. 1996
D. 1990

90. The eye condition for which the World Bank assistance was provided to the national programme for control of blindness (1994-2001) is:
A. Trachoma
B. Cataract
C. Vitamin A deficiency
D. Refractory errors

Answers

I A	2 B	3 C	4 C	5 B	6 D	7 C	8 A	9 C	10 C
11 A	12 B	13 C	14 E	15 A	16 C	17 E	18 D	19 C	20 A
21 B	22 C	23 D	24 E	25 B	26 E	27 B	28 A	29 D	30 C
31 E	32 A	33 B	34 C	35 D	36 A	37 E	38 D	39 A	40 D
41 D	42 C	43 B	44 E	45 C	46 D	47 A	48 B	49 C	50 B
51 D	52 C	53 D	54 E	55 C	56 A	57 C	58 D	59 E	60 B
61 C	62 D	63 A	64 B	65 A	66 C	67 B	68 D	69 C	70 B
71 D	72 B	73 C	74 D	75 A	76 B	77 C	78 A	79 D	80 A
81 B	82 A	83 B	84 A	85 A	86 A	87 C	88 D	89 A	90 B

C·H·A·P·T·E·R **NINETEEN**

Health Education and Communication

DIRECTION: Following MCQ's are provided with a few suggestive answers/completions. Only one answer is correct. You have to identify the *BEST* one in each case.

1. **"A state of complete physical, mental and social well-being and not merely the absence of disease or infirmity." This statement defines health is given by:**
   - **A.** WHO
   - **B.** UNICEF
   - **C.** UNESCO
   - **D.** International Red Cross
   - **E.** Indian Red Cross
2. **The objectives of health education is:**
   - **A.** Informing people
   - **B.** Motivating people
   - **C.** Guiding into action
   - **D.** All of the above
   - **E.** Both A and B above
3. **"Health education" is a process that improves motivate and helps people to adopt and maintain healthy practice, and lifestyles, advocate, environmental change as needed to facilitate this goal and conduct professional trainning and research to the same end. This definition is adopted by:**
   - **A.** Government of India
   - **B.** National Conference of PSM in USA
   - **C.** WHO
   - **D.** UNESCO
   - **E.** International Red Cross
4. **Which of the following statement is/are true?**
   - **A.** The object of health education is "to win friends and influence people"
   - **B.** Health education is concerned with promoting health as well as reducing behaviour-induced disease
   - **C.** Health education is change in belief, attitudes and habits of people
   - **D.** Both A and C but not B above
   - **E.** All of the above
5. **The 1st directive of health education is:**
   - **A.** Immunization and treatment of disease
   - **B.** To inform people or disseminate scientific knowledge about prevention of disease and promotion of health
   - **C.** To appoint health educator liberally
   - **D.** To provide job of paramedical staff
6. **Following are the recognised approaches to public health:**
   - **A.** Regulatory approach
   - **B.** Service approach
   - **C.** Educational approach

D. All of the above
E. Both A and C but not B above

7. **Regarding "health education" all the following are recognized features, *except* for one:**
A. Appear to reason
B. Disciplines primitive desires
C. Knowledge is actively acquired
D. Develops reflexive behaviour
E. The process is behaviour centred

8. **Following health problems can only be solved through education:**
A. Nutritional problems
B. Infant and child care
C. Personal hygiene
D. Family planning
E. All of the above

9. **For the adoption of new ideas and practices the following stages are involved in health education:**
I. Awareness
II. Interest
III. Evaluation
IV. Trial
V. Adoption

Select the true response from the code given below:
A. I and II only
B. I, II and III only
C. I, II, IV and V only
D. II, III and V only
E. I, II, III, IV and V All true

10. **In what respect health education differ from health propaganda?**
A. Appear to emotion
B. Develops reflective behaviour
C. Makes people think for themselves
D. Develops individuality, personality and self-expression

11. **Health education is:**
A. A part of only rural health care
B. Job of health educators
C. Job of paramedical staff
D. Duty of every health worker to make the people aware about disease

12. **The objective of health education is to:**
A. Impart knowledge regarding health to those who are illiterate
B. Effect change in health practices of people and in the knowledge and attitude related to such changes
C. Teach personal hygiene to people
D. Teach school children subjects like anatomy and preventive medicine

13. **Accidents are a feature of modern life, and can occur in the following situations:**
A. Home
B. Road side
C. Place of work only
D. All of the above
E. Both B and C above

14. **Mental health is of great importance in the following situations:**
I. Mother after child birth
II. Child at entry into school
III. Decision about future career
IV. Starting a new family
V. At the time of widowhood

Select the true answer as per code given below:
A. I, II and III only
B. I, II, III and IV only
C. I, II, III, IV and V All
D. I, III and V

15. **The predominant factor in accidents is:**
A. Lack of cleanliness
B. Carelessness
C. Faulty machine
D. Very bad employee management
E. All of the above

16. **Currently, family health care programme embraces:**
I. Human growth and development
II. MCH care
III. Human reproduction and family planning

IV. **Population dynamics**
V. **Immunization and nutrition**

Choose the false answer as per following code:
A. I only
B. II and IV only
C. I, II and III only
D. I, II, III and IV only
E. None of the above

17. **Consider the following statement about principles of health education:**
I. **Health education brings together the art and science of medicine, and the principles and practice of general education**
II. **The link is to be found in the social and behavioural sciences—sociology, psychology and social anthropology**
III. **Psychologists have given a great deal of attention to the learning process**
IV. **Learning and teaching is a two-way process of transactions in human relations, between the teacher and taught**
V. **Learning takes place not only in the class room, but also outside in the wider world**

Choose the correct answer as per code given below:
A. I, II and III only
B. I, III and V only
C. I, II and IV
D. I, II, III, IV and V All
E. II, IV and V only

18. **Which of the following is the key word in health education?**
A. Interest
B. Participation
C. Known to unknown
D. Comprehension
E. Reinforcement

19. **Following can provide oppurtunities for active learning *save* for one:**
A. Lectures
B. Workshop
C. Group discussion only
D. Panel discussion only
E. None of these

20. **In health education, "Teaching should be within the mental capacity of the audience". It is called as:**
A. Known to unknown
B. Motivation
C. Comprehension
D. Reinforcement

21. **In health education, what is called as "booster dose"?**
A. Motivation
B. Reinforcement
C. Leadership
D. Good human relations
E. None of these

22. **"If I hear, I forget; if I see, I remember, If I do, I know"—This proverb has come from:**
A. American people
B. British people
C. Chinese people
D. German people
E. Indian people

23. **Following visual aids are not requiring projection:**
A. Flannelgraph
B. Models
C. Posters only
D. Specimens
E. Epidiascopes only

24. **Following visual aids require projection:**
I. **Slides**
II. **Film strips**
III. **Overhead projectors**
IV. **Silent films**

Select the true answer as per following code:
A. I and IV only
B. I, II and III only

C. I and II only
D. I, II, III and IV All

25. Statement (S): Audio-visuals aids are increasingly being used in modern education.

Reason (R): Because they make learning more permanent.

Select the true answer as per code given below:

A. Both (S) and (R) are true and related to cause and effect
B. Both (S) and (R) are true but not related to cause and effect
C. (S) is true, (R) is false
D. (R) is true, (S) is false
E. Both (S) and (R) are false

26. Which of the following auditory aids are extensively used as teaching aids?

A. Microphones
B. Amplifiers
C. Taperecorders
D. Earphones only
E. All of the above

27. The most widely used method of teaching is:

A. Film and charts
B. Lectures
C. Group discussion
D. All of the above
E. Both A and C above

28. Statement (S): Lectures are not a good method of educating people.

Reason (R): Because communication is mostly "one-way".

Choose the true answer as per code given below:

A. Both (S) and (R) are true and related to cause and effect
B. Both (S) and (R) are true but not related to each other
C. (S) is true, (R) is false
D. (R) is true, (S) is false
E. Both (S) and (R) are false

29. A very effective method of health teaching is:

A. Lecture
B. Group discussion
C. Panel discussion
D. Symposium
E. Workshop only

30. Regarding group discussion, which of the following statements is/are false?

A. It is a two-way communication system
B. This method is useful when the groups have common interests and similar problems
C. The group should comprise not less than 10 and not more than 25 people
D. There should be a group leader who initiates the subject, helps the discussion in the proper manner prevents side conversations, encourages every one to participate and sums up the discussion in the end
E. None of these

31. "Four to eight persons who are qualified to talk about the topic sit and discuss a given problem, or the topic, in front of a large group or audience" such type of discussion is called as:

A. Group discussion
B. Panel discussion
C. Symposium
D. Workshop

32. Consider the following statements:

I. In panel discussion the panel comprises, a chairman or moderator and from 4 to 8 speakers

II. The success of panel depends upon the chairman

III. After the main aspects of the subject are explored by the panel speakers, the audience is invited to take part

IV. Panel discussion can be an extremely effective method of education provided it is properly planned and guided

Choose the correct answer as per following code:

A. I, II, III and IV All
B. I and IV only
C. I, II and III only
D. I, II and IV only
E. I, III and IV only

33. When a series of speaks are delivered on a selected subject, this is called as:

A. Lectures
B. Symposium
C. Panel discussion
D. Group discussion
E. Workshop

34. In a symposium:

A. Each person or expert presents an aspect of the subject briefly
B. There is no discussion among the symposium members unlike in panel discussion
C. The chairman makes a comprehensive summary at the end of entire session
D. None of the above
E. All of the above

35. Learning takes place in a friendly, happy and democratic atmosphere, under expert guidance in which method of group health education?

A. Group discussion
B. Workshop
C. Symposium
D. Panel discussion

36. In America, which of the following method of group health education has become a tradition?

A. Programmed instruction
B. Institute
C. Workshop
D. Demonstration

37. The most common objective of an institute is:

A. To present information
B. To create interest
C. To create awareness
D. All of these
E. Both B and C above

38. A variety of techniques are used in an institute:

I. Lectures
II. Panels
III. Group discussions
IV. Symposium

Choose the correct answer from the code given below:

A. I and IV only
B. I, II and III only
C. I, II, III and IV All
D. II, III and IV only
E. IV only

39. In role playing or sociodrama, the size of the group is thought to be best at about:

A. 10
B. 15
C. 20
D. 25
E. 50

40. Which of the following methods of group health education is particularly useful educational device for school children?

A. Workshop
B. Lectures
C. Programmed instruction
D. Demonstration
E. Role playing

41. Statement (S): Practical demonstration is an important technique of health education.

Reason (R): Because a demonstration leaves a visual impression on the minds of the people and is more effective than the printed word.

Select the true answer as per following code:

A. Both (S) and (R) are true and are related to cause and effect

B. Both (S) and (R) are true but are not related to cause and effect
C. (S) is true, (R) is false
D. (R) is true, (S) is false
E. Both (S) and (R) are false

42. The method of teaching based on the "Socratic method" of advancing by easy stages is:
A. Simulation exercise
B. Programmed instruction
C. Role playing
D. Demonstration
E. Institute

43. In which of the following method of health education, the learning steps are called instructional "frames"?
A. Workshop only
B. Institute only
C. Programmed instruction
D. Symposium
E. Simulation exercise

44. Which of the following itself is regarded as one of the simulation exercise?
A. Role play
B. Frames
C. Institute
D. Demonstration only
E. None of these

45. For educating the general public, the most potent of all media is:
A. Radio
B. Television
C. Film
D. Health magazine

46. Statement (S): Mass media are generally less effective in changing human behaviour than individual or group methods.
Reason (R): Because in Mass media communication is "one way".
Select the true answer as per following code:
A. Both (S) and (R) are true and are related to cause and effect
B. Both (S) and (R) are true but not related to cause and effect
C. (S) is true, (R) is false
D. (R) is true, (S) is false
E. Both (S) and (R) are false

47. The Ministry of Health established a school health education division in the central health education bureau in which year?
A. 1971
B. 1947
C. 1958
D. 1968
E. 1978

48. The International Union for Health Education has been founded in which year?
A. 1951
B. 1961
C. 1971
D. 1981
E. 1991

49. The central health education bureau was established in the Ministry of Health in the year?
A. 1947
B. 1956
C. 1965
D. 1971
E. 1981

50. Which of the following agency are engaged in health education work?
A. Directorate of Advertising and Visual Publicity (DAVP)
B. Press Information Bureau (PIB)
C. All India Radio (AIR)
D. All of these
E. Both A and B above

51. Consider the following statements:
I. Evalution should be made along practical link and in terms of specific objective

II. The CHEB was established in the Ministry of Health in 1956 at Delhi with the assistance of the Technical Cooperation Mission of the United States

III. In 1971, it was suggested that each state should establish Health Education units at the district level

IV. Voluntary agency like Indian Red Cross are also engaged in health education activities

Select the true answer as per following code:

A. I and II only
B. I and III only
C. II and III only
D. I, II and III only
E. I, II, III and IV All

52. Transplantation of Human Organs Act was passed by Government of India in:

A. 1996
B. 1993
C. 1994
D. 1998

53. The information technology has revolutionized the world of medical sciences. In which year the Information Technology Act was passed by the Government of India?

A. 1998
B. 2000
C. 2001
D. 2003

Answers

1 A	2 D	3 B	4 E	5 B	6 D	7 D	8 E	9 E	10 A
11 D	12 B	13 D	14 C	15 B	16 E	17 D	18 B	19 A	20 C
21 B	22 C	23 E	24 D	25 A	26 C	27 B	28 A	29 B	30 C
31 B	32 A	33 B	34 E	35 B	36 B	37 A	38 C	39 D	40 E
41 A	42 B	43 C	44 A	45 B	46 A	47 C	48 A	49 B	50 D
51 E	52 C	53 B							

C•H•A•P•T•E•R TWENTY

Health Planning and Management

DIRECTION: Following MCQ's are provided with a few suggestive answers/completions. Only one answer is correct. You have to identify the *BEST* one in each case.

1. The orderly process of defining community health problems, identifying unmet needs and surveying the resources to meet them, establishing priority goals that are realistic and feasible and projecting administrative action to accomplish the purpose of the proposed programme. This definition of health planning is given by:
   A. W.H.O.
   B. National health planning
   C. National Conference on PSM in U.S.A.
   D. International Health Planning
   E. All of the above

2. "Target" in health planning means:
   A. Degree of achievement
   B. Purpose of initiating activities
   C. Sequence of activities designed to implement policies
   D. Ultimate end towards which all resources are directed

3. Which of the following words, are used to describe the end results of planning, has been drawn from military and sporting terminology?
   A. Objectives
   B. Targets only
   C. Goals only
   D. All of the above
   E. Both A and B but not C above

4. An important element of planning is the setting of clear-cut objectives, targets and goals.
   A. True
   B. False

5. Statement (S): An objective is a planned end point of all activities.
Reason (R): Because it is either achieved or not achieved.
   A. Both (S) and (R) are true but are not related to each other
   B. Both (S) and (R) are true and (R) is the true explanation of (S)
   C. (S) is true but (R) is false
   D. Both (S) and (R) are false

6. Goal is defined as the:
   A. Goals are constrained by time or existing resources
   B. Goals are necessarily attainable
   C. Ultimate desired state towards which objectives and resources are directed
   D. All of the above
   E. None of the above

7. A plan consists of following major elements:

I. Objectives II. Policies
III. Programmes IV. Schedules
V. Budget

Select the true response from the code given below:

A. I, II and III only
B. I, III and V only
C. I, II and V only
D. I, II, III and IV only
E. I, II, III, IV and V All

8. Which of the following statement is/are true?

A. A programme is a sequence of activities designed to implement policies and accomplish objectives
B. A programme gives a step-by-step approach to guide the action necessary to reach a predetermined goal
C. A schedule is a time sequence for the work to be done
D. All of the above
E. Both A and C but not B above

9. All the following are the important preconditions for planning, *except* for one:

A. Government interest
B. Legislation
C. Organization for planning
D. Administrative capacity
E. None of these

10. In planning, the correct sequence of steps is:

I. Assess resources
II. Analyse problem
III. Set priorities
IV. Check implementation

Select the true response from the code given below:

A. I, II, III and IV
B. II, I, III and IV
C. II, III, I and IV
D. III, II, IV and I

11. A sequence of activities designed to implement policies and accomplish objectives is called:

A. Plan
B. Schedule
C. Programme only
D. Target only
E. Goals only

12. Which of the following is NOT a management technique?

A. Work sampling
B. Model
C. Cost accounting
D. Evaluation only
E. None of the above

13. In a programme, results are analysed in comparison to cost is known as:

A. Cost accountancy
B. Cost benefit analysis
C. Cost effective analysis
D. Management by objectives

14. "To match the limited resources to accomplish a defined objective by eliminating wasteful expenditure in the shortest possible time". This is the definition of:

A. Planning
B. Management
C. Organisation
D. Evaluation
E. None of the above

15. The step in the process of evaluation are:

I. Determining the measurement yardsticks of the objectives
II. Pretesting of the yardsticks of measurement
III. Defining the objectives
IV. Identifying the goal achieving activities

Select the true sequence from the code given below:

A. III, I, II and IV
B. II, I, IV and III

C. III, II, IV and I
D. II, I, III and IV

16. Evaluation of a programme can be done by:
A. Surveys
B. Expert groups
C. Committees and commissions
D. All of the above
E. Both A and C but not B above

17. Steps in planning involved may be:
I. Establishment of objectives
II. Assessment of resources
III. Analysis of health situation
IV. Prepare alternate plans
Select the true sequence from the code given below:
A. II, I, III and IV
B. III, I, II and IV
C. I, II, III and IV
D. III, II, IV and I

18. The management functions can be carried out effectively by adopting:
A. Performance appraisal
B. Public relations system
C. Concurrent supervision
D. I.E.C. programme
E. Management information system

19. "Action methodology" is the most important characteristic of which of the following?
A. Policy
B. Procedure
C. Plan
D. Schedule only
E. Programme only

20. "Action sequence" is the most important characteristic of one of the following:
A. Plan only
B. Programme only
C. Schedule only
D. Procedure only
E. Any of the above

21. "Timing of actions" is the most important characteristic of which of the following?
A. Schedule only
B. Plan only
C. Policy only
D. Procedure only
E. All of the above

22. "Work rules" is the most important characteristic of which of the following?
A. Plan
B. Procedure
C. Programme
D. Schedule
E. Policy

23. "Guiding principle" is the most important characteristic of:
A. Schedule
B. Procedure
C. Policy
D. Plan only
E. Programme

24. "Authority" is the most crucial factor for the:
A. Decision making
B. Modification of action
C. Responsibility of results
D. Flexibility

25. "Responsibility for results" is an inbuilt factor with:
A. Authority
B. Accountability
C. Flexibility
D. Decision making
E. Any of the above

26. "Modification of actions" is closely linked with:
A. Authority
B. Responsibility in an operation
C. Accountability
D. Flexibility

27. Which of the following preconditions of pre-planning under which the MTP Act (1971) has been included by the Indian Parliament to protect the health of mothers?
- **A.** Government interest
- **B.** Legislation
- **C.** Administrative capacity
- **D.** Organization for planning

28. Unless objectives are established, there is likely to be:
- **A.** Haphazard activity
- **B.** Uneconomical use of funds
- **C.** Poor performance
- **D.** All of these
- **E.** Both A and C above

29. Following is the 1st step in Health Planning:
- **I. Analysis of the health situation**
- **II. Establishment of objectives and goals**
- **III. Assessment of resources**
- **IV. Fixing priorities**

Select the correct response from the code given below:
- **A.** Only I
- **B.** I, II and III only
- **C.** I, III and IV
- **D.** II, III and IV
- **E.** I, II, III and IV

30. Statement (S): The plan must be complete in all respects for the execution of a project.

Reason (R): Because for each proposed health programme, the resources required are related to the results expected.
- **A.** Both (S) and (R) are true and related to each other
- **B.** Both (S) and (R) are true but not related to each other
- **C.** (S) is true but (R) is false
- **D.** Both (S) and (R) are false

31. The 2nd most important step in planning is:
- **A.** Analysis of health situation
- **B.** Assessment of resources
- **C.** Establishment of priorities
- **D.** Establishment of objectives and goals

32. Following are true in respect of plan formulation:
- **A.** The plan must be complete in all respects for the execution of a project
- **B.** Each state of the plan is defined and costed and the time needed to implement is specified
- **C.** The plan must contain working guidance to all those responsible for execution
- **D.** All of the above
- **E.** Both B and C but not A above

33. At which stage that shortcomings often appear in practice?
- **A.** Planning
- **B.** Policy making authorities
- **C.** Implementation
- **D.** Programming
- **E.** All of the above

34. Following are the main considerations at the implementation stage:
- **A.** Definition of roles and tasks
- **B.** The selection, training, motivation and supervision of the manpower involved
- **C.** Organization and communication
- **D.** The efficiency of hospitals or health centre
- **E.** All of the above

35. "A continuous process of observing recording and reporting on the activities of the organization or project." This is the definition of:
- **A.** Plan
- **B.** Monitoring
- **C.** Objectives and goals
- **D.** Fixing priorities
- **E.** Evaluation

36. Which one of the following "measures the degree" to which objectives and targets are fulfilled and quality of the results obtained:
A. Evaluation
B. Management
C. Planning
D. Monitoring
E. All of the above

37. Following are related to evalution:
I. Measures the productivity of available resources in achieving clearly defined objectives
II. Measures how much output or cost-effectiveness is achieved
III. Makes possible the reallocation of priorities and of resources on the basis of changing health needs
Select the true response from the code given below:
A. I only
B. I and II only
C. I, II and III All
D. II and III
E. I and III

38. "The purposeful and effective use of resources—manpower, materials and finances for fulfilling a pre-determined objective." This is the definition of:
A. Planning
B. Objective and goals
C. Evaluation
D. Management
E. None of the above

39. Management consists of following four basic activities:
I. Planning
II. Monitoring (Controlling)
III. Communicating
IV. Organizing
Select the correct sequence from the code given below:
A. I, IV, III and II
B. I, II, III and IV
C. IV, I, II and III
D. II, I, III and IV

40. "Management techniques" are quite familiar in:
A. Industry
B. Business
C. Defence only
D. All of the above
E. Both A and B above

41. "Management techniques" are based on following principles:
I. Qualitative methods
II. Behavioural sciences
III. Quantitative methods
Select the true answer from the code given below:
A. I, II and III
B. II and III
C. I and II
D. I and III only

42. Quantitative methods are derived from the field of following, *except* for one:
A. Operation research
B. Budgeting only
C. Economics only
D. None of these

43. A management technique which has attracted the widest attention for application in the health field is:
A. Cost-benefit analysis
B. Cost-effectiveness analysis
C. Cost-accounting
D. Input-output analysis

44. Statement (S): Cost-effectiveness analysis is a more promising tool for application in the health field than cost-benefit analysis.
Reason (R): Because it is similar to cost-benefit analysis except that benefit, instead of being expressed in monetary terms is expressed in terms of result achieved.

A. Both (S) and (R) are true but (R) is not the true explanation of (S)
B. (S) is true but (R) is false
C. Both (S) and (R) are true and (R) is correct explanation of (S)
D. Both (S) and (R) are false

45. Which of the following is regarded as the basic concept of management science?
A. Cost-benefit analysis
B. Model
C. Cost-accounting
D. Input-output analysis
E. None of the above

46. In health field, "INPUT" refers to all health service activities which consumes the following?
A. Manpower
B. Money
C. Materials only
D. Time
E. Any of the above

47. Following statements is/are true about Network analysis:
A. It is a graphic plan of all events and activities to be completed in order to reach an end objective
B. It brings greater discipline in planning
C. The 2 common types of network technique are PERT and CPM
D. All of the above
E. Both A and B but not C above

48. "PERT" stands for:
A. Programme evalution and review technique
B. Programme execution and related task
C. Programme elimination and Rosenberg technique
D. Programme evaluation and rescue tank

49. "CPM" stands for:
A. Community Measures
B. Critical Path Method
C. Crucial Path Measurement
D. Community Preventive Medicine

50. PERT is a useful management technique which can be applied to a great variety of projects, *except:*
A. It aids in planning, scheduling and monitoring the project
B. It allows better communication between the various levels of management
C. It does not identify potential problems
D. It furnishes continuous, timely progress reports
E. It forms a solid foundation upon which to build an evaluation and checking system

51. The essence of PERT is to construct:
A. An arrow diagram
B. A dumpbell diagram
C. A figure of eight
D. A pyramid diagram

52. Critical path method (CPM) is .... path of the network.
A. Shortest
B. Longest
C. Most cost productive
D. Dearest
E. None of the above

53. Systematic observation and recording of activities of one or more individuals is called:
A. System analysis
B. Network analysis
C. Work sampling
D. Decision making

54. The time taken for any project can be determined by which of the following?
A. Work sampling
B. System analysis only
C. Input-output analysis
D. Network analysis only

55. PPBS stands for:
A. Preventive Paediatrics in Bachelor Science
B. Planning Programming Budgeting System

C. Preventive Paediatrics Budgeting System
D. Planning Paediatrics Building System

56. Which of the following statement is/are true?
A. The PPBS does not call for changes in the existing organization
B. The PPBS calls for grouping of activities into programmes related to each objective
C. Zero budget approach means all budgets start at zero and no one gets any budget that he cannot specifically justify on a year to year basis
D. All of the above
E. Both B and C above

57. Work sampling studies have been done on following categories of medical personnel:
A. Doctors only
B. Nurses only
C. Pharmacists
D. Technicians only
E. All of the above

58. Following statements are true about work sampling:
I. Provides quantitative measurement of the various activities
II. Permits judgements to the appropriateness of current staff job description and training
III. Helps in standardising the methods of performing jobs and determining the manpower needs in any organization
Select the true answer from the code given below:
A. I and II only
B. II and III only
C. I, II and III All
D. I and III only
E. None of the above

59. Which of the following resembles the basic discipline of D/d in medical practice?
A. Input-output analysis
B. Network analysis
C. Work sampling
D. Decision making

60. In the health sector, decisions have to be made about:
A. Development of resources
B. Optimum workload for medical and paramedical staffs
C. Strategies for providing health care
D. Both A and B above
E. All of the above

61. In which year, the Ministry of Health and Family Welfare, Government of India, has evolved a National Health Policy keeping in view the national commitment to attain the goal of Health for All by the year 2000 AD?
A. 1981
B. 1983
C. 1985
D. 1993
E. 1995

62. Which of the following goals for Health and Family Welfare in India at current level is almost near to the target set at 2000 AD?
A. Pre-school (1-5) mortality rate
B. Infant mortality rate
C. Crude death rate
D. Perinatal mortality rate

63. Selected goals for Health and Family Welfare in India by 2000 A.D.
I. I.M.R. — < 60
II. Crude death rate — 9.0
III. Net. reproduction rate—1.48
IV. Family size—2.3
Select the true response from the following code:
A. I, II and IV
B. I, III and IV
C. I, II and III
D. II, III and IV
E. I, II, III and IV

64. The Government of India in which year appointed a committee popularly called as the "Health Survey and Development Committee"?

A. 1943
B. 1946
C. 1952
D. 1962
E. None of these

65. The concept of Primary Health Care (PHC) was given by which health committee?

A. Kartar Singh Committee
B. Bhore Committee
C. Mudaliar Committee
D. Mukerji Committee

66. Who is related with "Health Survey and Development Committee"?

A. Shrivastava
B. Kartar Singh
C. Mukherji
D. Sir Joseph Bhore
E. Dr N Jungalwalla

67. Which committee includes 3 months training in PSM to prepare "Social Physicians"?

A. Mukherji Committee
B. Kartar Singh Committee
C. Bhore Committee
D. Shrivastava Committee

68. Following are recommendations of Mudaliar Committee:

I. Constitution of an All India Health Services on the pattern of I.A.S.
II. Strengthening of district hospital with specialist service
III. To improve the quality of health care
IV. Each PHC not to serve > 40000 population

Select the true answer from the code given below:

A. I and II
B. II and III
C. III and IV
D. II, III and IV
E. I, II, III and IV

69. A "long-term programme" of Bhore Committee was suggested as or also known as:

A. Three million plan
B. Health survey
C. Multipurpose
D. Both B and C above
E. All of the above

70. "Health Survey and Planning Committee" has been given by whom?

A. Sir Joseph Bhore
B. Dr AL Mudaliar
C. Mukerji
D. Dr N Jungalwalla
E. Kartar Singh

71. Which committee gives the concept of "Basic health service"?

A. Bhore Committee
B. Mudaliar Committee
C. Chadah Committee
D. Mukerji Committee

72. The concept of "Multipurpose Workers" has been recommended by which committee?

A. Kartar Singh Committee
B. Mudaliar Committee
C. Chadah Committee
D. Shrivastava Committee

73. Which committee defined "integrated health services"?

A. Mudaliar Committee
B. Bhore Committee
C. Mukherji Committee
D. Kartar Singh Committee
E. Jungalwala Committee

74. "The Committee on Multipurpose Workers under Health and Family Planning" was given by whom?

A. Shrivastava

B. Bhore
C. Kartar Singh
D. Chadah
E. Jungalwalla Committee

75. Which committee gives the concept of "Group on medical education and support manpower"?
A. Shrivastava
B. Bhore
C. Chadah Committee
D. Kartar Singh
E. Jungalwalla Commitee

76. The recommendations of the Kartar Singh Committee were accepted by the Government of India to be implemented in a phased manner during the:
A. 2nd five year plan
B. 3rd five year plan
C. 4th five year plan
D. 5th five year plan

77. Chadah Committee primarily dealing with the following:
I. Integrated health services
II. Vigilance operation of National Malaria Eradication Programme (NMEP)
III. Changes in medical education
IV. Development of PHC

Select the true answer from the code given below:
A. I only
B. II only
C. I, II and III
D. I, II, III and IV

78. The unipurpose workers were reoriented as MPW or health workers (HW) on the suggestion of:
A. Kartar Singh Committee
B. Bhore Committee
C. Chadah Committee
D. Jungalwalla Committee

79. Multipurpose workers (MPW) are posted at:
A. Primary health centre
B. Subcentre
C. Village
D. District hospital
E. None of the above

80. All the following category of personnel are trained to become health workers, *except* for one:
A. Malaria surveillances workers
B. Vaccinators
C. Sanitary inspector
D. Health education assistants

81. According to Kartar Singh Committee, each subcentre should serve a population of:
A. 10,000
B. 5,000
C. 3,000
D. 1,000
E. None of the above

82. "Referral Services Complex" was recommended by which committee?
A. Mudaliar
B. Bhore
C. Kartar Singh
D. Shrivastava
E. None of the above

83. The concept of "Rural Health Scheme" was given by which of the following committee?
A. Jungalwalla
B. Bhore
C. Chadha Commitee
D. Mudaliar Committee
E. Shrivastava Committee

84. For planning health sector has the following divisions, *except* for one:
A. Indigenous systems of medicine
B. Family Planning

C. Water supply and sanitation
D. None of these

85. The current five-year plan (1992-1997) is:
A. Fifth
B. Eight
C. Sixth
D. Seventh

86. The international drinking water supply and sanitation decade is:
A. 1951-60
B. 1961-70
C. 1981-90
D. 1971-80

87. In India HFA by 2000 AD is to be achieved through which of the following?
A. Primary health care
B. Referral services
C. Community health centre
D. Social medicine
E. Indigenous system of medicine

88. According to 8th five-year plan, universal immunization of expectant mothers and eligible children is to be achieved by:
A. 1993
B. 1994
C. 1995
D. 1997
E. 2000

89. To give effect to a better coordination between the Centre and state governments, a bureau of planning was constituted in which year?
A. 1950
B. 1952
C. 1965
D. 1971
E. 1981

90. The broad objectives of the health programmes during the five-year plans include:
I. Control or eradication of major communicable diseases
II. Strengthening of the basic health services through the establishment of PHCs and subcentres
III. Population control
IV. Development of health manpower resources

Select the true answer from the following code given below:
A. I, II, III and IV All
B. I and IV
C. I, II and IV
D. I, II and III
E. I, III and IV

91. Statement (S): In India, PHC has been established in each block to provide comprehensive health services.

Reason (R): Because, block is the unit of rural planning and development.
A. Both (S) and (R) are true but (R) is not the true explanation of (S)
B. Both (S) and (R) are true and (R) is the true explanation of (S)
C. (S) is true but (R) is false
D. Both (S) and (R) are false

92. By the end of the 8th five-year plan (1992-97), it is envisaged that the infrastucture for PHC as required on present population norms would be fully operational with regard to:
A. Village health guides
B. PHCs and subcentres
C. Multipurpose health workers
D. All of the above
E. Both B and C above

93. The 8th five-year plan envisages the following:
I. Universal immunization of expectant mothers and all eligible children by the year 1997
II. Couple protection rate of 56% by the end of 8th plan
III. Increased emphasis on female education and MCH services

IV. To provide adequate drinking water facilities for the entire population both in urban and in rural areas

V. Sanitation facilities for 80% of the urban population and 25% of the rural population

Select the true answer from the code given below:

A. I, II and IV
B. I, II, III and IV
C. I, II, III, IV and V
D. II, III, IV and V

94. By the end of 7th five-year plan, the total number of medical colleges in India was:

A. 42 only
B. 106
C. 125
D. 148
E. 200

95. During 1st plan (1951-56), the total number of medical colleges in India was:

A. 42 only
B. 106
C. 125
D. 148
E. Only 24

96. During 1st plan (1951-56), the total admissions annually in medical colleges in India was:

A. 1,000 only
B. 3,500
C. 8,000
D. 11,389

97. During 1st plan (1951-56), the total number of allopaths in India was:

A. 6,500
B. 65,000
C. 297,228
D. 394,088

98. By the end of seventh plan (1985-90), the total number of allopathic doctors in India was:

A. 6,500
B. 65,000
C. 297,228
D. 394,088
E. 5 lakhs

99. The official "organs" of the health system at the national level consists of:

A. The Ministry of Health and Family Welfare
B. The Director General of Health and Family Welfare
C. The Central Council of Health and Family Welfare
D. Both A and B but not C above
E. All of the above

100. The functions of the Union Health Ministry are set out in the 7th Schedule of which Article of the Constitution of India?

A. Article 24
B. Article 26
C. Article 246
D. Article 426
E. Article 642

101. The principal advisor to the Union Government in both medical and public health matters is:

A. Union Health Minister
B. DGHS
C. Health Secretary
D. All of the above
E. Both A and C but not B above

102. The Directorate of Health Services comprises following:

I. Medical care and hospitals

II. Public health

III. General administration

Select the true answer from the code given below:

A. I, II and III
B. I only
C. I and II only
D. II and III only

103. In which year, the Central Bureau of Health Intelligence was established in India?
A. 1951
B. 1961
C. 1971
D. 1981
E. 1991

104. The Central Bureau of Health Intelligence has the following units:
I. Epidemiological unit
II. Health Economics unit
III. A national morbidity survey unit
IV. Man power cell

Select the true answer from the code given below:
A. I only
B. I and II only
C. II and III only
D. I, II, III and IV

105. The Central Medical Library of the DGHS was declared the National Medical Library in which year?
A. 1956
B. 1962
C. 1966
D. 1976
E. 1986

106. The Central Council of Health was set up by a Presidential order on 9 August, 1952 under which article of the Constitution of India?
A. Article 103
B. Article 263
C. Article 363
D. Article 463

107. Who is appointed as chairman of the Central Council of Health?
A. Health Secretary Government of India
B. Prime Minister
C. Union Health Minister
D. State Health Minister

108. The first milestone in state health administration was which year, when the states (then called provinces) obtained autonomy, under the Montague-Chelmsford reforms, from the Central Government in matters of public health?
A. 1919
B. 1929
C. 1931
D. 1935
E. 1941

109. The "State" list which became the responsibility of the state included the following:
A. Provision of medical care
B. Preventive health services
C. Pilgrimages within the state
D. All of the above
E. Both A and B but C above

110. Which of the following statement is/are true?
A. The principal unit of administration in India is the district under a Collector or D.M.
B. There are about 593 districts in India
C. Most districts in India are divided into 2 or more sub-divisions
D. A tehsil (taluka) usually comprises between 200 to 600 villages
E. All of the above

111. Each district in India has been subdivided into 6 types of administrative areas:
I. Sub-divisions
II. Tehsil
III. Blocks
IV. Municipalities and corporations
V. Villages
VI. Panchayats

Select the correct sequence in descending order:
A. I, II, III, IV, V and VI
B. VI, V, IV, III, II and I
C. I, II, IV, III, V and VI

D. I, II, V, IV, III and VI
E. I, II, III, V, IV and VI

112. "Community Development Programme" was launched in India in which of the following year?
A. 1951
B. 1952
C. 1953
D. 1955
E. 1961

113. The urban areas of the following district are organized into the following institutions of local-self government:
A. Town area committee (in area with population ranging between 5,000 and 10,000)
B. Municipal Boards (in areas with population ranging between 10,000 and 2 lakhs)
C. Corporation (with population above 2 lakhs)
D. All of the above
E. Both B and C above

114. Which of the following statements is/are true?
A. The Municipal Boards are headed by a Chairman/President, elected usually by the members
B. The term of municipal board ranges between 3 to 5 years
C. Corporations are headed by Mayors
D. All of the above
E. Both A and C but not B above

115. "Panchayati Raj" at village level consists of all the following, *except* for one:
A. Panchayat Samiti
B. The Gram Sabha
C. The Gram Panchayat
D. The Nyaya Panchayat

116. Following are true regarding Gram Panchayat *save* for one:
A. It is executive organ of the Gram Sabha and an agency for planning and development at village level
B. Its strength varies from 30 to 50
C. The members hold office for a period of 3 to 4 years
D. Every panchayat has an elected president called as Sarpanch or Sabhapati or Mukhia
E. The powers and functions of Mukhia covers the entire field of civic administration including sanitation and public health and socio-economic development of the village

117. The following may be true of Gram Sabha:
I. The assembly of all the adults of the village
II. Meets at least twice a year
III. Considers proposals for taxation
IV. Discuss the annual programme
V. Elects members of the Gram Panchayat
Select the correct answer from the code given below:
A. I, II and V
B. II, III and V
C. I, II, III, IV and V All
D. III, IV and V only
E. I, II, III and IV only

118. Under Integrated Rural Development Programme (IRDP), following are usually provided, *save* for one:
A. Resources
B. Bank loans
C. Subsidies
D. Employment

119. The target families under IRDP are generally:
A. Agricultural labourers
B. Shopkeepers only
C. Land owners
D. Anganwadi workers
E. All of the above

120. Each "Gram-sevak" appointed for rural development caters to how much of population?
A. 3000 people
B. 5000 people
C. 7500 people
D. 10000 people
E. Only 1000 people

121. Following are facts about the Block:
I. Consists of 100 villages and a population of about 80,000 to 1,20,000
II. The Panchayati Raj agency at the block level is the Panchayat Samiti/ Janpada Panchayat
III. The Panchayat Samiti consists of all Sarpanchas of the village in the block, MLAs, MPs in the areas plus representatives of women, ST and SC and cooperative societies
IV. Mukhia is the ex-officio secretary of Panchayat Samiti
Select the true answer from the following code:
A. I and IV only
B. I and II only
C. I, II and III
D. I, II, III and IV

122. Who is the ex-officio secretary of the Panchayat Samiti?
A. MPs residing in the areas
B. BDO
C. Mukhia
D. MLAs residing in the areas
E. All of the above

123. In Zila Parishad, who is a non-voting member?
A. MPs only
B. MLAs only
C. Collector or D.M.
D. Two persons of experience in administration, public life or rural development

124. In which state in India, the District Health Officers and the District Family Planning and MCH officers are under the control of the Zila Parishad?
A. Gujarat
B. Bihar
C. West Bengal
D. Delhi only
E. All of the above

125. Which Programme was hailed as a programme "of the people, for the people, by the people" to exterminate the triple enemies of poverty, ill health and ignorance?
A. IRDP
B. Community development programme
C. Village level worker programme
D. All of the above

126. Following are true about community development blocks (CD blocks), *except* for one:
A. Each block consists of approx. 100 villages
B. Each block has a population of 1 lakhs
C. Each block is headed by a BDO
D. There are about 10,000 CD blocks in the country

127. The CD programme was launched in India in which of the following year?
A. 2nd October 1952
B. 2nd January1952
C. 3rd December1952
D. 5th June 1952
E. 7th April 1952

128. Following are recognised facts about the CD blocks:
I. Each block passed through 2 stages of development stage I (5 years) intensive development followed by stage II (5 years)
II. The Central Government supported the programme substantially by providing funds to the tune of Rs. 12 lakh during stage I and Rs. 5

lakh during stage II phases of development

III. By the end of 10 years the CD blocks entered into post stage II phase and then State Government has to bear the financial requirements

Select the true answer from following code:

A. I, II and III All
B. I and II only
C. I only
D. I and III only

129. In which year IRDP was launched in India?

A. January 1978
B. February 1978
C. April 1978
D. August 1978
E. April 1988

130. The target families under IRDP is:

A. Agricultural labourers
B. Small cultivators
C. Village artisans
D. Craftsmen
E. All of the above

131. Following are true about the village level workers, *save* for one:

A. Each VLW is incharge of 10 villages
B. Each VLW attends to 5 to 6 thousand people
C. He probes into their "felt needs"
D. In a nutshell, he functions like a unipurpose worker

132. Steps in process of evaluation includes:

I. Collection of data or information
II. Analysis of results
III. Reevaluation of health services
IV. Establishment of standard and criteria
V. Planning the methodology

Select the correct sequence from the given code:

A. IV, V, I, II and III
B. I, II, III and IV
C. I, II and III only
D. I, II, IV and V
E. II, III, I, IV and V

133. The following are recognised barriers of the accessibility but one:

A. Physical only
B. Economic
C. Social and Cultural
D. None of these

134. Following examples are included under efficiency (elements of evaluation), *but* one:

A. Male sterilization
B. The % of bed occupancy
C. Cost per day in hospitals
D. Cost per patient treated

135. Which of the following statements are true?

A. Medical education was introduced in the ancient universities of Taxila and Nalanda, leading to the titles of Pranacharya and Pranavishara
B. A hospital system was developed during the reign of Rahula Sankirtyana (son of Buddha) for men, women and animals
C. The Unani system was introduced by Muslim rulers
D. All of the above
E. Both A and C but not B above

136. Following are the important milestones of public health in British India, *except* for one:

A. The quarantine act was promulgated (1825)
B. Appointment of Sanitary Commissioner (1864)
C. A public health commissioner and a statistical officer appointed (1869)
D. The Birth and Death Registration Act promulgated
E. None of these

137. The following events occurred in 1881:

I. The 1st Indian Factories Act was passed
II. The Vaccine Act was passed
III. The 1st All India Census was taken
IV. The Epidemic Disease Act was promulgated

Select the true answer from the code given below:

A. I and II only
B. I and III only
C. I, II and III
D. I, II, III and IV All

138. In which year, the Drugs Act was passed, and drugs were brought under control for the 1st time?

A. 1940
B. 1950
C. 1960
D. 1970
E. 1980

139. In which year, the Applied Nutrition Programme (ANP) was launched in India

A. 1947
B. 1984
C. 1963
D. 1973
E. 1983

140. In which year, the Bhopal gas tragedy occurred?

A. 1983
B. 1984
C. 1985
D. 1986
E. 1987

141. In which year, the ICDS renamed as Integrated Mother and Child Development Services?

A. 1990
B. 1992
C. 1994
D. 1995
E. 1996

142. Following events taken place in 1996, but one:

A. Pulse Polio Immunisation
B. Family planning programme made target free
C. Prenatal Diagnostic Technique Act 1994 came into force
D. Malaria action plan

143. Which is not a source of manager's power?

A. Efferent
B. Legitimate
C. Coercive
D. Reward

144. Under National Health Policy (2002), the following are the goals to be achieved by 2005, *except:*

A. Eradicate polio and yaws
B. Eliminate kala-azar
C. Eliminate leprosy
D. Establish an integrated system of surveillance, national health accounts and health statistics

145. Under National Health Policy (2002), the following goals are not to be achieved by 2010:

A. Malaria and other vector and water borne diseases
B. Reduce prevalence of blindness to 0.5%
C. Increase state sector health spending from 5.5% to 7% of the budget
D. Reduce IMR to 30/100 and MMR to 100/lakh

146. Under National Health Policy (2002), which of the following goals to be achieved by 2007?

A. Eliminate lymphatic filariasis
B. Further increase of health budget to 8%
C. Eliminate kala-azar
D. Achieve zero level growth of HIV/AIDS

147. The current five-year plan (2003-2007) is designated as:

A. 7th plan

B. 8th plan
C. 9th plan
D. 10th plan

148. **The monitorable targets for the 10th five-year plan includes all, *except:***
A. Reduction of MMR to 1
B. Reduction of IMR to 45
C. All children to complete 5 years of schooling by 2007
D. Reduction of poverty ratio by 5% points by 2007

149. **Following health sector parameters are achieved during the 10th plan *save* for one:**
A. PHC—229,367
B. Community health centres—3,076
C. Health visitors—12,000
D. Health workers male—71,053

150. **Following medical and health education parameters are achieved during 10th plan, *except:***
A. Total number of medical colleges in India—222
B. Total annual admissions in medical colleges in India—19,000
C. Total number of allopathic (MBBS) doctors—575,600
D. Total number of hospital beds—500,000

151. **ICMR (Indian Council Medical Research) in New Delhi was founded in:**
A. 1900
B. 1911
C. 1947
D. 1950

152. **In which year the state health administration then known as provinces obtained autonomy, under the Montague-Chelmsford reforms, from the Central Government in matters of public health?**
A. 1919
B. 1935
C. 1947
D. 1957

153. **The Government of India Act provided further autonomy to the state in respect of health in:**
A. 1925
B. 1935
C. 1947
D. 1950

154. **By 2001, how many districts are founded in India?**
A. 500
B. 550
C. 593
D. 690

155. **In which Indian state, the district health officer and the District Family Planning and MCH officers are under the control of the Zila Parishad?**
A. West Bengal
B. Gujarat
C. U.P.
D. M.P.

156. **During 9th plan (1997-2002) IRDP was implemented through the following existing schemes:**
I. **Training of Rural Youth for Self Employment (TRYSEM)**
II. **Supply of improved toolkits to rural artisans (SITRA)**
III. **Development of Women and Children in Rural Areas (DWCRA)**
IV. **Ganga Kalyan Yojna (GKY)**
Select the true answer from the code given below:
A. I only
B. I and III
C. I, II and IV
D. I, II, III and IV All

157. **Each gram sevak is in charge of how many villages?**
A. One
B. Three
C. Five
D. Ten

158. Which article of Indian Constitution covers all the health subjects?
A. Article 146
B. Article 246
C. Article 300
D. Article 13

159. In India, BCG vaccination programme was launched in which year?
A. 1897
B. 1947
C. 1951
D. 1958

160. In India, the Epidemic Diseases Act was promulgated in which year?
A. 1897
B. 1907
C. 1930
D. 1948

161. The 1st step towards decentralisation of health administration in India occurred in:
A. 1912
B. 1919
C. 1935
D. 1947

162. In India, the Drugs Act was passed in:
A. 1919
B. 1935
C. 1940
D. 1948

163. Following events ensued in 1948:
I. **India joined the WHO as a member state**
II. **The ESI Act was passed**
III. **The report of the Environmental Hygiene Committee was published**
IV. **Ministries of Health were established at the Centre and states**

Select the true answer from the code given below:
A. I only
B. II and IV
C. II, III and IV
D. I, II and III

164. In which year Revised National TB Programme with DOTS introduced as pilot project in the country?
A. 1993
B. 1995
C. 1997
D. 2001

165. In which year ICDS renamed as Integrated Mother and Child Development services (IMCD)?
A. 1993
B. 1995
C. 1996
D. 2000

166. In which year, the legislation on transplantation on human organs was enacted to regulate the removal storage and transportation of human organs for therapeutic purposes and for prevention of commercial dealings in human organs?
A. 1992
B. 1994
C. 1995
D. 2001

167. From which year prenatal diagnostic technique (Regulation and Prevention of Misuse) Act 1994 came into force?
A. December 1994
B. January 1996
C. April 1997
D. March 2000

168. In which year RCH (Reproductive and child Health) programme was launched?
A. 1993
B. 1994
C. 1995
D. 1997

169. Following events occurred in 1998-99:
I. **National Family Health Survey-2 undertaken**

II. NMEP renamed as National Anti-Malaria Programme

III. Phase II of National AIDS Control Programme became effective

Select the true answer from the code given below:

A. I only
B. II and III
C. I, II and III All
D. III only

170. In which year India staged the last decadal census of 20th century?

A. 1901
B. 1951
C. 1991
D. 2001

171. In which year India staged the 1st decadal census of 21st century?

A. 1991
B. 2001
C. 2002
D. 2000

172. PERT is a type of:

A. Input output analysis
B. System analysis
C. Network analysis
D. Work sampling

173. ROME scheme was introduced consequent to the recommendation of:

A. Shrivastava Committee
B. Mukherjee Committee
C. Chaddha Committee
D. 20-point Programmee

174. The concurrent list of the Constitution of India list the following function, *except:*

A. Prevention of extension of communicable disease
B. Administration of hospital and health services
C. Collection and compilation of health services
D. Labour welfare

175. The objective of National Population Policy 2000 is to bring down the TFR to:

A. 1.5 by year 2010
B. 2.1 by year 2010
C. 2.6 by year 2010
D. 2.9 by year 2010

176. The National Health Policy of India (2002) sets out the following goals to be achieved, *except:*

A. Zero level growth of HIV/AIDS by 2007
B. Elimination of kala-azar by 2007
C. Elimination of leprosy by 2005
D. Eradication of polio by 2005

177. The National Health Policy (2002) India includes the following goals, *except:*

A. Eliminate lymphatic filariasis by 2015
B. Eradicate polio and yaws by 2005
C. Achieve zero transmission of HIV/AIDS by 2007
D. Reduce IMR to 30/100 and MMR to 100/lakh by 2007

Answers

1 B	2 A	3 D	4 A	5 B	6 C	7 E	8 D	9 E	10 B
11 C	12 D	13 C	14 A	15 A	16 D	17 B	18 E	19 C	20 B
21 A	22 B	23 C	24 A	25 B	26 D	27 B	28 D	29 A	30 B
31 C	32 D	33 C	34 E	35 B	36 A	37 C	38 D	39 A	40 D
41 B	42 D	43 A	44 C	45 B	46 E	47 D	48 A	49 B	50 C
51 A	52 B	53 C	54 A	55 B	56 D	57 D	58 C	59 D	60 E
61 B	62 C	63 A	64 A	65 B	66 B	67 C	68 E	69 A	70 B
71 D	72 C	73 E	74 C	75 A	76 D	77 B	78 A	79 B	80 C
81 C	82 D	83 E	84 D	85 B	86 C	87 A	88 D	89 C	90 A
91 B	92 D	93 C	94 D	95 A	96 B	97 B	98 D	99 E	100 C
101 B	102 A	103 B	104 D	105 C	106 B	107 C	108 A	109 D	110 E
111 A	112 B	113 D	114 D	115 A	116 B	117 C	118 D	119 A	120 B
121 C	122 B	123 C	124 A	125 B	126 D	127 A	128 A	129 C	130 E
131 D	132 A	133 D	134 A	135 D	136 E	137 B	138 A	139 C	140 B
141 D	142 D	143 A	144 B	145 C	146 D	147 D	148 A	149 C	150 D
151 B	152 A	153 B	154 C	155 B	156 D	157 D	158 B	159 C	160 A
161 B	162 C	163 D	164 A	165 B	166 C	167 B	168 D	169 C	170 C
171 B	172 C	173 A	174 B	175 B	176 B	177 D			

C·H·A·P·T·E·R TWENTY-ONE

Hospital Waste Management

DIRECTION: Following MCQ's are provided with a few suggestive answers/completions. Only one answer is correct. You have to identify the *BEST* one in each case.

1. **Sources of health care waste includes:**
   I. Hospitals, clinics, nursing homes, dispensaries
   II. Medical research and training establishments
   III. Mortuaries
   IV. Blood banks and collection centres

   Choose the correct answer from the code given below:
   A. I and II
   B. I, II and III
   C. I, II, III and IV All
   D. I, II and IV

2. **Biomedical waste means any waste which is generated during the diagnosis, treatment or immunization of human beings or animals or in research activities pertaining thereto or in the production or testing of biologicals. This definition is given by management and handling rules of BMW in:**
   A. 1998
   B. 1999
   C. 2000
   D. 2001

3. **Recognized characteristics of health care waste includes:**
   A. It contains infectious agents
   B. It contains toxic and hazardous chemicals or pharmaceuticals
   C. It contains genotoxic and radioactive substances
   D. It contains sharps etc.
   E. All of these

4. **Waste types not to be incinerated are all, *but* one:**
   A. Pressurized gas containers
   B. Reactive chemicals, silver salts
   C. Photographic and radioactive waste
   D. Linen cotton gauge etc.

5. **To burn infectious health care waste which incinerators are used?**
   A. Double chamber pyrolytic incinerators
   B. Single-chamber furnaces with static grate
   C. Rotary kilns
   D. All of these

6. **A technology by which the waste is reduced by 80% in volume and by 20 to 35% in weight is known as:**
   A. Incineration

B. Screw feed technology
C. Microwave irradiation
D. Wet thermal treatment

7. A technique used to dispose by causing decomposition of genotoxic substances and heat-resistant chemicals is:
A. Double chamber pyrolytic incenerators
B. Microwave irradiation
C. Rotary kilns
D. Screw-feed technology

8. Blood, urine, stoods or hospital sewage are most suitable for:
A. Incineration
B. Microwave irradiation
C. Land disposal
D. Chemical disinfection

9. Microwave irradiation are mainly used to disinfect:
A. Microbes
B. Blood and urine
C. Chemicals
D. Genotoxic materials

10. Most microwave utilizes following frequency and wavelengths to kill the micro organisms:
A. 1200 MHz and 6.12 cm
B. 2450 MHz and 12.24 cm
C. 600 MHz and 3.3 cm
D. All of the above

11. The treatment and disposal of category 1 waste (human anatomical waste like tissues, organs, body parts) includes:
A. Incineration and deep burial
B. Microwaving
C. Chemical treatment and mutilation
D. Disposal in municipal land

12. Cat 1, 2, 3 and 6 wastes are carried in which colour plastic bags?
A. Red
B. Yellow
C. Blue/white
D. Black

13. Cat 5, 9 and 10 (solid) wastes are carried in which colour container?
A. Yellow
B. Black
C. Red
D. Blue

14. Colour coding for Cat 3 and Cat 6 wastes include:
A. Blue
B. White
C. Yellow
D. Red

15. A typical proportion of mixture (inertization) includes all, *except:*
A. Pharmaceutical waste—65%
B. Lime—15%
C. Cement—10%
D. Water—5%

16. Biomedical Waste (Management and Handling) Rule 1998 prescribed by the Ministry of Environment and Forests, Government of India has come into force on:
A. 26th January 1998
B. 26th February 1998
C. 26th April 1998
D. 28th July 1998

17. The Least component of hospital waste in India is:
A. Glass
B. Sharps (metal)
C. Plastics
D. Rags only

18. What is the colour-coding of bag in hospitals to dispose off human anatomical wastes such as body parts?
A. Yellow
B. Black
C. Red
D. Blue

Answers

1 C	2 A	3 E	4 D	5 A	6 B	7 C	8 D	9 A	10 B
11 A	12 B	13 B	14 D	15 C	16 D	17 B	18 A		

C·H·A·P·T·E·R **TWENTY-TWO**

Disaster Management

DIRECTION: Following MCQ's are provided with a few suggestive answers/completions. Only one answer is correct. You have to identify the *BEST* one in each case.

1. **"Any occurrence that causes damage, ecological disruption, loss of human life or deterioration of health and health services on a scale sufficient to warrant an extraordinary response from outside the affected community or area" is the definition of:**
   A. Disaster
   B. Hazard
   C. Both of the above
   D. None of the above

2. **Any phenomena that has the potential to cause disrsuption or damage to people and their environment is:**
   A. Disaster
   B. Hazard
   C. Both of the above
   D. None of the above

3. **Morbidity which results from a disaster situation includes:**
   I. Injuries
   II. Emotional stress
   III. Epidemic of disease
   IV. Increase in indigenous diseases

   Choose the correct answer from the code given below:
   A. I and II
   B. I and III
   C. I, II and III
   D. I, II, III and IV All

4. **Victims of earthquake at night mainly gets injuries like all, *but* one:**
   A. Head injury
   B. Fracture pelvis
   C. Fracture of thorax
   D. Fracture of spine

5. **The only approach that can provide maximum benefit to the greatest number of injured in a major disaster situation is:**
   A. Search, rescue and 1st aid
   B. Triage
   C. Field care
   D. All of these

6. **The most common classification uses the internationally accepted 4 colour code system:**
   I. Red indicates high priority treatment or transfer
   II. Yellow signals medium priority
   III. Green signals ambulatory patients
   IV. Black indicates dead or moribund patients